There A Place For Us 1991 - 2021

Thirty Years History of the
Wokingham Mental Health
Crisis House
Told Through Stories And Songs

by

Pam Jenkinson

Illustrations by Anna Felice Cook

The June Press

First published in 2021

by The June Press Ltd

UK distributor
The June Press Ltd
PO Box 119, Totnes
Devon TQ9 7WA
Tel: 44(0)8456 120 175
Email: info@junepress.com
Web: www.junepress.com

ISBN 978-0-9927501-8-3

Contents

Sequel to 'Triumph and Tragedy'
1991 - 2016
The Twenty-Five Year History

Part One

The History of the Station House

Part Two

Part Three

Part Three

Further Success Stories

Further Poignant Stories

Further Funny Stories

Further Tragic Stories

Part Five

Children, Sadness, And Premature Deaths

Part Six

Obituaries 2016 - 2021

Part Seven

Part Eight

Update On Our Services

Part Nine

Our Ongoing Campaign For Mental Health Education - Through Letters To The Press

Part Ten

Students At The Crisis House

Part Eleven

Annual Reports

Part Twelve

Benefactors

Part Thirteen

Visitors To The Crisis House 2016 - 2021

Part Fourteen

Reminiscences

Somewhere

There's a Place for Us
Somewhere a Place for Us.
Peace and Quiet, and Open Air
Wait for Us Somewhere.
There's a Time for Us,
Someday There'll be a Time for Us –
Time Together, with Time to Spare,
Time to Learn, Time to Care.
A Place Somewhere.
We'll find a new way of living.
We'll find a way of forgiving.
Somewhere!
There's a place for Us.
A time and place for Us..
Hold my hand and I'll take you there.
Somehow! Someday! Somewhere!

Introduction

There's a place for us. Somewhere, a place for us

It is now, five years, since the publication of '*Triumph and Tragedy*' –
the twenty-five year history of the Wokingham Crisis House. So what
has happened, in the ensuing five years - which now mark the thirty-year
history? We have gone on flourishing. We have had further spectacular
success stories, and, inevitably, some tragedies, as well. Our drop-in
centre is busier than ever, and we have developed, significantly, our
Advocacy Service - as the Government's shake-up of the Benefits System,
has greatly increased the numbers of mentally ill claimants, who require
advocacy - help with form-filling and preparation of the papers, and our
volunteers, to accompany them, to Tribunal Hearings. Throughout the
five years, we have continued to be grateful to our benefactors - who,
through their generosity - have enabled us, to keep our services going. In
particular, we have received grants, to help us relieve isolation and
loneliness. There has also been, significant development, in the
placement of students at the crisis house. There was a simpler time in
our history - when a student would just telephone, and ask if they could
come to us, and we would simply reply - 'Delighted, I'm sure!' Not any
more. We now have a formal Placement System, whereby we usually
accept three, second year, undergraduate, psychology students, and three
Master's, psychology students - on placement with us - in each academic
year. The placements, form an, integral part, of their degrees, and we
have to mark them. We are only too happy - thus to contribute to the
education of young people - who will be our future in the delivery of
mental health services - once the current generation has retired. An old
chestnut, frequently voiced - particularly at times, when there didn't,
currently, appear to be too much, else, to worry about, is, 'Who will take
over the crisis house, once you are no longer able to run it?' My answer
is, invariably, 'The Young!' There is no point, whatsoever, at this,
present, juncture, in my trying to train a middle-aged/elderly, person, to
succeed me, when I have, as yet, no idea of how long I can continue -
because, when I am geriatric, they may, by then, be geriatric, as well!
Give young people good training, and experience, and they, when the
time comes, will take over, successfully At least, one effect, of the current

coronavirus pandemic, is that people are, firmly focussed, on surviving, in the present, and so are, not worrying, about the future!. I recall, once buying a ticket for a concert - at which Rubinstein was to play Chopin. When I arrived, they were apologetic, and explained that Rubinstein was ill, so they had asked Daniel Barenboim, to play, instead. 'Were we happy with this?' We were. Rubinstein was ever so old, and ever so good at playing Chopin. Daniel Barenboim, at the time, was ever so young, and ever so good at playing Chopin. So, it will always be with everything, and with both performers, it would always be a case of 'Music, Maestro, Please!' Music, therapy for all one's mental distress - whether it be for the lovelorn, like the person in the following song, or for any other trauma - music hath charms - to soothe the troubled breast!

A table near the band, A small one.
Tonight I mustn't think of her -
Music, Maestro, Please

Finally, in our five years, we have continued, of course, to keep the enemy at bay! Perhaps surprisingly, there have still been attempts to undermine us, but we have defeated them all! As with *'Triumph and Tragedy'* - where I included quotations from twenty-five of Agatha Christie's books - to mark the twenty-five years, in which I used her psychology, to help run the crisis house, I now include dozens of, further quotations, from her books - to mark the thirty-year anniversary. I have also, brightened up, this history, with more than a hundred cheerful songs, most of them, shortened, so that only the words that are most relevant to the text, are included. What then, can, the highly cultured, Dame of Letters, Agatha Christie, with her brilliant insight, into human nature, possibly share, with the cynical wit, of old, cockney, music hall songs? The answer is - realism. Both, perceive, and, incidentally, love, human nature, as it really is, and not, through the, rose coloured, spectacles, of idealism.

Rather than re-writing them, in the narrative, I have included numerous letters - just as they were published, over the last five years - since this is a, more authentic, way of recording history, and gives a better insight into the way that we have been operating over this period. As well as letters, contributing to the mental health debate, and published in the local paper, I have included - with all names changed - letters exchanged as part of our, most important, and growing, Advocacy Service.

'*There's a Place for Us*' – this is the, most apt, title, of our thirty-year anniversary publication. What mentally ill people need, above all else, is a place to come and talk. May 2019, saw Mental Health Awareness Week, and this need, for a safe place, to come and talk, was highlighted by everyone involved - including Royalty, and other, notable, public figures. Thus, Agatha Christie writes, in '*Death in the Clouds*', Hercule Poirot says to Jane:

'Everyone likes talking about themselves.... It is based on a fundamental need of human nature - the need to talk - to reveal oneself.'

I shall never forget, an incident - though it took place more than thirty years ago - when, at MIND in Bracknell - an occupational therapist - given the title of 'Dopey Dora' by service users, told us, that, if we wanted to talk about, what we were talking about, [I can't remember what it was], then we would have to go elsewhere! We did! To prevent freedom to talk, is a direct contravention, of the first law of mental health psychodynamics! A mental health centre, which denies people the opportunity to talk, becomes redundant overnight - which hers did! MIND in Bracknell, has, long since, been consigned, to the dustbin of history! In order to prevent, such an outrage, happening to us again, is one of the reasons why we have banned, all mental health professionals, from our Association.

Members of the Royal Family, are doing excellent work, in trying to dispense with the stigma of mental health problems, and I have confidence in their achieving, at least a measure of success, in this campaign. Nevertheless, some stigma is bound to persist, so all names of service-users - throughout this sequel - have been changed completely - to ensure their anonymity, and thus, their protection. Volunteers, many of whom, are former service-users, are mentioned by, first names, only. Dignitaries, patrons, and benefactors, are the only ones, referred to, by their full names, and titles. I hope that readers will enjoy this sequel as this new book, takes us into the Wokingham Crisis House's fourth decade. When writing her '*Autobiography*', Agatha Christie said, that a good time to stop, was when she was seventy-five. I agree with her. I celebrated my seventy-fifth birthday on 27th October 2020, and I also consider this, to be a good time, to stop writing the history, of the Wokingham Crisis House. Agatha Christie, went on to live for a further ten years, and I hope that we also, will continue, for many years to come.

Acknowledgements

This book is dedicated to all those people, who, through self-help, and the support of the Wokingham Crisis House, have turned their lives around, for the better.

Foreword

By Christopher Hoskin

My interest in mental health arose, because, early in my life, I had problems which were successfully dealt with, by a private psychoanalyst, and, later on, I realised that my good fortune was not shared by those who were dependent on the State mental health services. I wrote a book on the subject, and, in doing so, I came across an article by Pam Jenkinson. I got in touch with Pam, and I have been going to the crisis house, on a regular basis, ever since. The crisis house is furnished like a private house. It is decorated with plenty of china ornaments and pictures. It has a cat, a fish tank, and a budgerigar. The atmosphere is the complete opposite of clinical. It is non-threatening, and designed to make people feel at home. Mental health professionals are banned from the crisis house. The people with problems, who drop in, come into a relaxed place, where they are accepted, for who they are, and there is no pressure on them, of any kind. They can be sociable, or not, as they please. In all the time that I have been coming to the crisis house, there has never been any violence, or unpleasantness, from anybody. There is a bar open, at lunchtime, where everybody, is allowed, one alcoholic drink. Upstairs, there is a room, where people can play snooker, a library, and another room - where they can go, to be quiet. Pam has fought like a tiger, for the crisis house, and has, constantly, been willing, to do the work, necessary, to keep the place as it is. She has also been, ever ready, to help those who come to the crisis house, in practical ways. She will help them to fill in their statutory forms, to secure the benefits, to which they are entitled. Unlike most people, she is unfazed, by the authorities, and is, ever willing, to think outside the box. Her achievement, in creating, and running, the crisis house, is all the greater, in that, over the whole country, it is, probably, unique. During the year 2020, there was a Lockdown, enforced by the Government, due to the coronavirus. Pam kept the crisis house open, for all who wanted to drop in, refusing to be scared, by the virus, and declaring, that it was an essential service, for those who use it. She thus provided, a lifeline, for the, extremely vulnerable, users of it, and, quite probably, prevented them, from suffering extreme depression, and, maybe, committing suicide. She thus, once again, turned up 'trumps'. I am sure that you will enjoy this, second book, of hers. It is, really descriptive, of the activity of the crisis house, in the years after, that described, in the first book. I am sure that you will come to admire, both Pam, and the crisis house, as do I, and many others.

Christopher Hoskin has a degree in philosophy from Cambridge University, and is a published author on a number of subjects of social importance.

PART ONE

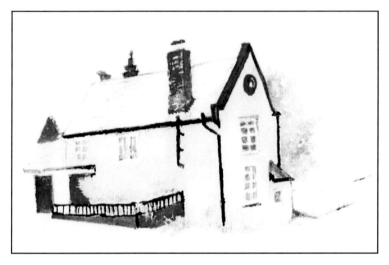

The History Of The Station House

Peace, and quiet, and open air wait for us somewhere.

Chapter 1

First Setting Foot In Station House - Reliving History

When I first set foot in Station House, Wokingham, on 7th March 1987, I experienced a familiar warm feeling of recognition; I was at home! This was because, Station House, was built at exactly the same time, in the nineteenth century, as the house in which I spent my childhood. Where you have spent your childhood, will always be home, and normality, for you. People, as diverse, as the crime writer, Agatha Christie, and Derek, a paranoid schizophrenic, of my acquaintance, have both said the same thing. In her '*Autobiography*', Agatha Christie says, that Ashfield, the house in Torquay, in which she grew up, would always be home to her. In contrasting circumstances, the schizophrenic said, that when, as an adult, he went to prison, he was immediately at home, and happy. It was the adult version of the children's home, in which he had lived, from the age of three. If you have grown up in an institution, then an institution is home to you. Amazingly, the late Princess Margaret, sister of the Queen, maintained, in a television interview, that Buckingham Palace, was a cosy home! Prisoner - or Royalty - what you are used to, is home!

Victorian houses have recognisable characteristics - the most noticeable of which, is solidity. The house of my childhood had great thick floorboards, and thick, solid, wooden doors. Fittings, like the letterbox, were made of cast iron. The door-knobs were of solid brass. There wasn't as bit of plastic in the place. There wouldn't be. It hadn't been invented! The 'plastics revolution', of the twentieth century, was hailed, at the time, as great technological progress. Now, we are attempting to rescue the environment - especially ocean fish - from the damage that plastics cause! Victorian rooms had great, high ceilings. In their centre was a beautiful, plaster cast, 'rose' - from which was suspended the gaslight. I would swear that the cast iron cistern, in our outside lavatory, dated from the building of the house, itself. The chain was of solid, indestructible, metal, and the seat was a great, solid, piece of wood - replaced in the Nineteen-Fifties - by the, then, fashionable, black plastic. When we arrived at Station House, it had the Fifties, black plastic toilet seats, so evidently, a small amount of modernisation, but not much, had taken place. Victorian rooms were huge. In our largest bedroom, it would have been easy, to fit in three double beds. The basement kitchen was also huge. It was where the family gathered. The sitting room, or 'parlour', was largely kept for visitors, and in the times before the modern 'funeral parlours' - for laying out the dead!

The kitchen had a 'range' - which you polished with blacklead. The range had a main oven - in which you roasted the Sunday joint, and two side-compartments - in which you baked cakes, and in which you placed the Yorkshire puddings, to rise. There was a big, white wooden table - which you scrubbed with a scrubbing brush, and adjacent to the kitchen was a scullery - which housed the copper and the mangle - for doing the laundry. No washing machines in those days!

No doubt, Station House would have boasted all these Victorian features, when it was occupied by the Station Master, and his family. When we arrived, it had been converted into scruffy little offices, for the local mental health team, and the Wokingham Volunteer Centre, but the basic features - thick floorboards, solid brick walls, and wooden sash windows, remained. A shame - the lack of vision in the statutory social services! The building had, such potential, as a mental health crisis house - and they just set up scruffy offices here! At a later date, when we were doing some refurbishment, and removing an old, wooden, lean-to, the wood being removed, looked like that from a battleship! The water-pipes in Station House, are external, and visible. The original building would not have had running water. There would have been a pump in the yard. By 1987, central heating had been put in, and the fireplaces boarded over, but they are still there, and the house has chimneys - as did all Victorian houses - which were heated with coal fires, and lit by oil lamps. Electricity did not come to Wokingham until 1924. Country areas were generally served with this, much later than were big cities. I noticed this, particularly, when I moved from London - to college in Saffron Walden, in rural Essex - in 1965. Saffron Walden, then, would have been very similar to Wokingham - a small, rural, town - about forty miles from London. In 1965, it had no street lighting, at all. After dark, one went out with a torch. Contrast this, with Newcastle, home of the inventor of the electric light bulb. It had electricity in the nineteenth century! In 1878, Sir Joseph Swan, invented a durable incandescent lamp – with a carbon filament. By 1881, he was an established electrical manufacturer, in Newcastle, and he later patented lamps - with long-lasting cotton filaments. In the early 1880s, the American inventor, Thomas Alva Edison, fought him, over infringement of electric lamp patents, but in 1883, the two inventors, joined forces, to form, the prosperous, Edison and Swan United Electric Light Company. This relative privilege of big cities - as compared with rural areas - persists to this day. People have a pastoral, idyllic, image of the country, and believe that, all the problems, are in inner cities. Not so! Research indicates that, the worst, educational standards, are to be found among white boys, in rundown seaside towns - while, 'deprived', inner cities, can achieve very high standards indeed - especially where there are large Asian populations!

Recently, I shared, happy reminiscences, with Don, one of our services users. He was, born and bred, in Newbury, in West Berkshire. Though quite a few years younger than me, he can remember gas lighting - with the old, fragile, gas mantels. Make a clumsy movement, and they would be crushed to powder! He can remember coal fires, and the coalman, with a black face, tipping sacks of coal into the coal cellar - which was part of the house, but had a separate entrance - outside. He remembers the old black kitchen range - where you cooked the Sunday joint in the central oven, and cooked the Yorkshire puddings, and the cakes for tea, in the compartments on each side - relying on the heat from the fire, to make them rise. It is a fact, that rural areas, achieved modernisation, much later, than did big cities. Don feels completely, at home, in Station House - as I do myself!

Chapter 2

The Station House Through Time

This chapter records the history of a station House, through time, itself. So let us, at this juncture, pause for a time, from recording personal history, and the history of our Association, and turn to, the earlier history, of Station House. Our building is, physically attached, to one of the outbuildings of the 'Station Tap' Pub - proudly re-opened, as such, on Monday 30th April 2018. Originally, it was called the 'Railway Tap', and then, the 'Molly Millar' Pub. Briefly, in the 1990's, it was called 'Big Hand Mo's', and then it reverted, once again, to being the 'Molly Millar'. 'Big Hand Mo's' did not go down, at all well, with Wokingham - which is proud of its rich history. The 'Molly Millar' was much more suitable, and, originally, the pub sign, depicted pretty Molly, in a white starched cap. She was a local girl, and the King used to gallop over from Windsor to visit her - hence the name, of the local road, called, to this day, 'The King's Ride'. Unfortunately, when 'Big Hand Mo's' took over, the lovely pub sign disappeared, and was not restored when the name, 'Molly Millar' was resumed. The 'Railway Tap' was a Commercial Hotel. This was built in the mid-nineteenth century - to serve the new railway. The original line, which ran only from Reading to Redhill, was built by the Reading, Guildford, and Reigate Railway, and was opened in stages. The first sections - from Reading and Farnborough North, which included a station at Wokingham, were opened on 4th July 1849. The Staines, Wokingham, and Woking Junction Railway, opened between Staines and Wokingham on 9th July 1856. The London and South Western Railway was authorised to run over the South Eastern Railway, and this, gave Wokingham, a direct route to London Waterloo. With the coming of the railway to Wokingham, and the London line, in particular, there was a huge upsurge in commercial travelling. Trains now replaced stage coaches, and facilitated this - hence the need for a Railway Commercial Hotel.

Records reveal that, in 1850, the 'Railway Tap' was run by Publican, William Monk - with the help of his daughter, barmaid, Mary Monk, his son, John Monk - who was a commercial traveller in wines and spirits - and Eliza Butler - who was their servant - a housemaid. By 1861, James Lane was Publican - helped by his servant, Ellen Long. By 1871, Martha Roberts was Hotel Keeper, and then, Thomas Burge, who was Hotel

Keeper in 1881, continued throughout the rest of the nineteenth Century. By 1901, John Cox had taken over this position. Wokingham, is an historic market town in Berkshire - thirty-nine miles West of London, and, seven miles, Southeast of Reading. In the nineteenth century, country girls, could be found, easily, for employment in domestic service - since their other opportunities, were very limited. It was not only the, 'Station Tap', that changed with the changing years. Wokingham Station changed as well. The original Victorian Station was a beautiful structure, but, in 1973, it was demolished. Because of the heavy increase, in road traffic, throughout the twentieth century, the, former, Berkshire County Council, had proposed to build an Inner Distributor Road - a link to the motorway. In 1973, British Railways replaced Wokingham's Victorian Station with a hideous, temporary, prefabricated structure - with a view to the building of the new road. In 1976, Berkshire County Council bought, on a Compulsory Purchase Order, a number of buildings which lay on the proposed route of the new road, and so were due for demolition. Then, in 1979, the Council, changed political colour. At a meeting, in February 2020, I met a former Conservative Councillor, who said that, he had actually been there, when the Inner Distributor Road Project, had been agreed. But, the new, Liberal Democrat Council, scotched the plan. They claimed, that the Council did not have, the thirty-eight million pounds, required for the building of the Inner Distributor Road - so the Scheme was abandoned. The Council sold as many of the properties as it could, but both the Molly Millar Pub, and Station House, remained, empty and derelict, for a time. In the early 1980's, the Molly Millar reopened as a pub, and was certainly most flourishing, as such, when I first, set foot, on Wokingham soil, in March 1987. Some of the other, redundant buildings, were put across, for use, by various social services. Houses on the Reading Road - some of which, have now, been demolished - became a Youth Centre, an Old Folks' Centre, a Centre for the Unemployed, and a Mental Health Day Centre. Station House, accommodated the Wokingham Volunteer Centre, and the statutory Mental Health Team.

Although the original Inner Distributor Road Scheme had been abandoned in 1979, a modified version, for eventual implementation, always remained on the cards. When we moved into Station House - in March 1991, we were advised to do nothing to improve the building - since it would be demolished within a year! We knew that it would not. It would be demolished, eventually, maybe, but not within a year. Nevertheless, we lived with the knowledge, that our crisis house was temporary, until redevelopment of the whole Wokingham Station area went ahead - in 2013 - when both the 'Station Tap', and Station House, escaped the bulldozers. Temporariness, in its day, did not bother us unduly, because a crisis house, by definition, accommodates temporarily, so those who benefited from short stays, would still have benefited, and turned their lives around - even if the building were to be demolished eventually. Nevertheless, it is good, now that we have secure occupation of Station House, for as long as we wish to run it. In August 2013, the new station footbridge, was opened to the public, and in October 2013, the station building, itself was opened. The original footbridge, which was built in 1886 - following two accidents at the level crossing at Barkham Road - was constructed from old stock of rails and sleepers, and has been preserved by the Wokingham Society. As recently as September 2020, attempts to modernise the footbridge, have been resisted.

The Wokingham Society approved of the new name for 'The Molly Millar' - 'The Station Tap'. Thus, history repeats itself, and my letter on the subject was published in *The Wokingham Paper* (29th March 2018). I asked readers who wished to contribute to the history, to contact me. Nobody local, contacted me, but I was pleased, and very surprised, on September 11th 2020, to receive the following missive, from Brazil! I replied, promptly, with a copy of my chapter, entitled, 'A Station House Through Time', and informed Eric Schlosser, that *'There's A Place For Us'*, would be published by The June Press, in April 2021, to mark our thirty year anniversary, and would, like *'Triumph and Tragedy'*, be available, on Amazon.

Eric Schlosser's Letter.

Dear Mrs. Jenkinson,

This might reach you as a bit of a surprise, but I've been doing some research and ran into your article from The Wokingham Paper *of 2.5 years ago, named "What's in a name?".*

You mention that you planned to do some research on the old Molly Millar Pub, now renamed the Station Tap, and I was curious if you ever got down to it. My great-great-great-grandfather was James Henry Cordery (1834-1914) who used to run the "the Railway Tap", the pub at the back of the Railway Hotel. I have managed to find an old picture which shows both the pub and the hotel, and have attached it to this message.

I don't even know if this email will reach you, but in case it does I would be quite grateful if you could share any additional information you might have on the family or the pub from those times.

James Henry's son, my great-great- grandfather Daniel Edwin Cordery (1861-1924) was a Regimental Sgt. Major in the 7th Dragoon Guards (India), and his son Edwin John Walter Cordery (1891-1964) came out to Brazil around 1915 as a teacher. His daughter Alice May Cordery (1918-1989) was my grandmother. So you see, this side of my family has been in Brazil for just over a century.

I live with my family in São Paulo, Brazil, and we have relatives spread out all over the place, including the US, Spain and Canada.

I apologize for this message 'out of the blue', but look forward to hearing from you.

Thanks and best regards,

Eric Schlosser

Chapter 3

Spade Work For The Crisis House

So how did the creation of the Wokingham Crisis House, come about? From December 1986 to December 1989, Wokingham District Council, employed, on a three year fixed-term contract, a social worker, named Joan, to work with volunteers in the community. Her brief was to get them setting up voluntary mental health services. Joan knew me, because she had attended some of my, mental health, educational events, and since Wokingham is fairly near to Bracknell, where I live, she asked whether I would be willing to be involved. She had set up a committee that was endeavouring to establish a Wokingham MIND Association, but was failing to get it off the ground. They enquired whether, instead of MIND, they could join up with my Schizophrenia Fellowship Group. Since schizophrenia is so specialised, and, a general, mental health association, is needed everywhere, I suggested that, instead, I come over to them, and get a MIND Local Association going. They were pleased with this arrangement, but I warned them, that it would be separatist. I refused to be involved with Social Services. They agreed, but I don't think that they really believed, that I meant what I said. This is why there are no other user-run crisis houses. They won't do, the one thing, that you have to do - get rid of the statutory authorities. They believe that everyone should work together. Extraordinary, is it not? They all say, that main-stream services - even main-stream voluntary services -

are oppressive, and demeaning. They all say, that they do not provide, what service users need, so, presumably, they know what they need. Why not, then, set this up for themselves - excluding their demeaning oppressors?

The original committee hadn't been, totally, without local achievement. They had done a certain amount of spade work, and had approached the local branch of the British Red Cross - with a view to holding, a drop-in, at their Denmark Street Headquarters.

At first, the British Red Cross Committee refused - because they thought that our mentally ill people, might present a threat to their own service users - some of whom are in wheelchairs, but after we ran a, successful, Mental Health Education Programme, for them, they changed their minds, and we set up our Drop-In, at the British Red Cross, in June 1989. At first, we met only on Tuesdays, and quickly achieved an attendance of thirty people. We had only been at the British Red Cross for a short time, when we were informed that the local mental health team - who had been based in Station House - were moving to Wokingham Hospital, and that we were being offered a Lease on Station House, as our base, with minimal funding - three thousand pounds per year - to run it. Our members were worried. We had, barely started, at the British Red Cross, and they felt that we were not ready to take on something bigger. I reassured them. Knowing bureaucracies, the way that I did, it would be at least, another year, before the thing happened. Sure enough, the mental health team didn't move out until 29th March 1991, and we then moved into Station House. But I also was worried, very worried - for other reasons. I had witnessed what had happened to Bracknell MIND. We were, at that time, still in the process of forming our Association, and preparing for affiliation to MIND - so I called a meeting of the members, and proposed that, we vote, to ban all mental health professionals - including social workers - if you wish to dignify them with the term - 'professional' - in the Rules and Constitution of our Association. Some doubts were expressed, but I said, 'Look, a number of you, have used the mental health services directly, and others, have experience of them, as relatives, of the mentally ill. You know, none better, how awful, and deficient they are. If we get involved with them, our service, will be awful as well.' There was also the point, that, if we ever felt a, desperate need, to have their involvement, we could always call a general meeting of the Association - to change our Rules and Constitution. The power would still be in our hands. But, as I learned, to our cost, in Bracknell, once they are in, you never get rid of them. Our members always could reverse the vote, but I knew that they never would! They knew what the mental health services were like - for both patients and relatives, and they knew, that I was right.

The vote went through unanimously. All thirty of us, voted to ban them, and, boy, did I go out celebrating, on the night that I got that vote through! Into our neighbouring pub, the 'Molly Millar', now the 'Station Tap', I sailed, in triumph, and the landlord - with whom we were friendly - gazed at me curiously. 'Pam, what has happened? he asked. You are ecstatic. You look like someone who has lost a penny piece, and found a million dollar bill!' Outsiders don't understand psychopolitics, so I simply replied, 'Have one on me; I have never been happier in my life!'

Chapter 4

Planning The Services

As well as planning to ban the social services, during the year, in which we had time, to consider, the services that we would offer, once in Station House, we planned what we would do. Station House had been a conventional, Victorian, dwelling house. Downstairs, it had one large room, and two medium sized rooms, a passage with a scullery sink, and a back door, which led to, what had been, two outside toilets, but which were now in a covered area. Upstairs, it had, four, medium sized, rooms. Before we moved in, the Wokingham Volunteer Centre, had occupied the large downstairs room - and a dire state it was in. It had grimy, yellowish, old wall paper - that was peeling off the walls, and a dirty old brown carpet - that was covered in water marks. Evidently, they had had, a flood, at some time. The rest of the house was occupied, as scruffy offices, by the local Mental Health Team. As you entered the front reception room, the first thing that you, as a depressed, and distressed, mental patient, saw, was a large splodge of dirt on a bare wall - where now hangs a good copy of a famous work of art! I used to think, ruefully, that 'dirt' would be the, newly arrived, patient's, lasting memory, of his introduction to this mental health 'service'! A large computer was looking you, threateningly, in the eye, and the shelves were full of patient files. Although computers were, by this time, in use, we were still in the days, before all records, were computerised! The second, downstairs, smaller room, was the Senior Social Worker's Office - with typical office furniture, and the, 1950's style, toilets, were shared - by service users, the mental health team, and the Volunteer Centre, staff. Upstairs, two of the rooms were offices - with social services' employees - sitting - looking like bookends - at computers. One room was a very basic kitchen, and one was a drop-in lounge, for the mentally ill - which would have accommodated, eight people, at the most! The whole house looked, very dirty, and neglected, and where filing cabinets had been moved out, dirty black rectangles were visible on the grimy walls.

What did we do as soon as we moved in? Clean of course! Scrub away the grime of years, and scrub away the grimy, 'profession', of social work with it! Then we painted, and decorated. There is nothing like fresh paint - to get rid of the smell of neglect. Did not, the late, Margaret Thatcher, say, to one of, the first, families, to avail themselves of her, 'Right to Buy Council Houses', Policy? 'You need a lick of paint!'? In other words, 'Get on your bike! Help yourself. This is your chance to go up in the world!' For the first two years, of our occupation, the Wokingham Volunteer Centre remained with us, so we had to wait until 1993, to clean up, and re-decorate - what then, became our main lounge. When we moved in, we had already decided, to restore the house, to residential use. We would have mental health beds, in the upstairs bedrooms. We would install, ensuite bathrooms, for our guests. One, upstairs room, would be their, shared, kitchen, and, the fourth, would be a mental health library. We considered this to be very important. We could have used this room as, a third, bedroom, but, because it was situated, between the other two bedrooms, it allowed guests, to have a degree of privacy – which is so important for mental health. Quality, not quantity, every time! Our library has a very good collection of books on all aspects of mental health, but it also has a very fine collection of English Literature classics. Read up on mental health, by all means, but develop other interests, as well!

Since, for our first two years of occupation, we still shared the building with the Wokingham Volunteer Centre, we were able to have only one bedroom - the other proposed bedroom, being used as the drop-in lounge - for this initial period. Since, also, for those first two years, I was still engaged in the educational work for the National Schizophrenia Fellowship, we only held the, drop-in, on two days of the week. But, in April 1993 - we went full time - with two bedrooms, upstairs, and a four days, per week, drop-in service, downstairs. From first beginnings, our drop-in service was busy all the time, and our beds - always occupied.

Let us now have an update on our facilities. As more and more mental health facilities, close down, so the use of the crisis house, increases all the time. In 2018, we experienced what we described, affectionately, as 'The Reading Invasion'. The Reading, voluntary mental health service, was threatened with closure - due to withdrawal of funding - so their, former, service users, started coming to us, *en masse*! Not counting our downstairs kitchen, and the ladies' cloakroom, Station House has six rooms, and about forty chairs - in which people can be seated, comfortably, if necessary. It is a case of spreading out, and using all the rooms, if we are busy. We have six seats in our reception room, ten in our main lounge, and we can bring in three from the kitchen, when necessary, four in our games room [for spectators], five in our library, and three, in what we like to keep as a private counselling room, when possible. In September 2018, we opened up, the old upstairs kitchen - which - since closure of our beds - had simply been used as storage - as an additional games room, but this time, for table games, with four, comfortable, seats. The ladies' cloakroom, has seats for three, and there are four, additional chairs, in the area which houses our budgerigar, but we still stick to our philosophy, 'Small is Beautiful!' You don't need, bigger, crisis houses; you need more of them. We have done, all that we can, to encourage the mental health service users of Reading, to set up facilities for themselves, in their own town. But it is the old, old story. People always believe that you have to go to the statutory authorities, in order to get anything going. You don't! You need to get it going for yourself, and keep them out! In February 2019, a self-help mental health group, in Reading, finally signed the lease for a building in the Oxford Road - to set up as a centre for themselves, and its Opening Ceremony was held on 21st March 2019. They have named their centre - 'The Cuckoo's Nest'! To this day, people are still expressing the view, that people with mental illnesses can't run services, and must, recruit professionals, to do so. Nonsense! Of course services run by the mentally ill will be limited, but are you telling me, that services, run by professionals, are NOT limited? I wished, The Cuckoo's Nest, every success, and I had a wonderful vision of, Jack Nicholson, smiling at their initiative! Unfortunately, the project had to close after one year, but, no doubt, there will be future such initiatives, that will survive.

Chapter 5

Confronting The Enemy

Don't Fence Me In

Oh give me land, lots of land,
and the starry skies above
Don't fence me in.

How did social services take to being banned? Very badly. They are so used to bullying, and oppressing people, that I don't think that they could quite believe that we could actually be doing this to them! Who did we think we were? 'Democratic voters', was the answer. What we did locally, has resonances with what, democratic voters, did, nationally, in the BREXIT Referendum. It was, absolutely assumed, that we would vote to remain, but we didn't; we voted to leave! Politicians didn't like the result. Tough! That's democracy! Locally, social services didn't like being excluded. Tough! That's democracy!

By July 1991, Station House was looking very clean, and nice - with new carpets, pictures on the walls, nice homely furniture, and every appearance of success. It was then, that a social worker from the Mental Health Team, arrived, at the door of Station House. He told me that I was stupid to think that we could run a mental health crisis house, with no professional support at all. 'Crisis intervention, he claimed, is a very highly skilled branch of social work.' Since I consider social work to be a load of rubbish, his comments had a zero impact upon me, and I thought that it was his intelligence, that should be held, in question, and not mine! He then said that what we were doing was illegal, that we wouldn't be able to cope, and that the mental hospitals would dump people on us. No they wouldn't! While we retain all the power, and the say-so, WE decide whom we will, and will not, accommodate, and we can always send people, back to their referrers, if referrals prove to be unsuitable. I rather think, that what irked him, was that HE would not be able to dump people on us - as he had anticipated - when he assumed, that he would take us over - as soon as we were established in Station House. I found it interesting, as well, that he didn't appear to understand what a crisis house is. He claimed, defensively, bearing in mind that they had done, practically nothing, with Station House, when they occupied it, that social services had residences for, people with learning disabilities - all above board, and funded by Housing Benefit. From the beginning, we were adamant that we would not be funded by Housing Benefit. Crisis beds are just that - a place where you go, temporarily, to resolve a crisis. They are not meant to be long-term accommodation - on which you hold a Tenancy. Needless to say, we took no notice, whatsoever, of this social worker's opinions, and carried on as before. So what did they do? You've guessed it, they had a meeting! At the meeting - to which we were not invited - I suspect that they even considered turfing us out of Station House, but they could hardly come out with the truth - which was that they had, just assumed, that, once we were in Council-owned property, they could just come in, and take over, our Association, as they had done in Bracknell - having all the power for themselves, and relegating us, as free labour. Lest readers think that it is my paranoid imagination, I have proof, that this was the case. When we took over, I found, hanging in a key-cupboard at Station House, keys to other, local statutory facilities. People would not leave their keys in a place - unless they believed themselves, still to have free, and regular, access to it! When Wokingham District Council, employed a social worker, to work with volunteers in the community, to set up voluntary mental health services, they were, no doubt, looking for community care, on the cheap! They failed, to take on board, one fact. Voluntary work has a completely different basis, and philosophy, from statutory work, so, wise volunteers, do what we did - stay separatist!

Social services' resentment at their exclusion, hostility, and harassment of us, then continued, unabated, from 1991 - right through to 2007. At their first meeting, they, no doubt, assumed, that, within weeks, we would be failing to cope, and would be crawling on our knees to them - for support. It didn't happen. We had strict rules, ran our service in a very careful way, and only took on people, with whom we could cope, and for whom our service was suitable. Our beds were always occupied. By 1994, no doubt, through gritted teeth, the local Mental Health Team, were referring people to our beds - because nothing else was available. We still only had the, three thousand pounds, per year, funding - which was only for the drop-in centre, so we asked for more money - specifically for the beds, and were, grudgingly, awarded an extra, two thousand pounds, per year. As soon as this was awarded, they thought, that they then, owned the service, and made inappropriate referrals, immediately - which we refused. Nip it in the bud! Interestingly, no matter how much you trumpet the belief, that paid social work is rubbish, and that services are better run by volunteers, the conviction, that professional services, must be superior - because they are paid - persists intransigently - as illustrated by this exchange of letters in *The Wokingham Paper* (February 2019), Paul Farmer is a long-standing, mental health campaigner, in Reading, and is, incidentally, very well-liked, and respected, by Reading mental health service users:

Firstly, an excerpt from my letter of 24th January 2019:

'On the third subject, [the whole letter covered four topics], that of who should provide welfare services - the State - or individuals and charities - this is absolutely, a question of political belief. I believe that welfare should be provided by volunteers in charities, and that charitable service should be genuinely, voluntary, and not paid. By contrast, some people believe that welfare should be from paid staff in statutory services, and some, a mixture of both. One of our members feels that the whole idea of 'charity' was thought up by a clever capitalist - so that the State could avoid paying for any services at all. Despite all the hilarity, I am, nevertheless, relieved that this member is, at least, happy to avail himself of our own charity. However, even if all the work that charities do, is voluntary, buildings still need to be provided, and maintained, and bills still have to be paid, so on the fourth subject, that of the inadequacy of services, all our members are agreed. Mental Health Services, and provision for the homeless, are woefully deficient, and money needs to be put into better facilities for both.'

Now, Paul Farmer's response:

Positively Dangerous - (7th February 2019)
'I cannot agree with Pam Jenkinson [Your Letters: January 24], that 'All welfare, including mental health care, should be provided by volunteers.' I believe that could be positively dangerous. I do agree that volunteer groups and individuals, peer support, and charities, are vital and do build on professional input, as well as often providing what the latter cannot provide, or at least on a more regular/individual needs basis.'

My Response - 'Understanding Care':
'I read, with interest, the letter - 'Positively Dangerous' - February 7th]. This belief - that major services are only safe - if under statutory control - is very widely held, and I think it likely that more people agree with Paul Farmer - than with me. Nevertheless, facts disprove it!

Looking back, over decades of failure, Maria Colwell, Jasmine Beckford, Tyra Henry, Victoria Climbie, and Baby P. were not safe with statutory social services - nor were Dr. Harold Shipman's patients, safe, with the, highly regulated, medical profession. But the myth persists... This belief in professional 'magic' is widespread. The worried relative of a mentally ill person, will say, with relief, 'She has an appointment to see a social worker.' But frequently, all it amounts to, is precisely, that, seeing a social worker! We are never told what it is, that a non-medically trained professional, can do, in a mental health crisis, that a sensible, experienced, volunteer, cannot - because the answer is 'nothing', and all that even a, medically-trained, professional can do, is prescribe medication... I have known mentally ill people sit around for decades - waiting for the statutory mental health services to sort out their lives for them, and it never happens! Medication, counselling, befriending, and support, may help you along the hard, and stony, path, but the only person who is going to sort out your life for you, is yourself!'

Follow up Letter (February 28th) - 'Well done Pam'

'Given the appalling track record of Berkshire's remaining NHS mental health hospital, since its opening in 2003, and the more recent closure of all East Berkshire's NHS mental health beds, and the transfer of the few remaining beds to the aforementioned, already struggling, and inadequate, NHS mental health hospital, despite the almost one hundred percent opposition from the folk of Berkshire, it is hardly surprising that, currently, the hospital has a thirty-six percent shortage of qualified staff, and an overall staff shortage of twenty-two percent. So, thank goodness, for places like Wokingham's Crisis House, and folk like Pam Jenkinson - who continues to plug the gaps. It seems increasingly, that, all too often, the only way for local folk to get any help, support, or advice when in a mental health crisis, is to search out places, run by non-professionals, often untrained volunteers, and peers - such as the Wokingham Crisis House. We must all be very thankful for such places and individuals, despite their obvious limitations.'

So there you have the nub of the argument, and it is positively amusing, that the many who hold this view, cannot see its illogicality! Statutory services, are bureaucratic, unsafe, dirty, box-ticking exercises, and mostly operating under siege - while voluntary services are clean, welcoming, respectful to clients, and responsive to individual needs. But, in the view of the many, we are only plugging gaps - until the halcyon day arrives, when millions of pounds fall from heaven, and then statutory services can be as they should be! I can only quote the final sentence of the chapter that I wrote for a book, entitled *'This is Madness; A Critical Look at Psychiatry, and the Future of the Mental Health Services'*. My chapter was entitled - 'The Duty of Community Care - The Wokingham Crisis House', and I concluded it, by writing - 'If they are the professional experts, and we - the bungling amateurs, why are our services better than theirs?'

Nevertheless, I can't deny, that I find, most amusing, my mental image of the, rapacious, little old capitalist, sitting there, scratching his ear, and thinking up schemes - to get charities to provide for the whole of society's welfare - so that statutory, and tax-payer, funded, services, don't have to be provided.

Interestingly, as recently as Monday of this week, (11th March 2019), Joseph - for whom with his wife, Joan, we are providing advocacy, telephoned, to say, that the Care Co-ordinator, from the local statutory Mental Health Service, had, finally visited them - to assess Joan's needs. Now for the laugh! She said that she hadn't the resources to offer anything, but that she would visit them a few times! What's the point? If, as a result of their interventions, your health and life are no better, if they are not enabling you to get on, and progress along, the recovery path, what is the point of having them? With all the cuts in funding of public services, what has happened, is that we have ceased to provide the frontline services, and continued to fund the bureaucracy! We don't need them. Such money as there is, should be paying for practical facilities - staffed by unpaid volunteers!

In May 2019, we have seen the scandal of the staff at Cygnet Health Care Home - for people with learning disabilities, and autism - found guilty of taunting, demeaning, and abusing, their residents. Whistleblower, Colin Groombridge, gave evidence that Whorlton Hall Home, near Barnard Castle, in County Durham, was not fit for purpose. Eight years previously, he had resigned from another Cygnet Health Care Home - for the same reasons. In his evidence, he said that, the reasons, for the failure, were, firstly, a poor culture, secondly - lack of proper training - with people, being promoted, above their ability, and, thirdly, the failure to close big institutions - like Whorlton Hall - and replace them with small, local, person-centred services. Colin Groombridge is a person after my own heart! Did I not say in *'Triumph and Tragedy'*?

'Promote the development of small, local, volunteer-run, mental health crisis houses throughout the UK. If you are one of six, you are a person. If you are one of sixty, you are a number.'

Lead Inspector, Barry Stanley Wilkinson, also resigned, and also gave evidence - because the Care Quality Commission had not taken sufficient notice of his concerns about Whorlton Hall.

I elaborate on Colin Groombridge's first point - poor culture. Undoubtedly, there are people like Mrs Boynton, in Agatha Christie's novel, 'Appointment with Death' - described in 'The Agatha Christie Who's Who', as 'One of the most repellent characters in all of Christie's fiction, she had been a prison wardress, because, in Dr. Gerard's opinion, 'she loved tyranny and rejoices in the infliction of pain'. Dr Gerard said, 'What a horror of a woman!' Old, swollen, bloated, sitting there, immoveable - a distorted old Buddha - a gross spider in the centre of a web . . . small, black, smouldering eyes, they were, but something came from them - a power, a definite force, a wave of evil.'

One interpretation could be that - being a prison wardress - had turned Mrs Boynton into a sadistic monster, but Dr. Gerard thought otherwise. He thought that she had chosen such an occupation, because it gave her opportunities to act sadistically. She was incidentally, murdered, in the novel - by a dose of digitalin. This enabled her family to escape from her tyranny, and delighted Agatha Christie's readers!

True, some people may enter the field of learning disabilities or mental health 'care' for this reason, so that they can enjoy abusing the vulnerable. But I would say, 'not generally.' Most people enter the profession - well-meaning enough, and, as Colin Groombridge points out, mental health care IS a profession. But, a bad culture, produces bad practice. Where staff are valued - with good leadership, and management, and good working conditions, it is likely that they will do a good job for patients. On the other hand, if the culture demeans them, human nature being what it is, they may then be inclined to demean other people - and a ready target, are their service users. Then, Colin Groombridge's second point - 'inadequate training'. Good, well-managed, services, that value their staff, will attract the people with the best training and qualifications. Fail to value such people, and they will, easily, obtain employment elsewhere. Poorly run, and managed, services will then be left only with staff, with few, or no, qualifications - who can't get jobs elsewhere. As Reading mental health campaigner, Paul Farmer, says, repeatedly, this is, precisely, what has happened to Berkshire's, one remaining, mental hospital - Prospect Park, in Reading. This hospital was coping, reasonably well - until the Berkshire Health Authority, decided to save two million pounds - by closing the community mental health beds - at Slough and Ascot, and the dementia beds - at Maidenhead. These were, all transferred, to the now, overburdened, hospital - whose standards have declined, steadily, ever since! Two million pounds, is a lot of money, and it is ridiculous, to think that you can withdraw that kind of money from a service, and, still maintain, its former standards. Exhausted, overburdened staff, who are, inadequately trained, for the job, anyway, will probably, become stressed, and bad-tempered. To cope at all, they will, cut corners, with patient care. What you need in mental health services, is JOY! You need people, who enjoy, nurturing patients, and seeing their health improve, who enjoy, therapeutic activities - people who rejoice in recovery! Hearteningly, we have seen this joy, during the coronavirus crisis - as NHS staff applaud recovered patients, when they are discharged, from hospital. Colin Groombridge's final point, is my continual plea! Set up more small crisis houses - like ours, in Wokingham. It has worked well, for thirty years. It has received numerous awards - both national, and local! It works! Make others, like it, work in other towns! An example of 'Small is beautiful' is illustrated by the care home in Wokingham - to which Tommy Warfield moved in March 2019. [Please see: 'Success Stories Maintained'.] He is extremely happy there. Why? Because there are only six residents, and a very good standard of care. By contrast, I had a conversation - on 31st December 2019 - with Cathy, one of his carers. She said, that the staff, at Prospect Park Mental Hospital, are in despair. Morale, is at rock bottom; the place is being run like a prison, and patient care is abysmal.

So, we will always fight, to keep our beautiful, client enhancing, crisis house - which as it now enters a new, and fourth, decade – remains as a model of excellence for mental health services.

Chapter 6

An Update On The Wokingham Crisis House: 2016 - 2021

'*Triumph and Tragedy*', the twenty-five year history of the crisis house, was published in April 2016. Now let us look at some of the people described in the book, and see if they are sustaining their success. Of the 'Success Stories', we are still in, regular, touch, with half, of the people included. So far as we know, the others are continuing to be successful in their lives. Rob Jenkins and Malcolm Chase had, unfortunately, already passed away, when *'Triumph and Tragedy'* was published, but I included their success stories, to illustrate the fact, that even a few years, of happier life, can be accounted, a success, if previous times, were dire. Of those others, no longer in touch, it is simply likely that they continue to do well, and have no further need of involvement with us. They have crossed over - to the sunny side of the street!

> *'Grab your coat, and get your hat.*
> *Leave your worry on the doorstep.*
> *Just direct your feet,*
> *To the sunny side of the street.'*

PART TWO

Maintaining Success

Chapter 7

1996 – 1997: Jack Hayward: 'All Right In The Sanctuary'
Though not a frequent visitor, Jack drops in to see us occasionally. Twenty years on, he is still doing well, in his flat, and is continuing with his voluntary work. He also keeps us up to date with news of his mother - with whom, we were, at one time, very involved - and with the rest of his family. Jack is one of the lucky ones - who have a very supportive family. Our advocate, Tony, and I, just happened to encounter Jack, on 15th April 2019, and he told us that further progress has been made. He is now doing paid work. Jack is a success story, maintained.

1998 - 1999: Sadie Minton: 'She Ticks All The Boxes'
Sadie continues to visit us regularly, and continues to tick all the boxes. I have now been involved with her, and with her mother, since July 1987! You would not believe that Sadie reached her fifty-eighth, birthday in July 2020. She remains as glamorous as ever, and looks, a good twenty years, younger, than her actual age! She has been less

successful in working, latterly, but continues to cope, very well, with housework, cooking, shopping and gardening. Sadie suffers from chronic schizophrenia, but as I tell people, with wry humour, I know of plenty of people, who do NOT suffer, from schizophrenia, but are NOT good at cooking and cleaning, so Sadie is, definitely, a remarkable success story! Sadie has a penchant for buying, from charity shops, pictures, and lamps - some of them, very beautiful. She then, has no room for them, in her house, so she donates them, to the crisis house. Her most recent donation - in September 2020, was of a large consignment of handbags! These were, duly distributed, amongst appreciative service users. We have, getting on for eight hundred, pictures in the house, already, so I suspect that we shall, eventually, have to adopt, Michelangelo's venture, with the Sistine Chapel - and start having pictures, on the ceiling! Sadie is now more involved, as well, in giving more support to her partner, who has been suffering physical ill health, and her mother, who, in February 2019, moved into sheltered accommodation, for the elderly, and is now living nearer to where Sadie, herself, lives. Now, the boot is on the other foot! It is now - Sadie - who visits her mother - to make sure that she is eating, keeping her medical appointments, and, generally, looking after herself! Sadie's mother, also, still drops in to see us - and she visited on Friday 5th April 2019 - to tell us how she was settling into her new accommodation. Sadie is a success story, maintained.

Incidentally, in the summer of 2019, Sadie suggested that she should approach her, multi-millionaire, aunt and uncle - those who made sixty million pounds - through selling flight paths to foreign countries. Apparently, Sadie's mother, had encouraged, her brother, to apply for the top position at the Midland Airline, and, being successful, he proved to be, in the right place, at the right time. He made a killing! Sadie, wanted to see, whether they would like to make a donation, to the crisis house. I didn't hold out great hope of success - since I imagine that, multi-millionaires, experience many calls upon their purses, and there are, literally, hundreds of charities - just as worthy as ours - all seeking funding. However, Sadie's aunt telephoned me to find out more about our work, and, in August 2019, we did, indeed, receive a generous donation from them - [Please see our chapters on 'Benefactors']. Good for Sadie! On Friday 17th April 2020, Sadie telephoned the crisis house - to see whether we could provide her with a mask - since she would like to attend the drop-in centre, but was reluctant to do so, unprotected, during the coronavirus pandemic. We agreed to provide her with a mask - though, at present, the science on their efficacy, is inconclusive. If we all wear masks, I think that there will be psychological effects - both beneficial, and adverse. People will feel more protected, so they will resume normal business, in a more reassured, and cheerful way, But, we also, may become more complacent. If we are all wearing masks, we may, think it safe, to relax the social distancing rules, and there is, as yet, no scientific evidence, that ordinary masks, ensure, full protection, from the coronavirus infection. Now, at the end of May 2020, received wisdom, on the wearing of masks, appears to be, that they provide a very small amount of extra protection - so wearing them should be encouraged, but not made mandatory. June 2020, saw a further development in the saga of masks. From 15th June, it became compulsory to wear them on public transport, and, from 24th July, the wearing of masks, became compulsory, in all shops, and public buildings. We, of course, hastened to comply. Throughout the pandemic, I have been most impressed by the scientific, and medical advice, given, and even if, wearing masks, makes a minimal difference, this is better, than making, no difference at all, and any reduction in the risk of spreading the infection, is worth implementing. Interestingly, I have found that my own attitudes have changed, and developed, as knowledge about coronavirus, has changed and developed, over recent months.

1999 - 2000: Manfred Jameson: 'Whatever Love Is'

Manfred Jameson visited the crisis house in 2017 - to say that he is now retired, is doing charity work, and has taken up golf - at the local Billingbear Golf Course. When I heard that he had taken up golf, I asked whether he played at the Wentworth Golf Course - which is, just up the road, from us, at Sunningdale. When Agatha Christie, and her husband, Archie, lived in Sunningdale, Archie played golf on this course, and Agatha says, in her '*Autobiography*', that, although she did not realise it, she was gradually becoming a 'golf widow'. This golf course also features in a Tommy and Tuppence short story - 'The Sunningdale Mystery'. [Please see: '*Partners in Crime*'.] Manfred chortled at the idea, and said that, no, he was playing at Billingbear. Later, I found out why he laughed. A security guard, from Wentworth, happened to visit the crisis house in March 2019, and he explained, that the famous golf course, had been purchased by the Chinese, and that membership, now costs, one hundred thousand pounds per annum! Do some people have more money than sense? Or is it just - that if you are, literally, rolling in money - you might as well have the best, and the most expensive, of everything? Because it is true - you can't take your money with you.

Furthermore, I don't know, how much, is included in 'membership'. It might include drinks in the nineteenth hole, and other perks! Manfred had been working, as Treasurer, for a local Counselling Service, but this has closed down. He remains happily re-married, and his two sons, Luke and Ben, now in their thirties, are both doing well. Manfred is a success story, maintained.

2003 - 2004: Reg Gardiner: 'I Prefer To Work'
Reg Gardiner still uses the crisis house as a *'Poste Restante'* for his letters. He is very busy - working on building sites - so he is not a frequent visitor, but he has to call in occasionally - to collect his post! In March 2018, unseasonable snow, prevented work on the sites, so he was able to get in to see us, twice during that month. Although work on building sites, is casual, and so, regular employment, is not guaranteed, it is extremely well-paid, when available. This enables Reg to make most generous donations of cash to the crisis house. Like everyone vulnerable, Reg was in lockdown, from March 2020, but, as the restrictions eased, he was, in May, at least able to visit us, and collect what must have been, one hundred, items of mail! Reg is a success story, maintained. A further development to Reg's story occurred in July 2020. On Tuesday 28th, he called in, to say that he had just been discharged from hospital - having suffered congestive cardiac failure. With this health scare, continuing to sleep in his car, no longer seemed viable. I contacted Wokingham Borough Council, Housing Options Section, on his behalf. He was offered emergency accommodation in Reading, but turned this down, because he is paranoid about Reading - where he has been, Sectioned, in Prospect Park Mental Hospital. However, since Reg has now reached the age of sixty-five, he is eligible for sheltered accommodation for the elderly, and this is much easier to obtain, in Wokingham, than is, ordinary, social housing. The Housing Officer promised to assess Reg for this, by telephone, at the crisis house, on Friday 31st July. The assessment, was duly carried out, but Reg decided to opt, for the ordinary Housing Register, and not for the one for the elderly, so we had to see whether accommodation would be made available to him, in the near future. Evidently, the Housing Officer, herself, was not optimistic, because she also, suggested to Reg, the Deposit and Rent in Advance Scheme - whereby, the individual has to find, for himself, private sector, accommodation, and is then lent, by the Council, one month's rent, and a deposit, in advance. However, Reg was lucky. The Housing Panel, assessed him, as being homeless, and in priority need, and so he was offered a flat, in ordinary housing.

2004 - 2005: Sylvia Kann: 'I Want My Life Back'

Sylvia and her mother, who now run their nursing home together, always exchange Christmas cards with us. They are doing very well, and, now that mother must be getting towards retirement, Sylvia will, no doubt, in the near future, take over the nursing home, completely. She is a success story, maintained.

2007 - 2008: Nancy Shelton: 'Back In The Rhythm Of The Dance'

In the summer of 2016, Nancy, and her partner, visited, with her twin boys - Zac and Kai - beautiful babies. We could tell that Nancy was, idyllically happy, and fulfilled, as a mother, and appeared to be stable, and settled, with her partner, Mike. He runs a bathroom, and kitchen fitting, business, and they were, living successfully, in their home in Devon. Nancy, also, always exchanges greetings with us, at Christmas. Christmas 2019 was no exception. Nancy wrote to say that she was struggling. The relationship with Mike had ended, and he had moved back, to Sussex, in August 2019. Both twins have additional needs, but, fortunately, she has been able to obtain, Children's Disability Living Allowance for them, and had also applied, as a lone parent, for benefits for herself. So, although times are difficult, she is soldiering on. It is always very difficult to cope with children with special needs, but Nancy is determined to continue, so. Nancy is a success story, maintained.

2008 - 2009: Peter Black: 'Lonely No Longer'

June 2018, marked the twenty-year anniversary of the gay wedding, which we held, at the crisis house. Peter, and his partner, Ken, have now been happily married for twenty years, and their internet business is thriving and doing extremely well, financially. Almost incredible to think, that there was a time, when they appeared to have settled, for being permanent Benefits claimants! They are busy all the time, so we don't see much of them, but we keep in touch by telephone. I telephoned Peter during the coronavirus pandemic - to enquire as to how things were going, and how his business was affected. It is an ill wind, that blows nobody, any good! Their internet business, was flourishing, and things were, more hectic, than ever! Bored, self-isolators, were consoling themselves, and helping to pass the time, by buying, more enthusiastically, than ever, from the internet! I received a, seventy-fifth, birthday card from Peter - posted in Guernsey, so evidently, the successful partners, are currently enjoying, a well-earned holiday! Peter is a success story, maintained.

2009 - 2010: Kurt Haddow: 'Good With Computers'

My most recent update on Kurt Haddow - given to me by Ewan - was that he has moved to live with his father, in France, and is still doing extremely well with his computer work - evidently very deserving of his nickname - 'Computer Kurt'. Spectacularly intelligent, I always, held hope, that Kurt would make it, back into a normal life. Kurt is a success story, maintained.

2010 - 2011: Gavin Morton: 'Step By Step To Success'

Gavin Morton was over in England, and visited the crisis house early in 2018. He no longer works for the social services in Australia, but received, a generous, severance payment, from them. He was, at that time, suffering from a further bout of mania, but now, seems to have recovered, from this, so we are hoping that this was just a blip, and that Gavin will revert to being a success story, maintained.

2011 - 2012: Pamela McEllen: 'My Heart Is Singing Again'

Pamela keeps in regular touch with our befriender, Lucy, on Facebook. She is doing extremely well, but, is inevitably, extremely busy. She continues with her 'extra' acting parts, and has been sighted, for instance, in 'East Enders', in 'Father Brown', in 'Call the Midwife', and in 'Downton Abbey'. For relaxation, she frequents 'Nirvana' - the health club, that featured, so hilariously, in 'Twenty-five Funny Stories' - from *'Triumph and Tragedy'*. Pamela visited us - with her companion, Fiona - in April 2018 - when she needed some specific advice. Our charity, paid for Pamela, to see, a private Consultant, when she needed this help, and, more recently, she has been able to have one month's respite, in, the private, Cardinal Clinic - having, Health Insurance, to pay for in-patient care - on this occasion. She came out - fully restored to health, and the Insurance, has also covered, out-patient psychological therapy. So she needs our support from time to time, but, overall, Pamela is a success story, maintained.

What we find, all the time, at the crisis house, is that our service users need us - not so much to provide things for them, but to organise and engineer, so that they can access, specialist services. Pamela, simply didn't know, about her, Health Insurance, entitlements. I was able to contact the Insurance Company for her, and I discovered that she was entitled to one month's private inpatient care, and one month's outpatient care - with the premiums that she had paid. So I enabled her to avail herself of these services - with an excellent outcome! Pamela -

after a month's stay as an inpatient at the Cardinal Clinic, was looking like a million dollars - her mental health restored. I fear that I agree with her NHS Consultant Psychiatrist, that, the only alternative, seeking 'respite' in Prospect Park Mental Hospital, would not have achieved such a happy outcome! Like everyone, Pamela's success has, to some extent, been prejudiced by, the coronavirus, outbreak, [Please see: 'Advocacy'], but, also like everyone, we are hoping for a return to, and sustaining of, success, once the crisis is over. A step in the right direction, was achieved, in October 2020, when Pamela's 'extra' acting work, resumed. We consider it to be so therapeutic, for her, to be able to get out, and about, and to participate in this work, which she, greatly, enjoys.

2013 - 2014: Lucy Farmer: 'Back To Normality'

Lucy is visiting the drop-in centre on every day that we are open, and is an asset to the Association. [Please see our chapter on - 'Befriending']. She experiences problems, from time to time, but is, generally, a happy, contented woman. She finally qualified for her retirement pension in March 2018, so she can now devote all her time, to family, and also particularly, to grandchildren - with whom she is idyllically happy - and to befriending. I don't think that you can train people to befriend. It is an art! Lucy, just has, that ability, to involve, vulnerable people, in normal life, and so enrich it for them. Lucy is, naturally, sociable, so she is able to re-connect, isolated people, with normal social life. Currently, Lucy is befriending three mentally ill ladies. With the help of our Advocacy Service, Lucy also succeeded in getting Personal Independence Payment - her former benefit, Disability Living Allowance - having been discontinued. So, her personal financial circumstances, have now improved. Lucy positively relishes, having her three grandchildren, come to stay with her. They literally light up her life! Lucy is a success story, maintained.

Unfortunately, Lucy felt, in October 2019, that she could not attend our drop-in centre, 'for the foreseeable future', while Glyn continued to attend. Glyn has been with us for ten years - since he was discharged from prison, and is definitely becoming more and more paranoid - as the years go by. Some members, including Lucy, find his behaviour, threatening, though his aggression is only verbal, and not physical. We are monitoring the situation, carefully. No doubt, it would be much easier for me, just to ban Glyn from the drop-in centre, but I believe, that, within limits, we have to take the rough with the smooth. As Major

Despard says, in Agatha Christie's novel, '*Cards on the Table*',

'If I were only to dine in houses where I thoroughly approved of my host, I'm afraid that I should not dine out very much.'

I share, one hundred percent, Major Despard's point of view. If I only accepted into our service, people, of whom I, thoroughly approved, I fear that the service would be very limited indeed, and certainly, would not reach, many people who needed it - including Glyn. Just as Major Despard wished to kick, Mr. Shaitana, we may wish to kick Glyn, in our private thoughts, that is, but if we excluded him, from our service, he would probably die of exposure, and malnutrition, and, just as Major Despard had no desire to kill Mr. Shaitana, I have no motive for killing Glyn! As I explain to our service users, it isn't a question of whether I like or dislike people; it is a question of whether they need, and can benefit, from our service. All right, I agree, this is professional objectivity, and we are not a professional organisation, but, nevertheless, charities need to reach a wide community, and not just the people who appeal to those who run them.

Life is full of ironies. On the very day, (Monday 27th January 2020) that Lucy decided to venture back into the drop-in centre - probably having heard, on the grapevine, that Glyn was, at least temporarily, attending the local Salvation Army Centre, instead of the crisis house, a fresh problem was presented. Before our normal opening hour, Alec appeared. He was wearing a crown - complete with coloured glass, imitation, jewels, and was looking most bizarre. Alec, one of the 'Reading Invasion', had attended the drop-in centre, a few times, but I had never seen him, as deranged, as he was, on this occasion. He was extremely psychotic, and was speaking, absolute gibberish. Lucy complained, of not being able to hear herself speak, and I thought, with wry irony, that Glyn was a piece of cake - compared with Alec - whom I, nevertheless, warmly welcomed. This is what mental health services are for - to provide asylum for the psychotic, and what Alec proved to be, was an absolute gift from heaven, for our psychology students, on Placement. As I mention in '*Triumph and Tragedy*', for many years, I ran educational services for the National Schizophrenia Fellowship, and I believe in being, textbook accurate, when explaining things to young people. One of our Master's Psychology students, Danae, asked me this question, 'However can a person get into the state, that Alec is in?'

'The Schizophrenias, I explained - [they are a group of mental illnesses, and not just one specific condition], are stress-related biological disorders, with a genetic component. They are triggered by environmental stress, but will only be experienced by those, who have the genetic predisposition, to suffer from such disorders. They include - simple schizophrenia, a slow, mental deterioration, which develops over years - the kind of condition, often seen, in tramps, and vagrants. There is also hebephrenic schizophrenia - which is usually seen in young patients, and is characterised by irrational, giggling, behaviour. Then, there is schizo-affective disorder - which is a schizophrenia, but is sometimes confused with bi-polar affective disorder, because its sufferers experience mood swings. There is, also, paranoid schizophrenia. This tends to develop, later, than the other schizophrenias, and, interestingly, because its sufferers, have, already reached, some of the normal milestones in life, prior to becoming ill, they can be relatively normal - apart from their actual, paranoid, delusions. What you observe, in paranoid schizophrenics, are the positive symptoms of the illness, but not, the negative symptoms. They are not, usually, 'dilapidated', schizophrenics. Their self care, and maintenance of their households, are, frequently, normal, and many can behave, normally, in jobs - their paranoia, often being confined, to specific areas of life - such as jealousy, in relationships.' One of the ladies, Mary, whom Lucy befriends, is a typical example of the paranoid schizophrenia sufferer. Her house is immaculate, and she is a wonderful cook. But when her voices tell her to do so, she threatens to kill her daughter, and has also, on occasions, threatened to kill Lucy! Our service user, Elise, when observing Alec's behaviour, enquired as to whether, severe schizophrenia, was, in fact, a form of dementia - since she recognised, in his symptoms, some of those, exhibited, by a relative of hers - who was suffering from dementia. I then told her, that, interestingly enough, before the term 'schizophrenia', was coined, by the researcher, Kraepelin, early in the twentieth century, this condition was known as, 'dementia praecox' - 'early madness'.

Because we don't know Alec well enough, we don't know the stressors, that triggered his illness, but he is a perfect example of acute, imperfectly, treated, schizophrenia. I asked Alec whether he had been for his injection, and thus reminded, he then rushed off to receive it - much to my relief! Apparently, he is on Section 17 Leave, from Prospect Park Mental Hospital. This means that the, Sectioned patient, is allowed to live in his own accommodation, in the community, but is required, by law, to attend for his medication. If he fails to do, he will be recalled to hospital. The set-up, in essence, is not unlike 'parole' from prison - what is sometimes, termed, vividly, 'the long leash'! When Alec returned to our drop-in centre, on Tuesday 28th January, he was still thought-disordered, and talking gibberish, but was, noticeably, very much less agitated. The medication was doing its work! The absolutely, top-notch, psychiatrists, say - that, if you listen intently, you CAN work out, from the gibberish of untreated schizophrenia, known in the jargon, as 'Word Salad', what is that is distressing the patients. I don't doubt it, but for we, lesser mortals, I confess to regarding, effective medication, as a godsend! This experience, with Alec, also gave me, an opportunity, to point out to our students, the difference between the neurotic, and the, psychotic, disorders. You can sit down, with people, suffering from neurotic disorders, and discuss things with them. Together, you can identify the problems, and work out solutions. This is why, psycho-analysis, is a suitable treatment, for the neurotic disorders. Psychoanalysis, is not, generally, suitable, for people with the psychotic disorders. They are not in touch with reality, and are unable to discuss things rationally. There again, I believe that the, absolutely top, experts, disagree with me. They think that, psychoanalysis, can be achieved with schizophrenics. Yes, but probably with an, almost unbelievable, amount of time, patience, and expertise! It would be wonderful if we had the money to achieve such perfection in our mental health services, but, alas, we have not!

Over thirty years, I have observed, on numerous occasions, that people want the Wokingham Crisis House, for themselves, and on their own terms - to the exclusion of other people. They go away - thinking that we will change everything, to suit them, but we never do! It is a fact, that sometimes, as the following song states, they have 'stayed away too long', but, fortunately, Lucy, a valuable volunteer with us, came back, on our terms!

> *Have I stayed away too long?*
> *If I come home tonight,*
> *Would you still be my darling'?*
> *Or have I stayed away too long?*

Lucy made her second, return visit, to the crisis house drop-in centre, on Monday 24th February 2020, and Alec arrived, once again, as psychotic, as ever. Nobody took much notice of Lucy. The general consensus was, that she was as welcome, as anyone else, but no more welcome, than anyone else! I think that she realised, that everything had moved on, we had new people with us, and the entrenched position, which she previously enjoyed – being a long-term service user, no longer existed. The crisis house is a lovely place - cosy, comfortable, and welcoming. Such features, are particularly valued, by people, whose own home circumstances, are none of these things. But alas, we are cosy, comfortable, and welcoming, to people - with the full range of mental illnesses - including those with acute schizophrenia. Our service user, Don, and I, had a good laugh about the situation. 'Patsy, I said, left, because she couldn't stand Aileen. Aileen left, because she couldn't stand Patrick, Harold, and Glyn. Glyn left, because he couldn't stand being regarded as being mentally ill, though he is, actually, much more severely so, than are most of our service users! Lucy left, because she couldn't stand Glyn. Pamela will only attend, if Lucy isn't here!' Pamela was also most perturbed, when she attended the drop-in centre on Friday 14th February 2020, to find herself sitting next to Rosie. Apparently, they had clashed at another venue, in the past! More recently, in March 2020, Elise reported feeling, very uncomfortable, when Rosie attended the drop-in centre, and, in June 2020, there was an outright, clash, between Pamela and Phil. Pamela was very anxious to get support for some letters that she was writing, and felt that Phil, with his own problems, was diverting attention away from herself! In August 2020, Lucy had, an outright, clash with Des - because Des thought that, the Royal British Legion, had become a, 'jobs for the boys', organisation, while Lucy maintained that it was well-run, and their 'Poppy Appeal', a most effective, fund-raiser. How, Don and I, laughed! If we took note of all of it, and tried to act on it, we would have nobody left, but we take note, of none of it. Anybody who wishes to use our services, is most warmly welcome to do so, and anybody who doesn't wish to use our services, is equally welcome, not to! Despite this stance, remarkably, we are always very popular, and well attended. Exactly as predicted, after a few weeks of 'never coming here again', in February 2020, Glyn turned up, once again, and just like Lucy, behaved as though nothing had happened. Talk about - 'Leave them alone, and they will come home, wagging their tails behind them.' By late March 2020, the kaleidoscope had changed, once again. Everything, non-essential, had now closed. There are no social venues, no pubs, no cafes, and not even things like clothes shops - which one can, wander around, to help pass the time. Now, Lucy, is telephoning the crisis house, anxiously. 'Are we still open?' 'Indeed, we are!' Then, the relief. Lucy has said, herself, in the past, that if she had to spend all day, incarcerated, in her four walls, she would go stir crazy.

Now, the drop-in centre has become a vital place. Glyn is still attending - mainly for our refreshments, and to use our facilities - since he is still, street homeless, but his presence has ceased to irk. I have long held the view - that human beings are, remarkably good, adapting animals During the coronavirus pandemic, and, consequent, lockdown, Sadie's schizophrenic symptoms, have become florid - as they always do, when environmental stress, increases. The classic, textbook, definition is that 'Schizophrenia, is a stress related biological disorder, with a genetic component.' Come to the crisis house drop-in centre, during the current crisis, and you will see the proof of this definition, for yourself!. When visiting the drop-in centre, on Friday 29th May, Lucy appeared to be, much more relaxed and stable. With the gradual easing of Lockdown, she reported that she was now able to have, at least some, contact with her grandchildren, and since they are, undoubtedly, her *raison d'etre*, and lifeline, this was good news! As the clash with Des, in August, illustrated, there can still be, heated, exchange of opinions, but, overall, Lucy, now able, regularly, to have contact with her grandchildren, is restored to her position, of a success story, maintained.

2014 - 2015: Dan Kent: 'I Am Simply One In Four'

Dan Kent was very successful with his 'One in Four' campaign. For this, he produced sweat shirts, with a 'One in Four' logo - indication, that, one in four people, will suffer from a mental health problem, at some point in their life - so mental health problems are commonplace, and their sufferers, should not be the victims, of stigma! Dan also produced coffee mugs - with the design of the crisis house, decorating them. Then, he went away for some time. This was because, both his parents, were suffering from dementia, and he had the full-time job of looking after them. Dan returned to the crisis house, in October 2019. Both parents had now passed away; he, as a result, had become very depressed, and reclusive, but now, he was, once again, on the recovery path. Now, in 2020, Dan is fully integrated back with us, has ideas for the crisis house, and so he is a success story, maintained. From listening carefully, to Dan, I get the impression that, although neither acutely depressed, nor acutely, manic, he is wistful for the past - when he had, successful jobs, in engineering, and he also harks back, regularly, to when he received a Wokingham Town Council Civic Award, for his work at the crisis house. To meet his current needs, I therefore thought it appropriate, in March 2020, to invite him to become a Trustee of our charity, and he has accepted. This will be a further step in restoring his self esteem. On Friday 7th August 2020, I helped Dan to complete his application form for Personal Independence Payment. In November 2020, he heard that his application was successful, so a better financial position, will also help enable him to maintain his success.

2015 - 2016: Tommy Warfield: 'Why Not Enjoy Life?'
Tommy visits us, every day that we are open. He has now reached his seventy-eighth birthday, and certainly has some health problems, but he continues to enjoy life. In April 2018, his Consultant renewed his Section, now a Community Treatment Order - thus ensuring that he stays in staffed facilities, on account of his bi-polar disorder, and other health problems. Ill health does not prevent Tommy from partaking of a wide range of cocktails from our bar, and relishing every sip. He has enjoyed everything - from a Singapore sling to a White Lady - from a Ramoz Fizz - to a Strawberry Dawn! No doubt, eventually, he will have worked his way through the entire alphabet of cocktails - from an Amaretto, to a Zhombie! In May 2019, we counted up, and found that he had sampled, with relish, more than forty different cocktails from our book of recipes. Our book is a classic one - with recipes for things like 'sidecar', and 'Harvey Wallbanger'. If you want a 'Screaming Orgasm', you won't get one down at the crisis house bar - though I do have a recipe for 'A Slow, Comfortable Screw Against A Wall' - Southern comfort, vodka, and sloe gin - delicious! Fortunately, the company that run Tommy's nursing home, in Caversham, West Reading, opened, a similar facility, in Wokingham, in July 2018, so, in February 2019, he moved back - to be nearer to his ex-wife and daughter, and nearer to us. This is much better, and easier for visiting, and Tommy expresses himself, as being very happy, with this move back to Wokingham. He loves coming to the crisis house drop-in. The move has produced some hilarious situations. We are convinced that Tommy believes, that he is now discharged from prison. He detested his former hospital hostel - in Caversham - because it was very restrictive. The Wokingham home, is less restrictive, and Tommy fully believes, that he is back in the house, in Wokingham, that he owned before it was re-possessed - due to his manic illness, and that he is young, once again! In fact, he is still Sectioned, under a Community Treatment Order, but we believe that the authorities needed his place in Caversham, for an, even more severely, mentally ill, patient, and so have placed Tommy in a less restrictive home - but with an extra package of care, in place. Where other residents do their own cooking, for instance, Tommy has carers, coming in, to prepare his meals, but his daughter gets the food that Tommy chooses - vegetarian options - rather than having to accept the, standardised

menus, of his previous accommodation. Tommy objects strongly to our describing the staff as his 'carers'! They are not carers; I am their client', he avers! He can barely stand on his two feet, but he has re-applied for his Driving Licence! I reassured our members - not to worry - he won't be issued with it! But we don't live, do we - with what life is? We live, with what we perceive it to be! In his mind, Tommy is a young, man-about-town, once again, and happy with it. Now back in Wokingham, Tommy encountered, by chance, an old flame, Amanda. This renewal of friendship, has enhanced his life greatly. He sees her in the evenings, and, at weekends, they visit the Holme Grange Craft Centre, and go, for Sunday lunch, at the Old Leatherne Bottle. They have, particularly, enjoyed attending performances at South Hill Park Theatre, in Bracknell. They joined in an evening of Judy Garland songs, and a performance of 'The Elvis Story'. With the support of his carers, Tommy gets out and about, every day. He confided that his favourite film is 'My Fair Lady'. I had a CD of the original sound track, so, on Friday 31st January 2020, we decided to play this, and sing along to the songs. One of our favourites is, 'With A Little Bit of Luck'

The Lord, above gave man an arm of iron,
So he could do his job, and never shirk.
The Lord above gave man an arm of iron, but –
With a little bit of luck, with a little bit of luck,
Someone else will do the blinking work!

Tommy enjoyed every minute of our sing-song, and we agreed, that Audrey Hepburn - arrayed for the Embassy Ball, was the most beautiful woman - ever to appear - on the silver screen. No wonder that she wanted to dance all night!

I'll never know what made it so
Exciting, why, all at once,
My heart took flight.
I only know when he
Began to dance with me
I could have danced, danced,
Danced, all night.

Thus, still able to enjoy life, Tommy Warfield, is a success story, maintained.

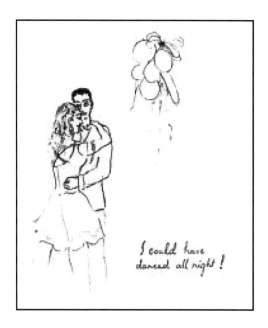

I could have
danced all night !

In March 2020, the Manager of Tommy's Care Home, took a decision, that he should self-isolate - being in the vulnerable group - aged, over seventy, and with underlying health conditions. We agreed that this was wise, though sad, of course, since Tommy enjoys coming to us, so much. As, with all, our elderly, members, who are self-isolating, we are keeping in touch, with Tommy, by telephone, and looking forward to the time when the current, necessary, restrictions are lifted, and we can welcome him back, into the drop-in centre. Fortunately, when I telephoned Tommy on Friday 27th March, he confirmed that he is still able to see Amanda - if less frequently. Tommy telephoned me, on Friday 3rd April, and stated that he was bored out of his skull. He is able to see his daughter, daily, but only through a closed window! I think that, a good idea, might be, to provide Tommy, with our student, telephone chat, service. A conversation, with someone, young and bright, will soon cheer him up. By the end of May 2020, some of the restrictions are easing, and we are hoping to have Tommy, back in our midst, as soon as circumstances, allow. It was good to hear, when Tommy telephoned on Tuesday 16th June, that he now able to go out with his daughter, so it looks as though a return to normality, is now, just around the corner.

On Friday 19th June, Tommy telephoned me - to say that he had been counting up, and that, in his lifetime, he had worked his way through two hundred girlfriends, and that he remembered, the names, of eighty-five of them! He added, 'And I've not stopped yet!' - what might be described as - 'There is still life in the old dog!' As Lockdown restrictions eased, Tommy was hoping to be back with us, in the drop-in centre, by July 2020. I discussed the matter with the manager of his care home, but her view, was that it was still, too early. to allow Tommy back - bearing in mind the risk to other residents, if he contracted coronavirus. However, the policy is being kept under review, and further relaxation of the rules, may be possible, once a vaccine is found. On Friday 7th August 2020, Tommy came up with a new initiative. He enjoys playing a game - whereby you are given a first name, and then have to identify, celebrities, with that first name. He has now, taken to playing it, over the telephone! There has been a further development in Tommy's situation. On Monday 14th September, his former wife telephoned, to explain that Tommy had attended a Mental Health Tribunal. He was represented by a very good advocate, and, as well as pleading, successfully, that, since Lockdown, he had been receiving, only five hours, per day, care - instead of the seven, allocated in his Care Package, he pleaded, successfully, that he should be allowed to return to the crisis house drop-in centre, which he values, so greatly, and misses so much. The Judge ruled in his favour, and is arranging for his care-co-ordinator to visit us - to ensure that we are complying with Covid Safety rules, which we are, and then he should be able to return to us - to our delight. Tommy visited with his daughter, but, to comply with the rules, until all is agreed, Patrick and myself, met them outside the crisis house. Tommy was looking very well, and this is a good development. On Friday 25th September, Tommy's Care Co-ordinator visited us - to look at our covid safeguarding arrangements, before Tommy's return. He explained that, as well as being under a Community Treatment Order, Tommy, has now, also been found to lack 'Capacity' - so extra care is required. We agreed, that when he returns, he should be accompanied by the regular carers from his home, and not by Agency staff - since their peripatetic service to care homes, has been, one, significant, way, in which the virus has spread. I had to laugh. Although the visit from Tommy's Care Co-ordinator, was amicable enough - [Please see the section on 'Comments from visitors to the crisis house'] - true to form, as soon as he was through the door, he was telling us how to run the place! As part of social distancing, he wanted Tommy to sit in Lucy's chair. She refused, firmly. Lucy also refused to wear the mask, that he was recommending for all service users! To date, I have made the wearing of masks, in the drop-in centre, optional. Some wear them; some don't. If masks in mental health centres, become mandatory, then we will all have to wear them - but not on the say-so of a local mental health professional! However, the good news is, that the Care Co-ordinator, evidently, reported, favourably, and Tommy returned to the crisis house drop-in centre, on Friday 16th October. He will attend, on every day that we are open, once this latest lockdown is over, and will relish, regular drinks, from our bar, once again!

The Crisis House Bar
There is no contest. Tommy is the most regular, and appreciative, user of our crisis house bar. It is, nevertheless, enjoyed by many, and appreciated - not just for its great variety of drinks - but for what it represents - respect, and adult status, accorded to the mentally ill. Human beings never fail to fascinate me. In our bar, we have the best single malt Scotch whisky - Haigs, and Taylor's vintage port. What do our service users opt for? American bourbon, and coca cola! It's damned unBritish of them! In Agatha Christie's novel, '*Dumb Witness*', like me, Miss Arundell wondered at the extraordinary preferences that people have. She writes:

'Her mind reverting to her niece's fiance, Miss Arundell thought, I don't suppose he'll ever take to drink! Calls himself a man, and drank barley water, this evening. Barley water! And I opened papa's special port!' My sentiments, precisely!

Our service users, themselves, like to see that we don't go short of drinks. Don, regularly, keeps us supplied with Smirnoff Vodka, and Dan Kent makes sure that the Harvey's Bristol Cream Sherry, is replenished, regularly. Bearing in mind his friend, Patrick's preferences, nor does he forget, donations of Kentucky Bourbon! Joseph, on a recent visit, supplied us with a large bottle of Bacardi - Lucy and Sadie's favourite, drink. Like the late Queen Mother, we are always in a position to enquire of visitors, 'What is your tipple, young man?' It is a standard joke, in the crisis house - that we are in crisis - if the number of bottles of alcohol in our bar falls too low.

I really miss my late Deputy, feisty old Scottish octogenarian, Frances - now, sadly, passed away. She soon put 'recovering' alcoholics in their place! 'I'm not doing without my lunchtime drink - just because you are an alcoholic', she would assert! True to Scottish tradition, her tipple was whisky - topped up with Drambuie - in fact, a 'Rusty Nail'. She expressed, our philosophy, perfectly. We are all about getting the mentally ill back into normal life - of which drinking alcohol is a normal part - for those who can do so safely. For those who can't, or for those who prefer soft drinks, we have a fridge full of soft drinks - and plenty of ice in our freezer! These have all been particularly popular in the hot summer of 2018, and even those who opt for alcohol, also like our wide range of fruit juices - as mixers. Always popular, are hot Drinks: We have the best Indian tea, and also Earl Grey, Lady Grey, and camomile. We have the best coffee – Carte Noir, and Kenco - both with caffeine, and decaffeinated. For those who prefer it, we also have cappuccino. In the winter, we offer various soups. Heartbreaking, is it not? Until recently, the local mental health team offices - which our members have to attend - provided no drinks at all. Finally, they actually got around to providing - just water! This is not a service at all. It is a soulless bureaucracy!

In the same way that I don't buy, Tiffany Lamps, from Tiffany's in New York, [Please see: 'More Funny Stories: Breakfast at Tiffany's'], neither do I spend, a fortune, on crisis house drinks. Instead, I always buy the best stuff, when it is on offer. I am like Mrs Hubbard – in Agatha Christie's novel, '*Hickory, Dickory, Dock*'. In altercation with the Mrs. Nicoletis, odious proprietor, of the student hostel, in Hickory Road, Mrs, Hubbard stuck to her ground. Mrs. Nicoletis had called her in, to complain about her household expenditure. Mrs. Hubbard explained that there had been some very good stuff going at Lampson's Stores - so she was taking advantage of this week's cheaper offers, and that the next week's shopping bill would be lower. Agatha Christie, presents Mrs Hubbard, as being like her sister, his efficient secretary, Miss Lemon - 'A Miss Lemon, softened as it were, by marriage and the climate of Singapore, but still having that sound core of sense'. This is the characteristic, which enables me to provide, the best of everything, for the people who use our services – without the Association going bankrupt!

PART THREE

Chapter 8

The Path To Recovery

In this chapter, I have included numerous quotations from Agatha Christie's novels - because so much of her work deals with what is PRESENTED, and not with actual reality.

She is the most superb, of natural psychologists - piercing the veneer of human behaviour, with consummate skill. People recovering from mental illness - or even remaining ill, but seeking a more normal life - have to learn to PRESENT themselves to the world, as normal, in order to achieve their goals. Look at some of the characters in Agatha Christie's books, and observe how different the mask can be - from the reality beneath it. Take, for instance, Neville Strange - in *'Towards Zero'*.

A similar mask can be observed, when Zachariah Osborne, the dapper little chemist, is exposed as a murderer, in *'The Pale Horse'* by Agatha Christie. Superb actor, Sir Charles Cartwright, also puts up a good show as Sir Bartholomew Strange's butler - only to be found out, by the astute Muriel Wills - in *'Three Act Tragedy'*. But, to me, Agatha Christie's *piece de resistance* - when it comes to people, not being what they seem – is achieved in her redoubtable play, 'The Mousetrap'.

Duchess of Cornwall, Camilla Parker-Bowles, is, currently, in 2020, involved in campaigning for the welfare of victims of domestic abuse - for both female, and male, victims. She is very conscious of the fact that nobody ever knows what goes on behind closed doors! Like mental illness, domestic abuse, permeates through the whole of society - from top to bottom The Duchess confirms, that officialdom, often fails to see, abuse, when it is cloaked in a disguise of respectability. Now, in March 2020, one of the problems arising from the closure of schools - due to the coronavirus pandemic, is concern for children who live in homes, where there is domestic abuse. Stress, and unwanted change - possibly compounded by financial problems - invariably makes such abuse worse, and more likely to occur. This is why Marcus Rashford's campaign to help families, has proved so vital. Nobody knows, what goes on behind closed doors, and when, as in this crisis, those doors are closed, virtually all the time, then the risk to the vulnerable, becomes much higher.

In the crisis house, the mentally ill can relax, and be themselves. We have eliminated all involvement from officialdom. People don't tell officialdom, what they are really thinking, and feeling. They tell them what they think they want to hear, and such is not therapeutic! When engaging with the world of work, and, indeed, with social life, generally, one has to put up a coping front. So people with mental health problems need, in addition, a place of complete, and stress-free, sanctuary. *'There's a Place for Us'* - never was a book more aptly entitled!

As I explain, regularly, to our service users, recovery of mental health, is achieved by struggling along a pathway, and, not, by a, dramatic, overnight, miracle. Furthermore, as our service user, Elise, says, 'The pathway isn't linear.' It has steps - both up, and down! In December 2019, Glyn happened to be in the drop-in centre with Elise, and said to her, 'The sooner you get back to work, the better!' I remonstrated with him. Elise has been struggling in jobs, for years. What she needs now, is a time of respite, and then, when she is ready, counselling, focussed on a career redirection, and probably, re-training. No such thing existed, when I was a youngster, so I had to work out my own salvation! When I was a youngster, and, due to adverse circumstances, had lost all my confidence, I determined to regain it, by taking on a job which was, generally regarded, as being very hard. If I could succeed in it, I reasoned with myself, and thus demonstrate my competence, then I would regain my confidence, and so find other things, easy. So I took on the job of nursing auxiliary. I did very well in this job, and the Matron of the hospital, was only too happy to re-employ me, during my vacations, and provided me with a glowing reference, when I was ready to move on. I recall, with wry humour, how I luxuriated in my recovery, at the time. I looked at, how little, by comparison, other people were required to do, and gloated. 'You would never cope, with what I can cope with!' I used to say to myself. But, note this important point. I wasn't really a nursing auxiliary; it was a mask! As Agatha Christie writes - in *'The Secret Adversary'*.

During the War, 'the talented Miss Cowley, [Tuppence], drove successively, a trade delivery van, a motor lorry, and a general. The last was the pleasantest. He was quite a young general!' 'What blighter was that,?' Inquired Tommy. 'Perfectly sickening, the way these brass hats drove from the War Office to the Savoy, and from the Savoy to the War Office.' 'I've forgotten his name now, confessed Tuppence . . .I fancy he keeps a bicycle shop in time of peace.'

This is the secret - that the recovering mentally ill, must learn, in order to survive. You must never, lose sight, of your own self esteem. Then you can, fit in, with all kinds of difficult situations. I believe that whom one marries, reflects one's true status, much more than any mundane job, that one may, temporarily, be doing. Agatha Christie may have been setting out to be whimsically amusing in her short story - 'The Girl in the Train' - from '*The Listerdale Mystery*', but it remains the case, that there is many a true word spoken in jest! Social status, and money, dictate most marriages! George Rowland had a rich uncle, and Lady Elizabeth Gaigh, had a title.

'H'm, said George. It will be one of those marriages made in Heaven and approved on earth.'

It is a fact of life, that money and social status, marry money, and social status. Just look at Jeff Bezos! 'Oh, Pam Jenkinson, are you a snob?' 'No, like Agatha Christie, a realist!' As recently as Friday 10th April 2020, I was advising Philip Worthing, that - lovely though it would be, if everybody were equal, unfortunately, they are not! [Please see: 'Poignant Stories - An Octopus's Garden']. I fear that we have to live with life as it is, and, not, with how we would like it to be! Furthermore, this point is important. To prove oneself, it is no good sticking out these menial jobs for three weeks! That proves nothing! I stuck it out for more than three years - for some months, before I started my degree course, and then for all my vacations, throughout the course - so that made a total time, of more than three years. I still recall, one morning in 1968, standing by a patient's bed, and having a thought - spontaneously crossing my mind - 'I don't need this any more!' Being so young, I didn't realise it, but I had successfully reached the end of the Recovery Pathway. I had regained, and, most important, SUSTAINED, my confidence. I never lost it again! This is what our service aims to do - to help people, step by step, to recover their confidence, and, thus, their ability to re-engage with normal life, and this, when achieved, is, invariably, done - slowly! So, I advise the Oxbridge graduates, and we have had some, staying in the crisis house in the past, 'adopt the attitude of Tuppence Beresford - described, above'. Accept a menial position for the time being - while you are getting over your breakdown; it won't be for life! I, also, advise people, to wait until they are recovered, before they start looking for a new partner. Then you stand a chance of finding someone of similar educational background, and social status, as yourself - of which unrecovered mental illness can, so cruelly, rob you!' It would be lovely, if everyone were equal, if all work colleagues, were sympathetic, and all jobs provided idyllic conditions, but they are not, and they don't. Idealism [due to lack of experience], and the harsh reality, are illustrated, beautifully, by Agatha Christie, in her novel, 'The Hollow'. Midge Hardcastle, young first cousin, of Lady Lucy Angkatell, was a poor relation of the family, and so was obliged to take a job in Madame Alfredge's, dreadful, dress shop. She was head over heels in love with Edward Angkatell, but, nevertheless, exasperated by his inability to grasp the realities of life. Furthermore, Midge also had to contend with young David - 'who preferred the contemplation of an Academic past, or the earnest discussion of a Left Wing future, and had no aptitude for dealing with a violent, and realistic, present.'

One thing that the coronavirus pandemic is teaching us, is that some, very menial, jobs, need to be done, in order for us, to survive. Of course, we need the front-line doctors, but we also, desperately, need the cleaners, the care assistants, the porters, the supermarket shelf-fillers, and the refuse collectors! However, I do not agree with the view, currently being expressed, that, this crisis, will change people's attitude, and that menial, but essential, occupations, will be valued, more appreciatively, and, consequently, become better paid. I fear not! Human nature, remains human nature, and is, by definition, competitive, and hierarchical. The reason that menial, but vital, jobs, are badly paid, is because any able-bodied person can do them. You don't have to be intelligent, or well qualified; you just have to be, physically capable, of performing a, mundane task. Doctors, engineers, and teachers, are well-paid, because, relatively few people, can do their jobs. If anyone suffers from the misconception that teaching is easy, and that anyone can do it, then I strongly recommend that they watch someone, who can't, and see what transpires. In her 'Autobiography', Agatha Christie describes, the chaos and mayhem, that reigned, when her own daughter, Rosalind, had been provided with an, incompetent, nanny, and, don't forget, this nanny, was only having to cope, with one child, from a good social background. 'Teaching is easy?' - try coping with forty pupils - from, a poor, social background! 'Children know authority' - Agatha Christie averred. She never spoke a truer word! One requires special gifts, in order to perform these, highly skilled, jobs, and it is the old, old, story - that it would be lovely - if everyone were equal, in ability, but they are not! It is good, that, in the current crisis, people are being, genuinely, appreciative, of all essential workers, but this is not a sentiment that will last. So many of the old war time songs, come to mind, at this time. We will bless them all, as the crisis comes to an end, and then, normal life, with its inequalities, and hierarchies, will resume.

Bless 'em all, bless 'em all,
The long, and the short, and the tall.

The following article appeared in *The Wokingham Paper* (25th March 2020). It was written by an Oxford University graduate, and former crisis house guest, who has now, achieved some recovery, and has got back into his writing.

Marking World Bi-Polar Day
'Monday 30th March is World Bi-Polar Day. [WBD], although few people know about it in the UK and Europe, not even my psychiatrist. It is an initiative of the international Bi-Polar Foundation, San Diego, the international Society for Bi-Polar Disorders, Chicago, and the Asian Network of Bi-Polar Disorder, Hong Kong. The date of March 30th was chosen, as it is the birthday of the Dutch painter, Vincent Van Gogh, who was retrospectively diagnosed to have this disorder, by various psychiatrists. The first world Bi-Polar Day was celebrated in 2014. Van Gogh was born in 1853, but only lived to be 37. On July 27th 1890, he walked into a wheat field, and shot himself, in the chest, with a pistol. He died a few days later. In Van Gogh's time, there was no access to any medication, to alleviate his condition. If there had been, he might have left a much greater collection of masterpieces. A high proportion of Bi-Polar sufferers commit suicide - as much as 15 percent, and many others attempt it. Those with Bi-Polar are often very creative individuals, who contribute a lot to society. Examples include, Stephen Fry, Mel Gibson, and Frank Sinatra. The aim of WBD is to increase the awareness of Bi-Polar Disorder, and to eliminate social stigma, as well as informing the world, about it. Bi-Polar is a brain disorder that causes unusual shifts, in mood, energy, activity levels, and the ability to carry out everyday tasks. Symptoms of Bi-Polar disorder, are severe, and different, from the normal, ups and downs, that everyone experiences. An estimated 1.3 million, people in the UK, suffer from Bi-Polar, previously known as

Manic Depression, according to the charity, Bi-Polar, UK. Diagnosis is not easy, and can take up to, ten years, or more. Most, are diagnosed, in their late teens, or early twenties. There are two main forms - Bi-Polar 1, and Bi-Polar 2 - with, the latter, having, less extreme, bouts of mania. About 5 percent of Bi-Polar 1 sufferers, only experience, manic episodes, and do not get depressed. What causes Bi-Polar, is unclear, although, genetic, and life circumstances, play a role. Some women can suffer from it, after childbirth. The Australian researcher, John Cade, had the first paper, published, in 1948 - showing that lithium carbonate, is, an effective, mood stabiliser, and anti-manic, agent. Danish researcher, Mogens Schou, subsequently, confirmed, the efficacy, of lithium, in further research, and it was introduced, into psychiatric practice. It became, widely used, from the late1960's, although doses have reduced, somewhat. It is not effective, for everyone, and can also, affect thyroid, and kidney, function. Studies in Texas, Austria, and Japan, have found, that high lithium levels, in the water supply, correlated with lower suicide rates, in the populations. Long-term exposure to lithium, increases grey matter - which is, generally, better for the brain, and also, possibly, helps with dementia. Professor Alan Young, Chair of Mood Disorders, at King's College, London, says there is no doubt, that lithium prevents recurrence, of manic episodes. It is, less effective, against acute depression. He is working on better lithium formulations, with less potential damage, to kidneys. Professor Young commented, that current treatments with lithium, and other products, show, nowhere near, the efficacy, and selectivity, of cancer treatment, and this is something that needs to be rectified. Current research efforts, focus on biological causes, new targets for drug treatment, better treatments, better diagnosis, genetic components, and strategies, for living well, with Bi-Polar Disorder. Some 300 delegates attended a conference, organised by Bi-Polar UK, IN London, on November 17th, last year - over half, of whom, were Bi-Polar. There was a Panel Session which was also filmed, by BBC TV's, 'Horizon', for a future programme, about the comedian, Tony Slattery, due to be broadcast, this year. The Panel of four, including Slattery, debated whether, they would prefer to remain, Bi-Polar, or turn it off, and eliminate the condition, permanently. All four acknowledged, that they owed their careers, and creativity, in part, at least, to being Bi-Polar. Bi-Polar UK took a poll of 85 Bi-Polar attendees, before the conference took place. Some 76 percent replied, that they would turn off their Bi-Polar, if they could. In a poll at the end of the Panel Session, some 65 percent of Bi-Polar attendees indicated, that they would prefer to, eliminate, their Bi-Polar condition. This suggests a substantial minority of sufferers, sees their condition, as providing, something positive, for their lives, despite, the considerable drawbacks, that come with it.'

Does not this, brilliant, and carefully researched, article, prove, the accuracy, of my argument. Despite suffering from a severe mental illness, the Oxford University science graduate, is still, really, an Oxford University science graduate - however humble the occupations, he may be required to adopt, while on the Path of Recovery. I am, particularly, interested, in the reference to Mogens Schou's work with lithium. In what was to be, one of my last international conferences, I brought Professor Mogens Schou, over from Denmark - to address a conference, on what, was then, called, Manic Depression. This was held, in Oxford, in November 1992. It was shortly after this, that running the Wokingham Crisis House, became a, full time, occupation, so I had to discontinue mental health education work. I have acknowledged Brendan's achievement in my letter to *The Wokingham Paper* (3rd April 2020) [Please see: 'The Campaign for Mental Health - Through The Exchange Of Letters'}.

As I have mentioned, currently, in January 2020, I am advising and supporting Elise. She hated her job as a Corporate Executive for a Car Company, and was demeaned, and bullied, by her boss. This exacerbated her existing mental health problems. When she is sufficiently recovered, I am recommending that she has specialist counselling - which will probably result in re-training, and a complete change of career direction. The car industry is chauvinistic, highly pressurised, and is certainly, not the place, for someone, with Elise's temperament. Psychotherapy enables the individual to look at both - his/her, strengths, and, his/her, vulnerabilities. Thus, I have advised Elise. 'You are intelligent, well qualified - with undergraduate, and Master's degrees in economics; you are personable, and well-presented. Those are your assets. But you are also, hypersensitive, vulnerable to depression, and anxiety, and thus likely to be the victim of bullying in the workplace - which, you have, indeed, been in the past. So you have to look at the type of future employment, in which your assets can be maximised, and your disadvantages minimised. This might mean leaving the Corporate World completely. You might find yourself, better suited, to more people-centred employment - such as that of a Housing Support Officer, for vulnerable people.' The great advantage of the crisis house, is that we have all the time, and space in the world, for people like Elise - thus to examine their situation, and plan, productively, for the future. 'There's a Place for us. There's a Time for us!' With a view to achieving the goals described, I wrote the following reference for Elise, and she started her initial training with Home Start in February 2020.

'Elise Sands joined the Wokingham and West Berkshire Mental Health Association, as a volunteer, in October 2019. She has a very pleasant, sympathetic, personality, and has proved to be invaluable, in her voluntary work with us. She makes a good contribution to our drop-in sessions - where she is mixing with people suffering from the full range of mental illnesses - including schizophrenia, bi-polar affective disorder, depression, anxiety, personality disorders, and addictions. She gets on well with all of them, and is completely unfazed by those displaying the more severe symptoms. During the time that she has been with us, Elise has also, working as a team with another of our volunteers, taken on the de-cluttering of a flat which is occupied by a lady suffering from a severe obsessional disorder, and requiring a great deal of support. The lady's own psychotherapist has commented on the huge amount of progress that has been achieved for this lady, by Elise and her colleague, in undertaking this task, and I, myself, have observed just how valuable it is, to have team work in such difficult circumstances. Elise has also, regularly accompanied, the lady to a support group for hoarders. She will be absolutely ideal in supporting your families who are experiencing problems, and struggling to cope with young children. Elise, herself, also has quite a bit of experience in helping out friends with young children, and has also done baby-sitting for another of our members, who has two young children, and doesn't get much of a chance to go out with her husband. Elise was working in the Corporate Sector - Car Sales, but she has expressed a desire to make a career change - into more, directly, people-centred employment - in the Care, or Mental Health, Sectors. Her step - in seeking voluntary work in such Sectors, is a sensible one - so that she can contribute, gain experience, and decide upon the client group with whom she is best suited to work - long-term. Elise will support families well, have a non judgmental, professional, attitude, and will respect confidentiality. She is highly intelligent, reliable, and has a good sense of humour, so I can recommend her unreservedly, as a volunteer, in your organisation.'

I am pleased to record, that Elise was accepted for the Home Start volunteering, and completed her training course, for this, on Tuesday 26th May. Due to the circumstances, some of the training had to be done, on line, but it did, at least, go ahead - in spite of the coronavirus pandemic. Finally, in October 2020, she was allocated an individual family - with whom to work.

Just look at some of our other success stories. Sadie Minton, for instance, had a history, of lasting, literally, for days, in a number of jobs. How was it, then, that she coped, successfully, for eleven solid years - cleaning a solicitor's office? This is why. Sadie suffers from schizophrenia, and so has very minimal social skills. She can't cope with people - particularly - not in the workplace. Schizophrenia is a stress-related disorder - so Sadie can't cope with stress - and, particularly, not in the workplace. She needs a predictable routine, and is unable to cope with change. Those are her disadvantages. Now, let us look at her assets. She is able-bodied, and quite intelligent. The solicitor leaves the office at 5pm, and Sadie has the key; furthermore, the office is near to where she lives, so she doesn't have the, additional, stress of travel. All Sadie has to do, is to spend two hours - cleaning the office, and then, lock up. Everything is always the same, and nobody is there, with her, so she doesn't have to cope with people, at all. Sadie is quite capable of routine cleaning, and if it takes her three hours, instead of two hours, nobody knows, or cares, and so won't be critical - provided that the job is done. Total employment success! So this is what the sufferer of mental health problems has to do - analyse strengths, and weaknesses, and then work out how disadvantages are to be overcome, and successful employment, thus maintained.

There is no doubt about it. Just as the, physically, disabled, are handicapped in the physical world, the mentally ill, are handicapped in the social world. Mentally ill people frequently talk of 'putting on a mask' - in order to cope with the mysteries of the social, and working, world. Sometimes, people will pierce the mask. Agatha Christie, as always, has her finger on the pulse. In 'N or M', she, thus reveals, that people who appear to be someone else, invariably ARE someone else! You are a cuckoo in the nest, and people, with animal instinct, can sense it! This was also the case with 'Anthony Browne' in Agatha Christie's novel, *'Sparkling Cyanide'*. Until he actually met 'Anthony Browne', Colonel Race thought that he had caught up with a master criminal, and murderer. But when he did meet him, he knew that he hadn't. In, 'N or M', at first, Tommy never suspected, for one moment, that Commander Haydock was anything other than a bluff, British Naval Officer. It was the Commander's manservant, who gave the game away. The supreme instance of people not being what they seem - is the whole thrust of Agatha Christie's novel – '*At Bertram's Hotel*'.

Interestingly, while, in Conan Doyle's '*The Red Headed League*', the ready, acceptance by an employee - to take half wages - made Sherlock Holmes smell a rat, in Agatha Christie's novel, '*The Pale Horse*', it is the opposite phenomenon, that arouses one's suspicion. The pay and conditions at C.R.C. [Customers' Reactions Classified], a market research company, were too good to be true. They led former employees to suspect that the company was a cover for something else. Indeed it was!

PART FOUR

Further Success Stories

Chapter 9

This sequel, follows this up, with further success stories - for the five, subsequent, years.

Tessa Kelly: 'A Grief Observed'

Tessa was our befriender, Lucy Farmer's neighbour. Tessa's husband had been in hospital, with depression, and, due to the pressure on beds, had been discharged, prematurely. One afternoon, Lucy observed Tessa, carrying a cup of tea to her husband, who was working in their garage. Then, Lucy observed her come out, go and get a knife, which she used to cut down his body. He had hanged himself in the garage! Thereafter, Tessa was in a state of trauma. She was unable to prepare meals, because she was terrified of knives! Lucy befriended her throughout this tragic crisis. A negligence case was pursued, and won - the Health Authority being found at fault on five points of negligence. Tessa received a small amount of financial compensation - though most of the money was swallowed up in Solicitors' fees. Furthermore, nothing could compensate for the loss of her husband. She was nevertheless, very disadvantaged, financially, so I applied for Benefits on her behalf, explained the extent of the trauma to the Benefits Officer, and so was able to obtain the money for her - without her having to endure the additional stress of a face-to-face interview. The great thing about Lucy's befriending, is that she is always on hand for the person, and it was lucky, in Tessa's case, that they were close neighbours - so Lucy could pop round at any time of day, or night, when needed. Slow step, by slow step, as it always is, Tessa rebuilt her life. She had a son, still at home, and a daughter. The daughter got married, moved to Buckinghamshire, and had a baby, so Tessa decided to sell up, buy a house near her daughter, and concentrate on being a grandmother. The baby was, literally, her emotional salvation. After Tessa moved, Lucy stayed regularly in touch, by telephone. Happily, in 2019, Tessa, always slim and attractive, revealed that she had a new romance in her life. Now, in 2020, Tessa continues to do well - though she is still under mental health treatment - which, fortunately, in her area, is of a good standard. Unsurprisingly, she feels unable, even to visit, Berkshire, but Lucy hopes to visit Tessa - once current restrictions are relaxed. A success story!

Tabitha Merton: 'Light At The End Of The Tunnel'
In August 2017, Tabitha Merton walked into the Station House drop-in centre - in a state of crisis. I had only met Tabitha, once before; she was a friend of Leona - who had stayed in the Crisis House from 2003 until 2005, and while staying with us, used to go to Tabitha's house to sunbathe. They had been pupils together at Wokingham's Holt School. The only occasion on which I had actually met Tabitha - was at a market stall - which we ran for our charity in 2004. Her mother was with her - on a rare visit home from Thailand! Tabitha explained the reasons for her distress. Her mother had abandoned Tabitha and her brother, when they were very young children, and had gone to live in Thailand. Their father was left to bring them up, and, understandably, found this extremely difficult. The family was very dysfunctional. From teenage years, Tabitha had to work - mainly in shops, and as a waitress. At the age of twenty-three, she gave birth to a son, Aaron, but her partner, and the child's father, also abandoned them, and went to live in New Zealand. Aaron suffered from Asperger's Syndrome, had to have special needs education, and bringing him up as a lone parent, caused Tabitha a great deal of stress - since she also, at her father's insistence, had to continue working. The last straw, when she came to us, was that her father, after suffering from diabetes, went on to be diagnosed with pancreatic cancer - a particularly nasty form of the disease, and, not one that responds best, to treatment. When terminally ill, Tabitha had to nurse him, full-time, because he refused to go into a hospice. Tabitha was overburdened with exhaustion and grief. She explained that he was 'green', and having to cope, caused her great distress - especially since

their relationship - from her infancy - had been so fraught and dysfunctional. [For comparison, [Please see: *'Triumph and Tragedy'* - 'Twenty-Five Poignant Stories - The Reversal of Fortunes']. Here, I describe the situation of Johnnie and Charles Hewitt. How can you nurse, compassionately, the parent, who, in the past, has bullied you? Tabitha's father died in June 2017. Then Tabitha went into crisis. We thought that she might benefit from private psychotherapy - which, though costly, can be accessed very quickly. No NHS Waiting Lists, in Private Practice, and we consider that paying for such therapy, for individuals, is a good use of our charity's funds. We followed our regular procedure of referring Tabitha to a top Consultant Psychiatrist at the prestigious Cardinal Clinic, a private psychiatric hospital, in Windsor. He then referred her to a Wokingham private psychotherapist - who specialised in treating patients with self esteem issues. Tabitha continued with this therapy throughout the remainder of 2017. In 2018, greatly recovered, she got her life back together, returned to paid work, and in fact, turned her whole situation around for the better. Now, in August 2020, three years after she came to us, in crisis, I get reports, from our members who are still in touch with her, that Tabitha is doing well, and this was reiterated by one of our service users, now, in November 2020. He said that Tabitha was flourishing. A success story.

Alistair Branson: 'Recovery - Despite All'

Alistair Branson was introduced to the crisis house drop-in centre by our service user, Neville, in August 2015. He was in an advanced state of alcoholism, and was homeless. He explained that he had been employed as a care assistant at Broadmoor Hospital, but had been dismissed - due to alcoholism. His second marriage had also broken down - for the same reason. Alistair became a regular user of our drop-in centre - as well as using the services of the local Salvation Army. He was very drunk all the time, and homeless, on the street. He made an attempt at residential rehab, but this failed. Eventually, the local Council provided him with a flat at Shinfield, but he was unable to cope there. His path to recovery was embarked upon, when he was provided with a place at Yeldhall Manor - which is a church foundation that offers residential rehabilitation - for both drug addicts and alcoholics. The initial programme requires residence in a tightly supervised environment, for a year - followed by residence in a move-on house. The move-on houses have various degrees of supervision - according to the progress made by the residents. Alistair made excellent progress through all the stages of the rehabilitation programme - which included group work, and counselling. By 2018, Alistair was completely free of alcohol addiction, and training to be a peer-supporter at IRIS, a drugs and alcohol rehabilitation service in Reading. He keeps in touch with the crisis house drop-in centre. On Tuesday 1st October 2019, Alistair dropped in to see us. – beaming with triumphant success! He was now working, in a paid post, with the Probation Service. What was formerly known as 'community service' is now called 'Pay Back'. Alistair was now working as a 'Pay Back' supervisor - overseeing the compulsory, unpaid, work of former offenders. Alistair illustrates the fact that I point to constantly. It is much easier for those who - either through psychiatric, or substance abuse, rehabilitation - get back to something that they have achieved previously, than, for those who suffer mental breakdown, or substance addiction, in early youth, and so have never made a start on life's path. The latter are starting from scratch. Alistair had years of experience, under his belt, as a care assistant at Broadmoor Hospital - dealing with the most difficult of mentally ill offenders. This experience must stand him in good stead for his work with the Probation Service. A success story.

Patrick Small: 'Work Wins'
When Patrick Small came to us, he was in a very depressed, and distressed, state. He explained that he had suffered two, major, adverse life events. Firstly, he had been made redundant from his job as a Technical Photographer, at Kew Gardens - where he had worked for the previous fifteen years - following fifteen years service in the Royal Air Force - from whom he had acquired his, excellent, Technical Photography, training. Since he had been grossly overworked at Kew, with far more work than any individual could possibly cope with, redundancy simply added insult to injury! To add to the trauma of redundancy, he had been obliged, like Tabitha, to nurse his, terminally ill, father, at home. Again, like Tabitha, the relationship between Patrick and his father, had always been fraught with problems. Patrick's mother had died, prematurely, from a brain aneurysm. Thereafter, Patrick's father experienced severe problems - including a failed relationship - in which the lady concerned, became his, abusive, stalker! When, later in life, Patrick's father became ill, he failed to accept the situation, and often rejected his son's offers of help and care. Such a situation is far more difficult for the carer - than is one where the patient co-operates. Once again, I bring Agatha Christie's, faultless, psychology into the equation. I am, currently, as I write this, in March 2019, having a 'Tommy and Tuppence' season. Never as popular with most Christie

fans, as Hercule Poirot, and Jane Marple, I, nevertheless, appreciate Tommy and Tuppence Beresford.

In her novel - '*By The Pricking of My Thumbs*', good old Agatha Christie, expresses exactly, the problems that people like Tabitha and Patrick, had to contend with! Chapter 3 of this book is entitled - 'A Funeral.'

'Funerals are rather sad, aren't they,' said Tuppence. They had just returned from attending Aunt Ada's funeral.'. . . 'I said funerals were sad,' said Tuppence when she reappeared a moment or two, later, wearing a brilliant cherry-red dress, with a ruby and diamond lizard pinned on the shoulder of it. 'Because it's funerals like Aunt Ada's that are sad. I mean, elderly people, and not many flowers. Not a lot of people sobbing and sniffing round. Someone old and lonely, who won't be missed much.' 'I should have thought it would be much easier for you to stand that, than if it were my funeral, for instance.' [said Tommy]. 'That's where you're entirely wrong', said Tuppence. 'I don't particularly want to think of your funeral - because I'd much prefer to die before you do. But I mean, if I were going to your funeral, at any rate, it would be an orgy of grief.'

Agatha Christie's points about death, bereavement, and grief are so pertinent. As Tuppence explained to Tommy, if someone whom you have loved for decades, dies, your grief is overwhelming, but straightforward. But if someone close to you, but who has given you a lot of trouble in life, dies, as was the case with Tabitha and Patrick's bereavements, you can't cope with your conflicting feelings, so you have a mental breakdown! There is also the point - that blood is thicker than water! The person who persecuted and abused you, was, nevertheless, your father - from whom you derived your existence! If Reg and Jean's funeral - which I attended in February 2019, [Please see: 'Obituaries'] - is anything to go by, Tuppence's idea of cheering things up, seems to have been taken on in modern times. Instead of singing 'Abide With Me', we sang 'Happy Talk' - from 'South Pacific'. Our local church, All Saints, Wokingham, has provision for the Aunt Adas of the modern world. The church has a team of volunteers, who will attend the funerals of old and lonely people - thus giving them a good send-off - in the absence of family and friends as mourners.

Patrick found it beneficial to attend our drop-in centre, for support, as he sorted out all his problems - both practical, and emotional. He never stopped working, altogether, and this is always a good ingredient on the path to recovery. Indeed, he continues to do part-time Consultancy work for Kew Gardens, and, in 2019, was invited to photograph the Graduation Ceremony of their horticulturists. In addition, he also undertakes private, photography contract work. Breakdown causes lack of energy, and resultant chaos in one's environment, but, step by step, Patrick is sorting things out, at home. The recovery process is slow. Indeed, at the time of writing this, in March 2019, it is now two-and-a-half years since Patrick was made redundant from Kew, and two years since his father died. Psychiatric rehabilitation takes years, but it is good to see it achieved, successfully. Patrick, is ,one such, success story.

Keith Rode: 'Music, Music, Music'
Keith first contacted us in 2017. His cousin, who lives in Kent, had, fortunately, discovered our website, and so was able to point him in our direction - in order to get a local service. That this proved to be highly beneficial to Keith, is described, in detail, in our chapter on 'Advocacy'. As a result, Keith is a success story. Because Keith's illness is an anxiety neurosis, the current coronavirus pandemic is causing him some, renewed, anxiety, but he is getting help with filling in the form, for his Employment Support Allowance Review, as well as receiving Elise's practical assistance, with collecting shopping, and medication - for which he is most grateful. I am keeping in regular, telephone, contact, with Keith, while he is self-isolating, and when I spoke to him, on Tuesday 14th April, he averred, once again, how marvellous, his advocate, Tony, was. His Employment Support Allowance Form, had now been completed, and Keith was now, much less anxious, as a direct result, of all Tony's assistance. Keith is a success story.

Joseph and Joan Allen: 'Money Speaks'
Joseph and Joan were referred by Joseph's sister, late in 2018. A lot of their problems were financial. As a result of our splendid Advocacy Service, their lives were transformed, for the better, and this is described, in detail, in our chapter on 'Advocacy'. Joseph and Joan are a success story. Likewise, Joseph and Joan were very happy to avail themselves of practical help - during the coronavirus pandemic. I spoke to Joseph, on the telephone, as recently as September 2020, and although there are still problems, both he, and Joan, are continuing to avail themselves of the help that we have found for them. Joseph visited the crisis house, on Tuesday 20th October. He explained that he and Joan were receiving

excellent help from their Support Worker, but that he was having problems with social services. Tell me something new! He pointed out that, as you walk into the crisis house, the doors are open, on the latch, and you walk into a pleasant, and welcoming, lounge. By contrast, when you enter the social services offices, there are several buzzers to press, as you negotiate, each part, of the entry system. I explained to Joseph, that the only place that I knew of, where that degree of security was necessary, was Broadmoor Hospital. Essential there, no doubt, but most off-putting, for mentally ill, but harmless, people, who need to access mental health services. It is true that, recently, a fairly new, user of the crisis house, asked if I would be 'all right', as he left, leaving me alone, and with the doors on the latch. My reply was that, my view was biased, because I had been 'all right', for the past thirty years! I advised Joseph and Joan, that they should continue to avail themselves of the excellent support from their support worker, but have no other involvement with social services, since they wouldn't change them.

Michaela West: 'No Place Like Home'
Michaela came to us, for help and advice, in February 2019. Our Advocate, Bev, gave her a lot of support. As a result of this, Michaela was able to get supported accommodation in Somerset. Her story is described, in detail, in our chapter on 'Advocacy. Michaela is a success story.

Further Poignant Stories

Chapter 10

There is a commonly held view that people in adverse circumstances have been unfortunate in life, and only need the right opportunities - in order to achieve better circumstances. True, in some cases, no doubt, but I have experience, and thus, sympathy, with the view expressed by Agatha Christie, in her novel, *'They do it with Mirrors'*. Miss Marple and Carrie-Louise are discussing Carrie's own daughter - Mildred - who it was thought, had had her nose put out of joint, by Gina - Carrie's adopted daughter, who was so much more attractive than Mildred.

'Perhaps, suggested Miss Marple, Mildred had cause not to be happy?' Carrie-Louise said quietly, 'Because of being jealous? Yes, I daresay. But people don't really need a cause for feeling what they do feel. They're just made that way. Don't you think so, Jane?'

Certainly, in its thirty years' existence, the Wokingham Crisis House has seen many spectacular successes, but we have also known of people who were living in a pigsty, were rescued by us, stayed in the crisis house, and were found, by us, a beautiful flat to move into, and so to get a fresh start in life. But they duly turned the flat into another pigsty! Nothing is more true than the old saying - 'You can take the people out of the slums, but you can't take the slums out of the people!' In 2019, we currently have a service user, who was provided with a council flat, and furniture. He had a bed, but, in the flat, he continued to sleep on the floor, and sold his, newly purchased, white goods - to buy alcohol. He failed to comply with the Job Centre's requirements, and so was 'sanctioned', that is, his Benefit was axed. He couldn't pay his bills, and so electricity, gas, and water supplies were cut off. Eventually, he relinquished the flat, and has gone back to living on the street - sleeping on a piece of cardboard against the car park railing, and foraging in bins for food! I have tried to advise this individual, but to no avail. 'If you only consume coffee and biscuits, I explained, you won't starve, but you will be malnourished, and so more liable to become ill. You need proteins, vitamins, carbohydrates, fats, and roughage.' The Wokingham Salvation Army is an excellent organisation, that provides a full, cooked breakfast on three mornings of the week, and a cooked, dinner, on the three alternate, evenings - all supplied, free, to the homeless. Even during Lockdown, they continued to supply food parcels, and now, hot, take-away meals. But this individual won't accept this service, because he is paranoid, and so is reluctant to get involved with institutions. Similarly, he ignored my advice to seek a place in the Salvation Hostel, in Reading, in the early Autumn - before it silted up for the Winter. Now, in February 2020, and back on the street for almost a year, apparently, he does turn up, occasionally, at the Salvation Army Centre, in Wokingham, has breakfast, and uses their shower facility. It is, probably, a case of desperation - driving him at accept, albeit in a limited way, their, quite excellent, services. I have given this man's situation, some thought. In conversation, he told me, that, at the age of nineteen, he entered into a, shared mortgage, arrangement, with a friend, so that they could purchase a property! At the age of nineteen, mortgages, were not on my agenda. I was studying, having a good time, and looking forward to travel! Thirty, was the age, at which, I was ready to take on responsibility - such as taking out a mortgage! It is true that, in my young days, couples were still running off to Gretna Green - to get married, at the age of sixteen! I thought it, quite mad, even then, and nowadays, it would be regarded, as ludicrous! I recall laughing, then, when a college friend of mine, who had just married, at the age of twenty, said, witheringly, 'I expect that Pamela will go staggering down the aisle, with some old professor, when's she's thirty.' What amused me, was that one could be perceived as 'staggering', at thirty! So, perhaps, what we are seeing here, with this man, is a reversal. He took on adult responsibilities, at a, much too young, age, and now, in middle age, he has discarded responsibility, completely. This seems to be the psychology, of the situation.

We have also known of people - whom we rescued from abusive situations - who, having stayed in the crisis house, then moved on to new, abusive, situations. Poignant it is, but we, nevertheless, rejoice in our many successes, and it remains a pity, that only lack of money, prevents us, from continuing, to provide, such valuable, residential, facilities. Our financial situation reminds me of that described by Agatha Christie, in her book, 'Taken at the Flood'. It is just after the end of the second world war, and times are very straitened. Lynn Marchant's mother, Adela, is bewailing the fact that they can no longer afford the things that they took for granted before the war. Agatha Christie writes:

'Lynn's thoughts were broken into. Dramatically, and with a trembling lip, Mrs. Marchmont produced a sheaf of bills.. . . Lynn took the bills and glanced through them. There were no records of extravagance amongst them. They were for slates replaced on the roof; the mending of fences; replacement of a worn-out kitchen boiler - a new main water pipe. They amounted to a considerable sum.'

Expensive up keep - our situation, exactly! Station House is more than a century and a half, old. Everything needs maintenance, and although we have generous benefactors, we are always in competition for grants - with all the other worthy causes! Equally pertinent, is Agatha Christie's short story, 'The Listerdale Mystery'. Mrs. St. Vincent is considering taking a lease on a very nice house, but she has reservations about the running costs. Agatha Christie writes:

'The servants, said Mrs. St. Vincent, pathetically, would eat, you know! I mean, of course one would want them to, but that is the drawback One can so easily just do without things - when it is only oneself!'

Crisis House guests would put on the heating in the Winter. They would use kettles, cookers, washing machines, tumble driers. Their presence would require more cleaning services, and there would be much more wear and tear on everything. You would want them to use the facilities, of course, but the costs involved, would be colossal, and it cannot be done without sustained, and predictable, funding. The two thousand pounds, per year, that we used to receive - specifically for the crisis beds - was nothing, in the Statutory Mental Health Budget, but it was everything to us. Have they been kicking themselves, ever since they axed this funding? Of course, they have. Two thousand pounds a year - for four crisis beds. What a bargain! Don't talk to me about slates on the roof! Some of ours, here in August 2020, appeared to have suffered a landslide - though, whether through vandalism, or just, bad weather, I hadn't established, but, our builder confirmed that it was vandalism. Like Lynn Marchant's mother, my lip trembled, at the thought of the cost to be incurred. So our very situation, is poignant, and there have also been some more individual, poignant, stories - which I now go on to describe.

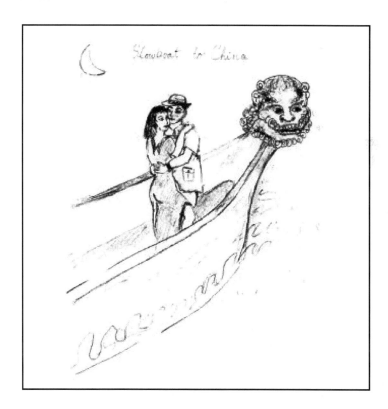

Poignant Stories

'I'd like to get you on a slow boat to China –
All to myself, alone!'

Aileen Brown: 'All To Myself, Alone'

Aileen telephoned in 2017 to explain that she had accessed our website, was a Reading resident, but was she eligible to use our drop-in service? As we are both, Wokingham, and, West Berkshire, Mental Health Association, of course she was eligible, so she started attending - at first, now and then, and then on all the days that we were open. She explained that she has suffered an abusive childhood, had cut all ties with her family, and lived, alone, in a flat. I would describe Aileen as the person-ification of a neurotic disorder - in fact - a narcissistic personality disorder - quite fascinating to observe. Lucy Farmer maintains that Aileen is a gift from heaven for our clinical psychology students! When I say that she never stops talking, I mean, never stops talking! This is usually a classic symptom of loneliness - which our drop-in centre is able to relieve, and where Aileen has expressed herself as feeling 'at home', but if one didn't take to interrupting, no-one else would ever get a word in edgeways! It is the same with attention. She demands this constantly, and one has to be firm - otherwise her neurotic illness would engulf the entire crisis house, and drive all other service users away. In fact, it has, with one service user! Aileen needed help on a number of fronts. We applied for Employment Support Allowance, and Personal Independence Payment, on her behalf. In addition to a severe neurosis, Aileen also suffers from vertigo, and balance problems - due to nerve damage sustained in a road traffic accident - which occurred when she was just seventeen. I suspect that a lot of this is 'conversion hysteria', but we, nevertheless, arranged adaptations to her current accommodation, and also applied for her to transfer to a bungalow - ground floor premises being more suitable for her - in view of her physical disabilities - even if they are exaggerated in her mind! She is terrified that she would not be able to escape from her third floor flat - if there were to be a fire in the block, and this terror is genuine enough - even if her physical disabilities are not! If anyone takes the view, that psychotic illnesses are more serious than neurotic illnesses, they may revise their views, after spending some days with Aileen.

I haven't visited Aileen's flat, but I have seen photographs - taken by two of our Association's befrienders - who have actually visited, and describe the clutter - the result of her obsessive/compulsive disorder, as 'incredible!' You can't sit down, and you can't move, for clutter! The last straw for our befriender, Lucy Farmer, occurred when Aileen got rid of her only chair - preferring to sit on the floor. Lucy has arthritic hips, so she can't sit on the floor, and so has ceased to visit Aileen's flat - though they do still meet up for coffee. I, in my naivete, tried to get a Reading Borough Council Personal Budget, for Aileen - to help clear the clutter, and to provide her with a regular, cleaning, service, but their Scheme doesn't include cleaning. They did arrange for her to be fitted with a chair in her bath - to make bathing safer for her - in the light of her physical disabilities. So it was arranged that this should be delivered and fitted, and that our befriender would be there when this was done. Imagine my amazement, when the bath seat turned up at the crisis house! The delivery driver explained that Aileen hadn't been there when he tried to deliver it, so she had telephoned, and asked him to deliver it to the crisis house. This is where we nip neurotic disorder in the bud! I sent the driver away with the seat - asking him to try, once again, to deliver it to Aileen's own address. 'I thought that, if it came here, someone with a car could bring it to my flat', explained Aileen. No, this was the beginning of the neurotic process, of Aileen filling up the crisis house, which she has now adopted as her home, with clutter, just as she has cluttered her flat. It is also a way of claiming 'ownership' of the crisis house. Needless to say, with thirty years' experience, we have observed this phenomenon before. Nip it in the bud! I refuse to house anybody's clutter in the crisis house - because I consider that keeping a clean, tidy, and well organised environment, is vital in maintaining mental health - especially because so many mental health service users - live - due to their illness - in squalid, and disorganised, environments. If we become squalid, and disorganised, as well, the problem is compounded. This experience of severe neurotic disorder, and how we handle the situation, is, as I have said, a gift from heaven for our current psychology students. It is something that they need to observe, in reality, and not just to read about, in a textbook. I highlighted the difficulty of getting appropriate Disability Benefits, for people as ill as Aileen, in the following letter – which was published in *The Wokingham Paper* (February 28th 2019).

The Reality of Being Fit for Work
'It is now being recognised - even by Government Ministers - that the reform of the Disability Benefits System is a complete fiasco - causing the disabled great distress, and a spate of suicides. This personal example illustrates just why. When my mother was old and ill, I bought

for her three new Mark's and Spencer's nightdresses, one more expensive than the others, and took them to her at the hospital. 'I'll keep the best one for when I see the Consultant', she said. Which nightdress, one wears, is of no relevance to the Consultant - who concerns himself, solely, with blood, breathing, and circulation, but this is human nature. Everyone, however ill, tries to look their best, when seeing someone important. So when the clinically depressed, and exhausted, mentally ill person, appears at the Disability Benefits Tribunal, they will have made a huge, one-off, effort - to appear clean, tidy, and presentable. The Tribunal then concludes that the person is able to look after him/herself, and so axes Disability Benefits. I think that people would be more accurately assessed in their own homes - where the chaos around them - frequently reflects - the chaos of the mental illness that they are suffering. But even then, I suspect that you would observe a similar phenomenon. The mentally ill person would be up all night - desperately trying to get the place into some kind of order - before the Assessor comes to see them, next day. In fact, it would be better, if the Assessor saw the reality caused by the disability. We have people who spend as long as they can at the crisis house - because it is much more of a home for them - than is the place in which they live - which can sometimes be in an, almost unbelievable, state of chaos, and I have always insisted that we provide an immaculately clean and tidy environment - undertaking a lot of the cleaning, myself, for that very reason. Their illness causes chaos. We aim to restore order to their lives. This very week, I said to our newest Master's Psychology student, 'You wouldn't think, would you, meeting these presentable, well-spoken, and well-behaved, people, that everyone of them has a serious mental illness? But they all have - because, otherwise, they would not come to a mental health centre!' The truth is, that most mentally ill people, are neither dangerous, nor dramatic. What they are, is dysfunctional in daily life, and that is why they need Disability Benefits. You cannot tell, how dysfunctional, a person is, from an hour's interview at a Tribunal. When people stayed in the crisis house for, say, three months, we were able to observe whether they cooked meals, did laundry, and generally looked after themselves. If they did, we got them into flats; if not, into mental health supported accommodation. But all of them required Disability Benefits - to help with the extra costs - inevitably incurred - by mental illness. Even the late Margaret Thatcher - not noted for a soft approach to life - stated, 'We have to look after the mentally ill.' And, much as I admire Theresa May, I do not agree with her statement that Disability Living Allowance is an out-dated Benefit. It will only be out-dated, when disability, itself, is out-dated, and I wish that these Conservatives would stick to their principles, and leave well alone! The ill-named, Employment Support Allowance, is another example. You cannot assess a person's capability for work in an interview. Capability should be assessed in proper Work Schemes – attendance at such schemes being a requirement for qualification for Benefits. People's capability to work, and, most important, to sustain effort, can then be assessed realistically. Once an acknowledgement of the actual disabling effects of mental illness, is restored, hopefully, it will put an end to the current chaos caused by such unrealistic reforms.'

As I have explained - both to our befrienders and service users - and to our psychology students - if you encountered Aileen, for half an hour, at a cocktail party - she would appear as being attractive, well dressed, charming, intelligent, and able to converse interestingly. You would never dream that she is seriously mentally ill. Over the years, she has worked her way through numerous people - all of whom, eventually, tire of her constant demands for attention, money, and tasks to be done for her. As a result, her life is both lonely, and limited. On 19th April 2019, we celebrated Tony's successful advocacy on Aileen's behalf - with champagne and hot cross buns - oddly assorted, but we always have hot cross buns at the crisis house on Good Friday! One of our members asked whether Aileen really was as intelligent as she appeared to be. This is the confusion that severe mental illness invariably causes. Of course she is very intelligent - so are numerous mentally ill people - especially those with a diagnosis of bi-polar affective disorder! Research indicates that this mental illness is found, most frequently, in people in classes One and Two of the Registrar General's Social Class Register - which is compiled through occupation statistics - and not through, inherited, advantages. Indeed, we have had Oxbridge graduates staying in the crisis house, and, in both cases, they had a diagnosis of Bi-Polar Affective Disorder. Mental illness inhibits functioning - so though the person is intelligent, they are unable to apply their abilities, while ill. This is very much the case, with Aileen. A poignant story!

Somewhere over the rainbow,
Way up high,
Are the dreams that you dreamed of,
Once in a lullaby.

People like Aileen, are always looking for the magic wand - the crock of gold at the end of the rainbow. Meanwhile, the years go by. You have tried every therapy under the sun - in your teens - in your twenties - in your thirties - and now - in your mid-forties! Her attitude caused some, understandable, friction in the crisis house drop-in centre. For instance, Pamela McEllen had dropped in - to explain that she was continuing, successfully, with her therapy with the Consultants at the private, and expensive, Cardinal Clinic. Aileen was sitting there, listening, intently. Then, she announced, 'I'm going to see these Consultants, and Therapists, as well - to get to the bottom of it.' I think that she assumed that we would pay for her treatment - just as we had for Pamela. But we would not. In Pamela's instance, her Health Insurance had run out, and it was a case of enabling her to continue, uninterrupted, a course of treatment, with a Consultant with whom she already had an, established, and successful, therapeutic relationship. By contrast, paying for Aileen to have a couple of appointments, would achieve nothing, since, in its own way, her illness is just as chronic, as is that, of some of our most chronic schizophrenics. Pamela was annoyed, because she thought that Aileen was encroaching upon her territory, but the Aileens of this world never take 'No' for an answer. Nothing loath, she persuaded a friend, who had recently come into some money, to pay for her treatment, and, as predicted, this achieved precisely nothing! Is not the truth to be found in Agatha Christie's novel, *'They do it with Mirrors'*. Miss Marple has been summoned by an old school friend, Ruth Van Rydock, to investigate what is going on in an institution for the reform of juvenile delinquents. This is run by a 'crank', Lewis Serrocold. Agatha Christie writes of him:

'He's bitten by that same bug of wanting to improve everybody's lives for them. And really, you know, nobody can do that but yourself.'

Lucy Farmer, who has befriended Aileen, is firmly of the opinion that - rather than chasing every therapy under the sun, she would be better advised to try to get her flat into order - and thus to create, a reasonably good living environment, for herself. There is no magic in mental health - no crock of gold at the end of the rainbow, but all that any building consists of - is floors, ceilings, and walls - so anywhere can be made habitable! Both Lucy, and I, had the female advantage. We were not captivated by Aileen's charms, but this was not the case with the male members of our association. The *'allumeuse'*, the *'femme fatale'*, or woman with magical powers of attraction, features regularly in Agatha Christie's works. For instance, there is Louise Leidner, in *'Murder in*

Mesopotamia.' Nurse Leatheran describes her, thus.

'She had that blonde, Scandinavian fairness that you don't see very often . . .Her eyes were lovely. They were the only eyes that I have ever come across that you might truly describe as violet.'

Then, in '*Peril at End House*', Hercule Poirot says - of Nick Buckley - 'That was her tragedy. She attracted people, and then they went off her'.

Such is the perfectly analysed, but nevertheless poignant, situation with Aileen Brown. As Racine would have it:

'Ce n'est plus une ardeur dans mes veines cachee.
'C'est Implacable Venus - toute entiere - a sa proie attachee'.

In September 2019, we were holding one of our regular 'Agatha Christie' Quizzes. These are great fun - as well as being good fund-raisers. Chris Hoskin always wins, of course, but everyone participates, and Aileen, in particular, is quite good with her knowledge of Agatha Christie. We currently have a homeless man, Glyn, who attends our drop-in centre. He is very thought-disordered, and paranoid, and so inclined to get into clashes with people - all over nothing at all! On Friday, it was over Glyn's cup of coffee. 'Had Aileen put poison in it?' You walk away, don't you? You take the heat out of the situation. Not Aileen. 'I'm going, I'm going!' she said repeatedly. She picked up her bags, made for the door, and then put them down again. A few minutes passed, and then, once again, she picked up her bags, and made for the door; then she put them down again.

To quote Racine, further:

'Elle flotte, elle hesite. En un mot, elle est femme.'

Aileen was obviously waiting for me to reply, 'Don't go. I'll get rid of Glyn'. Chris Hoskin tried to persuade Aileen to stay for the quiz, but I declined to do so. In more than thirty years, I can count on the fingers of one hand, the people whom we have had to ban from the crisis house. In a mental health centre, you must expect to encounter thought disorder, paranoia, and, in fact, the full range of psychotic and neurotic behaviours. So it has to be 'take it, or leave it!' No one can have the service on their own terms - which is precisely what Aileen wants. She flounced out, and members asked me what I was going to do. I replied that I was not going to do anything! Responding to such ploys, and rushing around after such people, would be playing right into their hands. Their personality disorder, would then, succeed in controlling you!

Little Bo-Peep has lost her sheep,
and she doesn't know where to find them.
Leave then alone, and they will come home,
wagging their tails behind them!

Three weeks after this incident, Aileen had not returned to the crisis house, and had also prevented her friend, over whom she has undue influence, from attending as well. I agree with Lucy Farmer that this is a sad situation, because the friend very much needs our services - which she describes as being therapeutic. Some of the men who attend the crisis house tried to persuade me to make efforts to get Aileen back, but I would not. 'Both Lucy and I have the advantage over you fellows', I said, 'Because - if you are of a classical turn of mind, you will be aware of what Racine says - or, if you are not of a classical turn of mind, to put things in a more prosaic turn of phrase, we can see Aileen's behaviour objectively - because - unlike you guys, we don't fancy her!'

Four weeks after the incident, Chris Hoskin came for his fortnightly visit, and requested an update on Aileen. I quoted Racine, and, of course, Chris took my point! I knew that he would. One always recognises the cultured, and educated, person. Thus, In Agatha Christie's short story – 'Sanctuary' – from '*Miss Marple's Final Cases*'. Bunch Harmon shares her suspicions about the people, claiming to be relatives, of the dead man in the church. Agatha Christie writes:

'It's all wrong', said Bunch 'The man who was there in the church, dying, knew all about 'Sanctuary'. He said it just the way that Julian, [her husband, and an Oxford scholar], would have said it. I mean he was a well-read, educated man . . .Those people, the Eccles, [who claimed to be the dead man's relatives], were quite different.'

To me, the needs of dilapidated schizophrenics, and alcohol - damaged paranoiacs, are just as important, and have to be provided for - as do those of beautiful, neurotic, women! What struck me in the last four weeks at the crisis house, is that Aileen's defection is still the major topic of conversation. One almost feels that narcissistic personality disorder, is so strong, that it continues to control, everyone, even when the sufferer has ceased to be present! Just look at how much space she has taken up in this book - as compared with other, equally important, people!

Now, three months on, the kaleidoscope has changed again. New people have joined our ranks - who never knew Aileen - and she has ceased to be a topic of conversation. But, the subject of Aileen, was raised, once again, during the coronavirus pandemic. I gathered that she had started to attend a, relatively new, mental health drop-in centre, in Wokingham, Prior to coming to us, Elise had attended this centre, and was not impressed by it, but Aileen tried to dissuade her, from trying our service, instead - because of her difficulties, with Glyn. Elise took no notice of this advice, and came to us, anyway - not experiencing any difficulty with Glyn. However, the new drop-in centre closed during the crisis - as did all pubs, cafes, and social centres - upon which, Aileen had, previously, relied. Her advocate, Tony, wanted me to contact her, because she was in a bad place, but I doubted the wisdom of doing this. These are, very difficult, times, and we need to maintain as much stability, in our services, as we can. However, in June 2020, Aileen telephoned me, and this was the first occasion on which I had spoken to her, since 6th September 2019. She explained that she needed my help. She lives on the third floor of a block of flats, the lift had broken down, and, due to her physical, disability, she was unable to get up and down the stairs, with shopping. I agreed to speak to the Housing Association, and to the Lift Repair Company, to get it fixed, and I also suggested, that Elise, who had been shopping for others during Lockdown, should get Aileen's shopping - just until the lift was fixed. This was excellent experience, for Elise, because she saw how quickly she could become Aileen's latest servant - if she didn't limit her involvement, just to this one, essential task. Elise coped splendidly, and, all the time, she is building up a raft of experience, which will stand her, in good stead, for the future. On Thursday 18th June 2020, Tony e-mailed to explain that, since the lift wouldn't be fixed, for two or three weeks, Aileen had moved, happily, into temporary accommodation, until the repair was effected, so a good outcome was achieved, for all. Aileen participates in Tony's Zoom meetings - which enable, those still isolated, because of coronavirus, at least to have, video contact. Furthermore, he telephoned, in July 2020, to say that Aileen's latest Benefit Review had been successful - due to his advocacy, on her behalf.

Cecile: 'Talking To The Wall'

Cecile started coming, occasionally, to our drop-in centre in 2018. She knew some of our service users from attendance at other local mental health services. She explained that she was living in a very unhappy, and violent, situation - with a husband who physically, and mentally, abused her, and with a son, of thirty-six, who was also abusive. The obvious answer was, first, to move into a Women's Refuge, and then, to file for divorce. Cecile was entitled to a half-share of their house, and the sale could be arranged through a solicitor - so that she would then have the wherewithal to buy a smaller place for herself. Her abusive husband did not want to put the house up for sale - because he wanted a large place to accommodate his motor bikes! You would think that he could be overruled, on legal grounds, but none of it ever happens. When life at home becomes intolerable, Cecile goes off - to stay with friends, or with her daughter - and then goes back to the abusive situation - with nothing resolved! She resorts to alcohol as an anodyne for her pain. In April 2019, she came to the drop-in centre with two bottles of wine. She drank one, but, obviously in a drunken state, dropped and broke, the second. The drop-in centre was very busy on this occasion, so Cecile sat in the reception room - where it was quiet. She expressed a wish to talk, but then just went home! We are all agreed that constantly talking, and giving, unheeded, advice, can achieve nothing. I think that this inability to deal with a problem is analogous to failing to go to the dentist when you have toothache! The pain abates a bit, so you are lulled into a false assurance that nothing is wrong! But the tooth would not ache if nothing were wrong - and it will flare up again, if you fail to get treatment. In Agatha Christie's novel, '*One, Two, Buckle my Shoe*', this is the wise advice given to key character, Mabelle Sainsbury-Seale! The whole plot revolves around dentists and dentistry! Agatha Christie writes:

'At the Glengowrie Court Hotel, South Kensington . . . Miss Sainsbury Seale was sitting, talking to Mrs. Bolitho. . . Miss Sainsbury Seale said, 'You know, dear, it really HAS stopped aching! Not a twinge! I think perhaps I'll ring up' - Mrs. Bolitho interrupted her. 'Now don't be foolish, my dear. You go to the dentist, and GET IT OVER!' . .

Also, in Agatha Christie's novel, '*Four-fifty from Paddington*', Dr. Quimper describes this phenomenon which, as a doctor, he encounters, frequently. Agatha Christie writes:

'Quimper finished his evening surgery . . . he looked tired, and depressed. 'Poor devils', he said, as he sank down in a worn easy chair. 'So scared, and so stupid. No sense. Had a painful case this evening. Woman who ought to have come to me a year ago. Now, it's too late. Make's me mad. The truth is, people are an extraordinary mixture of heroism and cowardice. She's been suffering agony, just because she was too scared to come and find out what she feared might be true.'

Cecile is only going to get older, not younger; the people she stays with are only going to get more impatient, not less impatient! Left as they are, things are only going to get worse, not better! It is the usual situation of wanting a magic wand! We all fear that things will just go on as they are - with Cecile continuing to put sticking plaster on the cancer - by escaping, every now and then, for short stays with relatives and friends. It could all end one day in a most extreme, or even, fatal, violent incident. Cecile visited us on 27th December 2019. Christmas is always a particularly stressful time, so we enquired as to how hers had gone. Awful, with husband and son, at home, but good, subsequently, staying with her daughter. Cecile then explained that she had been offered sheltered accommodation for the elderly, by Wokingham Borough Council, but had declined the offer, because she did not want to lose her share of her house - which was owned, jointly, by herself and her husband. All very well, but you can't take your share of your house with you! Would it not be better to spend one's twilight years in safe, stress-free, and civilised peace?

Don: 'From Dukes To Dustmen!'
Don Harris first came to us some twenty years ago. He suffered from bi-polar affective disorder, and this caused the breakdown of his marriage. He stayed, briefly, in the crisis house. Eventually, his accommodation was organised - he, retaining tenancy of the marital home - because of his mental health, but, being required to pay a sum of money to his ex-wife - in order to help with her resettlement. He recovered, sufficiently, to return to work. For years, we saw him only rarely. Don worked solidly for seventeen years - on the local dustcarts! He returned to our drop-in centre in 2019 - explaining that he was now aged sixty-five, had retired, and so was at a loose end. He no longer wished to get up at five in the morning, and continue working on the dustcarts, but neither did he want to sit looking at the wall, and twiddling his thumbs. What struck me, was that the sentiments, are exactly the same – almost literally 'from dukes to dustmen!' When our Patron, Lady Elizabeth

Godsal, retired as High Steward of Wokingham, in April 2018, she said that she didn't want to give up everything at once. We assured her that we would still like, very much, for her to continue as our Patron, and she has. Both dukes and dustmen would be in complete sympathy with the feelings of the, retired, Hercule Poirot – as described by Agatha Christie, in her novel, '*Mrs. McGinty's Dead*'. Agatha Christie writes:

'The truth is, Poirot reflected, my work has enslaved me, just as their work enslaves them. When the hour of leisure arrives, they have nothing with which to fill their leisure.' When Poirot arrived home, Superintendent Spence, of the Kilchester Police, was waiting to see him. He said to Poirot, 'I'll be retired in about six months. Actually, I was due for retirement, about eighteen months ago. They asked me to stop on, and I did.' 'You were wise', said Poirot, with feeling 'Was I? I wonder, I'm not so sure.' 'Yes, very wise', Poirot insisted. 'The long hours of *ennui*, you have no conception of them.'

Fortunately, Hercule Poirot was shortly to be relieved of his *ennui* once Superintendent Spence explained the reason for his visit, and so presented Hercule Poirot with a, particularly intriguing, murder mystery.

I advised Don, that a good plan, would be to return to a former part-time job of his - pushing the trolleys at Tesco's. He duly enquired about this, and was told that he had to apply 'on line'. This absurdity, in the way that technology has taken over our lives, made us laugh, but I said that our current psychology students would be, *au fait*, with the internet, and that they would help with this application'. A poignant story! Don is particularly grateful, that we are keeping the drop-in centre open, during the coronavirus pandemic. Having been so physically active, throughout his working life, and, furthermore, working, principally, as a gardener, and on dustcarts - out in the open air - being incarcerated, in four walls, is, to him, an unbearable prospect. Don is one - happy to avail himself - of telephone contact from one of our Placement students - particularly on the days of the week, when the drop-in centre is closed. When visiting the drop-in centre on Friday 10th April, Don, explained, whimsically, that, although he had access to a tiny patch of garden, and so could sit there - in order to get some fresh air, sitting, alone outside, wasn't really any better than, sitting, alone inside. His desperate need, is for some human company, and this is why it is so important for the drop-in centre to remain open - throughout the duration of the coronavirus pandemic. There are allotments in the area of Wokingham

- near to where Don lives, and I suggested, that renting one of these, may satisfy his need for occupation, but Don thought that an allotment, would be too much of a tie, and is still thinking in terms, of obtaining, a little, part-time, job - once the coronavirus crisis, is over.

Patrick: 'Avoiding A Bad Move, And Obtaining A Good Move'
It can't be, just chance, that Slough has now entered a higher risk category, for the spread of coronavirus. Overcrowding, and human beings, in too close a proximity, this is what causes the spread of infection. I am afraid, that poor old Slough, has never had the reputation of being a desirable place in which to live - witness John Betjeman's 1937 poem!

> *Come friendly bombs and fall on Slough!*
> *It isn't fit for humans now.*

Late in 2019, Patrick came into the drop-in centre, and said, 'I now have to go to Slough, for treatment.' It transpired that the Bracknell services had decided that Patrick's needs were too complex for them to provide – so they were referring him to Slough. I knew Slough well, some years ago, because I took over, as Voluntary Co-ordinator, of an existing National Schizophrenia Fellowship Group, in Slough, shortly after we moved to Berkshire in 1986. Even then, more than thirty years ago, it was a difficult place to get to, very bustling, and cosmopolitan, and hardly a suitable place for someone who is both physically, and mentally, disabled. Patrick suffers from cerebral palsy as well as post traumatic stress syndrome, and other mental health problems, so I agree that his needs are complex. Nevertheless, Slough is difficult to access by public transport - particularly for a person with physical disabilities. Because of this, eventually, the Bracknell Service referred him, instead, to Reading - which is much easier to access from his home in Bracknell. I advised Patrick to keep the proposed appointment in Reading, and thus to see if they were able to meet his needs adequately. Patrick has been using the health and social services since birth. Now, aged thirty-seven, you would think that they would have been able to provide for his needs in his own community. Fortunately, on Tuesday 7th January 2020, Patrick kept his appointment with the doctor in Reading - who was then to refer him to a specialist. I didn't like to think of him having to traipse all the way to Slough, for treatment, so I was pleased with this outcome. Many of Patrick's difficulties stem from the fact that cerebral palsy sufferers, have a depressed immune system, and so are less able than healthy people, to fight off infection. Furthermore, the medication that he takes for mental health problems, doesn't always interact successfully, with his other medication. As a fall-back position, I advised Patrick, if the Reading service proves inadequate, to seek treatment at the Radcliffe Hospital in Oxford. Having the world's experts, this hospital is unrivalled in its ability to treat complex cases. I cited the example of Norma - whom Patrick knew. Some years ago, Norma had called in at the crisis house - for me to complete a Disability Benefits Application Form. She was so ill, that she appeared to be near death's door. Some months later, she called in for an update, and was looking like a million dollars! 'I've been to the Radcliffe, to have treatment for brain aneurysms, and they have cured me', she said. That's the Radcliffe, for you. Brilliant! Incidentally, Patrick has been appointed as a Trustee of our charity. What qualifications are required for such a role? That you suffer from a mental health problem, and if you suffer physical problems, as well, then that makes you doubly qualified. Who knows best if the shoe fits? Answer - the one wearing it! A poignant story. In Patrick's case, he is probably wise, to self-isolate, during the coronavirus pandemic. Having been born with cerebral palsy, his immune system is weak, and he is very vulnerable to contracting infections. Knowing Patrick the way that I do, I am sure that he will keep in contact with people - through telephone, texting, and social media. He won't go short of his regular supply of alcohol. That's for sure. He will, probably, just order on line, and get it delivered straight to his flat! On Monday 6th April 2020, Patrick telephoned - to explain that his doctor had said that he wasn't in the 'high risk' group - for succumbing to coronavirus, and that, consequently, he could visit the drop-in centre. He attended on Tuesday 7th April , and proved to be, his old, jolly, self! Unfortunately, shortly after this visit, Patrick came into contact with a coronavirus - infected person, so after all, being in the 'vulnerable' group, he had to self-isolate, for twelve weeks. Patrick telephoned on Friday 5th June 2020, to explain that he was in a desperate state - due to enforced isolation, but that this should be ending, by 30th June. I commiserated, but encouraged him, by saying that this was not such a long way ahead, now, and that we were all looking forward to having him, back in our midst. Patrick, eventually, returned to us, in July - having, at last, been released from shielding. It was lovely to see him - back in our midst. Patrick, now back, in what is known in the new jargon, as our 'bubble', made one of his regular visits to the drop-in centre, in September 2020. I mentioned, to him, that a kind member of the local station staff, had given me a big bottle of Hand Sanitizer, and that I was advising people, that, if they wished to bring in their own, empty, bottles, I had a funnel, and could fill the bottles for them. Patrick replied, 'I am happy to rely on water, and soap!' A man after my own heart! During the pandemic, I have been washing my hands, a hundred times a day - with water and soap! As the following poem explains, you can't beat it!

Millionaires. Presidents, even kings,
can't get by, without everyday things.
If you wished to be clean, and you would, I hope,
you can't do better, than water and soap.

On Friday 9th October 2020, Patrick came into the drop-in centre, with the good news, that he had obtained a transfer to a, much better, flat. How we helped with this move, is also mentioned, in our 2019 - 2020, Annual Report. Moving house, is generally recognised to be, the third, most stressful, common experience that people can go through - after bereavement, and divorce. Sure enough, Patrick is, currently, extremely stressed, but we have carpeted his new flat, and arranged for his move to the new flat, on Wednesday 2nd December, so he should be feeling, more settled, by Christmas 2020.

The Parable of the Talents

She was a sweet little dicky bird.
Tweet, tweet, tweet, she went.
Sweetly, she sang to me
Till all my money was spent.

Hippie Jack: 'Till All My Money Was Spent'
Hippie Jack was one of the, 'Reading Invasion', who started coming to the crisis house in 2017. Then, in 2019, he got involved with the 'Cuckoo's Nest' Project, in Reading. I had hoped that this project would be successful, because I believe that the mentally ill of Reading, need a service in their own town. In December 2017, Hippie Jack was told that he was to receive an inheritance of two hundred and twenty-five thousand pounds - from the estate of a relative, who had just died. He had to wait for Probate, but the money became available, to him, in 2018. Then, he started spending it like water! He flung money here, and he flung money there. All the leeches came crawling out of the woodwork, and bled him white. At least, when he set up the 'Cuckoo's Nest', in March 2019, I thought that some of the money would be put to a useful purpose. Not a bit of it! He continued to fling money here

and there - so that, by late 2019, he was bankrupt! Until March 2019, Hippie Jack had been living in mental health supported accommodation, but he lost this - through continually breaking the house rules. The 'Cuckoo's Nest' had a flat above its shop - so he moved in there. Money continued to diminish, and, eventually, there was only enough left to pay the rent up until February 2020, so sadly, the 'Cuckoo's Nest', had to close down. At least, Hippie Jack, didn't have to be out on the street. Reading Borough Council provided him with a bedsitter in Whitley Wood. Hippie Jack attended the crisis house Christmas Party, on 23rd December 2019. He explained that he had no money left, at all, and no Benefits. He had no food, so we provided him with a Wokingham Lions' Club Christmas Food Parcel. In less than two years, two hundred and twenty-five thousand pounds, had gone down the drain - with nothing whatsoever to show for it! One of our members, Dolly, has socialist beliefs, and talks about the rightness of the redistribution of wealth. Hippie Jack is the living proof that it wouldn't work! Sometimes, I play this game with our members. I say - 'Suppose that I were in the happy position of being able to give each of you, one million pounds. Then I tell you to go away, and come back - five years later.' We then have fun - discussing what we would do with the money. The stark reality, is that - five years on - some people would have turned their million pounds into ten million pounds, some would have done nothing significant, but would, at least have some money left, and some, like Hippie Jack, would be bankrupt. It is absolutely, the Parable of the Talents! A poignant story - which, practically, qualifies as a Tragic Story!

Agatha Christie's works are always relevant, and the poignant story of Hippie Jack, is no exception. Among her works, one of Agatha Chrisie's own favourites was '*Crooked House*'. Murder victim, old Mr. Leonides, when, shortly before his death, writing to his solicitor, Mr. Gaitskill, says this:

'When I die, the burden I have carried must descend on someone else. Someone must be my successor . . .Only my granddaughter, Sophia, seems to me to have the positive qualities required.'

Then, later in the narrative, once Sophia has assumed control of the money, there is a description of an interchange between her fiance, Charles, and herself. Sophia says, of her mother,

'She'll be after me to put on the Edith Thompson one before you can turn round.' 'And what will you say? - If it keeps her happy', [said Charles]. 'I shall say, No! It's a rotten play, and mother couldn't play the part. It would be throwing the money away.'

I laughed softly. I couldn't help it. 'What is it?' Sophia demanded suspiciously. 'I'm beginning to understand why your grandfather left you his money. You're a chip off the old block, Sophia.'

Having had the sad experience of THREE of our members throwing their inheritance to the four winds, and also my own experience - of my guarding, our one major legacy, with my life, I couldn't agree more with Agatha Christie!

I was delighted, on Friday 7th February 2020, to receive a visit from Hippie Jack - together with Alec, and Dean - from the 'Reading Invasion'. Hippie Jack, confirmed, that the money had, indeed, run out, but he thought that there was, a possibility, that another tenant could take over The Cuckoo's Nest premises - with its, prime, High Street, location, and run it as a cafe. There would still be the annexe at the back of the premises, which might still be used as some kind of mental health facility. At least it seemed possible, that something can be salvaged from such a poignant story! However, on Monday 23rd March 2020, Annie, one of the 'Reading Invasion', telephoned, to find out whether we were remaining open during the coronavirus crisis, and, sadly, confirmed, that the Cuckoo's Nest, had closed down, completely. But readers should not be discouraged, and conclude that, just because this user-run service, did not succeed, none can. They can, and our thirty years, of running the Wokingham Crisis House, proves it!

I'd like to be, under the sea,
In an octopus's garden, with you.

Phil Worthing: 'In An Octopus's Garden'
I first encountered Phil, twenty-five years ago - in the summer of 1995. Even then, he was talking about wanting to buy a boat, and live, in seclusion, on the river. But he moved, from the crisis house, into a conventional bedsitter. Now, in March 2020, the block of bedsitters, is due for demolition, and, on Monday 9th March, he is due to move into a bungalow - an improvement, in my opinion. Phil was, particularly, stressed, on this occasion, so I reassured him, that moving house, is generally, recognised, as being one of the most stressful, life events, and

it would be, unnatural, for him not to experience stress, in the current circumstances. Another of our members, Marcus, has a bungalow - with a garden in which he can grow his own herbs, and vegetables. I suggested to Phil, that, once settled in, he could do the same. But, like the ancient fantasy of owning a boat, he retains a fantasy of buying a piece of land, being self-sufficient there - and growing all his own food. Phil is an aspiring vegan, and is certainly, at least, vegetarian, and seeking 'the good life'. In it all, can my readers not detect, that what Phil is really seeking, is the kind of asylum - described in Yeats's most famous poem? A poignant story.

> *I will arise and go now, and go to Innisfree,*
> *And a small cabin build there, of clay and wattles made:*
> *Nine bean-rows will I have there, a hive for the honey-bee,*
> *And live alone in the bee-loud glade.*

While Phil seeks asylum, and seclusion, he, nevertheless, also has the human desire for a female companion.

> *Woman needs man, and man*
> *must have his mate,*
> *That no one can deny.*

Phil has spoken to me a couple of times, since the onset of the coronavirus pandemic, and reports himself as being, 'Unbearably lonely.' When I spoke to him, on Friday 3rd April, I suggested that he come in, to see us, on Monday 6th April. He fits into the category, of those whom I mention, in my letter, entitled, 'Spot On, Brian' - published, in *The Wokingham Paper* (2nd April). He may, generally, be self-isolating, but we are still here, and he can come to see us, if this isolation, becomes unbearable. Phil telephoned, subsequently, to explain that there was a, further, complication. Neither buses, nor trains, were accepting payment, in cash, for fares. Only, payment by card, was accepted, and Phil, didn't have a card. He had some cash - because he was paid, compensation, for being required to move, so I suggested that he travel, by taxi; they still accept cash. Alternatively, he could cycle in.

Phil duly arrived, by taxi, on Tuesday 14th April. He was so relieved, to get some, human, company. He continues to seek a wife, and we continue, to laugh together, about his chances. 'When this crisis is over, I said, I have, advised you, before, Join the Wokingham Ramblers, and, who knows? You may find, a rambling rose.' Much more likely, by joining, he will encounter some congenial company, and this will help to relieve his isolation and loneliness. In the course of one of our, most recent, telephone conversations, Phil enquired, once again, as to whether there was, on that afternoon, anyone in the crisis house drop-in centre - whom he could marry? I had to reply, that, at that precise time, there was only myself, and the cat! Since I was already married, that just left the cat! I added this story, to those that keep Rosie, in fits of laughter, and, sure enough, when she heard it, she rolled around with mirth! A more serious matter arises, with Phil's objection to all medical treatment. He, in all the quarter century that we have known him, has always resisted the taking of anti-psychotic medication. He also believes in leaving his own immune system, to fight infection, and does not believe, in either taking antibiotics, or in having vaccinations. In current circumstances, the latter are vital. I explained to our service users, that they might feel slightly ill, after a 'flu jab', for instance, because the whole basis of vaccination, going right back to Louis Pasteur, depends upon the patient receiving a weakened version of the disease - which then enables him/her, to produce antibodies, to fight the disease itself! Was it not, in classical studies, observed, that dairy maids, who suffered from the mild disease, cowpox, never contracted, the fatal, disease, smallpox? Is not the word, 'vache', French for 'cow', and does not the term, 'vaccination', derive from this very word? I have advised our service users, strongly, to ignore Phil's stance, to have their 'flu jabs', and to accept vaccination against coronavirus, once this becomes available. If we could all fight off disease, by our own efforts, and with no treatment, we should have no need for a medical profession, at all! I loved the Press photograph of the Biontech Researchers, who, now in November 2020, have come up with the most promising vaccine, to date. The lady has her hair - all anyhow. Hairdressing is not important. Only research is important, and there is no time for anything else. They even spent their wedding day, in the laboratory. Laugh, yes, but as millions queue up for life saving vaccinations, take your hat off. These are the world changers! I have advised Philip, that once current restrictions ease, he would be wise to take my suggestion, and join Ramblers. He may meet not meet a rambling rose, but, at least he will be getting some human contact.

Rambling rose, rambling rose,
Why you ramble, no one knows.

Although Philip is desperately lonely, he also, desperately, seeks solitude. He regrets that, currently, he is unable to go metal detecting, with a group, but what he actually loves, is the beautiful, peaceful, and solitary, West Berkshire countryside. How he would love, to live, in solitude, there - with all the stresses of daily life, eliminated.

Here, in the country's heart,
Where the grass is green,
Life is the same sweet life,
As it e'er hath been.

Conversion Hysteria: 'Is It His Mind Or His Penis'

I had been expecting a new member - requiring advocacy, to visit the crisis house in March 2020, so when a new service user arrived, I thought that this would be the person. But no, it was somebody completely new - who asked to speak to me, in private. We duly moved into a private room – away from the busy, main lounge. He told me that he lodged in a local village - where another resident, a former nurse, aged seventy-seven, was pressurising him into having sex with her. He explained that he was aged, seventy-five, and could not have sex - because he was suffering from am enlarged prostate gland. He told me that he had been an alcoholic, but was cured of this. He had connections in Sweden, and had visited there - with an intention of committing suicide, but he had now decided to go to the West Country, and commit suicide there, by walking into the sea. He told me that his prostate problems were benign, and that he did not have a diagnosis of cancer, but that he could not pass urine, and dreaded dying slowly, in excruciating pain - hence the intention of committing suicide. I explained that my youngest brother had been diagnosed, with prostate cancer, eleven years ago, had an operation, and radiotherapy, and was absolutely fine, to this day. The man, who would not give his name, then said that he would not agree to surgery, for religious reason. 'Are you then, A Jehovah's Witness?' I enquired. 'No, I am a Quaker', he replied. I was puzzled. I had never heard, of Quakers, refusing medical treatment. 'But you must be under a doctor, I said. There is conservative treatment, for prostate problems, and catheterisation, if necessary'. He then said that his penis was so reduced in size, that he could not be catheterised. I advised him, not to go to the West Country, and commit suicide. Drowning, is, in any case, a particularly distressing, way to die. 'Come back, and see us again, on Monday', I said. He agreed to think about it, and said that he might come back, on Monday, or Tuesday. He said that I had been very kind, listening to him, and that he wanted to make a donation, to our Charity, but I suggested that he left this for a future occasion, since he was short of money.

Fortunately, all our five, current psychology students, were with us on Friday 6th March. I explained that it is best, to take what a person says, as the truth, until one has good reason to believe, otherwise. In this case, there may be no physical illness at all; the whole thing could be mental. On the other hand, his physical symptoms, may, be exactly, as he described them. But more likely, as in the case of Jimmy Jenkins [Please see: 'Triumph and Tragedy' - 'Round and Round in Circles' - from 'The Crisis House Today'], a small, physical problem, has been hysterically converted, by the mentally ill person, into a major, and even, life-threatening, illness. This was certainly, the verdict - reached, by the Consultant Psychiatrist, when we arranged for Jimmy Jenkins, to see him. Nor was this new, and anonymous, enquirer's situation, the first occasion, on which we encountered a mentally ill person, convinced that it was not his mind, it was his penis! [Please see, the story of Mark Runce, in 'Funny Stories', from 'Triumph and Tragedy'.] Even in our current collection of 'Poignant Stories', we have Aileen, whose problems, we believe, are principally, mental, but are hysterically converted, by her, into major, physical disabilities.

The man never returned, so we don't know whether, he indeed, committed suicide. A poignant story!

Paul Grenfell: 'I Never Promised You A Rose Garden'
Paul contacted me by telephone, and then, came to see me, at the crisis house, on Friday 10th April 2020 - Paul - being Delpha's son. He had explained, that, his grandmother, had died, and that there was a lot of family friction, and disagreement, about the funeral - at which he was scheduled, to deliver a Eulogy. Tell me something new! Poor Paul's family, is the quintessence of dysfunctionalism - as were its family members' families, before them! Paul is very intelligent, and, fortunately, retains a good sense of humour, despite everything! 'It would be lovely, I told him, if all families were harmonious, all marriages, blissfully happy, all love lives, wonderfully, fulfilling. It would be lovely, if we were all millionaires, all in robust health, and all, enjoying, marvellous, excellently paid, and fulfilling jobs! But we are not!' We laughed, together. Agatha Christie's character, Alexander Bonaparte Cust, who appears in, 'The ABC Murders' explains these facts, so realistically. He had got into conversation with a young man, who said, 'I don't hold

with wars.' Mr. Cust replied,

'I don't hold with plague, and sleeping sickness, and famine, and cancer . . . but they happen, all the same.'

Paul is due to celebrate his thirty-seventh birthday, later in April, and I first met him, when he was, a callow youth, of eighteen, having just completed his 'A' Levels'. As Agatha Christie, so correctly avers, 'Youth is the time of greatest vulnerability.' I remember, seeing Paul, sitting in the crisis house library, researching possible degree courses. I reminisced with Paul, poignantly. This was, just at that time, in late adolescence, when he most needed parental support - as he prepared to launch into the adult world. But he was deprived of this support - with, unfortunate, mental health, consequences. At the time, his mother and father, were pursuing a vendetta, against a psychologist, whom Delpha alleged, had abused her, in therapy. The, unfortunate, Paul, was sucked into the vendetta, with them, and said, how embarrassed he had felt - at being, at that time, forced to wear a tee shirt - emblazoned with the logo - 'Mum sued a psychiatrist, and won!' His father wore, an identical tee shirt - with the emblem - 'She sued a psychiatrist, and won.' Delpha, herself, wore one, emblazoned, 'I sued a psychiatrist, and won.' Paul achieved, in the words of his mother, 'only', three 'A' Levels - grades A, B, and C. - which I regarded as, jolly good, but mother thought, disappointing. What, one asks, is wrong with an 'A', a 'B', and a 'C'? The 'A' is for your best subject, and you go on to read for your degree in it. 'B' is for a subject, at which you are, also, quite good. 'C' is for the subject, at which you are least able, but a bit of hard work ensures respectability! Fortunately, Elise, happened to be in the drop-in centre, at the time of Paul's visit, so they were able to commiserate, together, about the unfortunate, mental health effects, of an, over-pressurised, academic education. Paul accepted a place at Warwick University, which I also regard as, jolly good, but, not surprisingly, he dropped out. It was then, the usual, sad, psychiatric, route. The happy side to this story, is that Paul has continued to receive, excellent support, from our befriender, Johnnie, and did, eventually, complete an Open University Degree. Coming back to the present problems, I advised Paul to avoid the funeral, completely, if there were to be violent scenes there. Apparently, his mother had threatened her sister-in-law, and there had, long been, wrangling over, what Delpha regarded, as the mismanagement, of her mother's Power of Attorney - by her brother. Alternatively, if he did decide, to attend, and there were ructions, I advised Paul, just to walk away from them. He also explained, that there were arguments about the eventual disposal of his grandmother's ashes. 'Ashes to ashes. Dust to dust.' It is true, that this is not the first occasion, on which I have heard, of disagreements, about a deceased person's ashes! Some people, wish to keep them, in an urn, on the mantelpiece. I have even heard, of people, who want to incorporate them, into a necklace, and wear it! It is not for me, to dictate, how people should deal with their grief; grieving is an individual thing, but I am, nevertheless, fascinated. When my mother was old, I used to take her, regularly, to Kew Gardens - which she described as being - 'the Garden of Eden'. I also, took her, to Hampton Court Palace - with its lovely gardens, and, regularly, for lunch, at an old coaching inn, in Kent. She loved all these outings. When she had died, and when the curtains closed, at the end of the funeral service, that was closure, for me. I asked the crematorium staff, to scatter her ashes in their rose garden, and I had no further involvement with them. It is what you do, for people, when they are alive, that matters - not a prolonged concentration on their death! Modern mourners, may opt for 'Love Is All Around' - to be sung at a funeral, but, with my mother, we chose tradition. We sang - 'The Lord's My Shepherd', 'O, God, Our Help, In Ages Past', and 'Abide With Me'. Known, by funeral directors, affectionately, as 'C and A', 'Crimond,' and 'Abide With Me', are chosen, by a majority of people, for funeral hymns - precisely, because they express, perfectly, their grief, helplessness, in loss, and turning to God, for support, and comfort. Additionally, 'Abide With Me', invariably, brings a, much needed, smile, to the faces of mourners - as they recall singing it, in happier times, at Football Match Cup Finals!

Crimond

Yea, though I walk in death's dark vale,
Yet will I fear no ill, for Thou art with me,
And Thy rod and staff, my comfort still.

Abide With Me

Abide with me, fast falls the eventide.
The darkness deepens, Lord, with me, abide.
Where is death's sting? Where, grave, Thy victory?
I triumph, still, if Thou abide with me.

O God, Our Help, In Ages Past

O, God, our help in ages past,
Our hope for years to come.
Our shelter from the stormy blast,
And our eternal home.

Fortunately, Paul now has, the advantage of, maturity, on his side. In conversation, with Elise, he said, in bitter/sweet, tones - 'I passed thirteen GCSE's' - and what job is he doing? A little, part-time gardening! There is no doubt about it, T.S. Eliot's assertion, that 'The Prize Awarded For The English Essay', is, of relevance, only, at the time that it is awarded, rings so true - as he considers, the nature of 'time', itself. But Paul, was greatly cheered up, by coming to see us, and promised to drop in again, after the funeral, to let us know how things went. He, duly, dropped in to see me, on Friday 17th April. He had given the Eulogy, and the funeral - which, due to current circumstances, was, in any case, restricted, in attendance, had gone off, without any unfortunate incident. Thank God! A poignant story.

Counter Therapeutic
Readers, would think, that, after all my decades, of experience, in the field of mental health, nothing could amaze me, but, on Friday 1st May 2020, Elise succeeded in doing so. I had been very pleased with Elise's progress, during the, six months, that she had been with us. She was proceeding, along the path of recovery, at a steady rate, and so, was regaining her health, and self confidence. Furthermore, the fact that she was doing, voluntary work, with a range of client groups, was providing her, with an excellent foundation, on which to build a future career, once she was ready to do so. But, on Friday, she was upset. Her psychotherapist, had said that, instead, she should be aiming to go straight back to work, and that she. was behaving, like a snail, hiding away, in her shell of a flat. I advised Elise, that her psychotherapist, was mistaken. When I worked as a volunteer, for the National Schizophrenia Fellowship, I made the acquaintance, of a top, rehabilitation psychiatrist, Dr. Roger Morgan. He ran a, highly successful, psychiatric rehabilitation hospital, St Wulstan's - which, incidentally, had the most beautiful setting that I have ever seen, for a mental hospital - up in the Malvern Hills. He said, that one must learn to discriminate, between the concept of 'rehabilitation', and the concept, of, 'resettlement'. 'Rehabilitation', is recovery, of one's mental health; 'resettlement', is, returning to full-time work, and

to a normal life, in the community. I don't expect, the man in the street, to appreciate, the difference, but one would expect, a psychotherapist, to be able to do so! Elise is, currently, in the, successful, process, of rehabilitation. Resettlement, will come later, and she, herself, realises, that she is not yet ready, for full-time, open market, employment. I have every confidence, that, properly supported, she will achieve this, eventually, but the path that she is currently pursuing, is the correct one, for the present, and she needs to be, firmly resolved, to stick with it, and to prevent anyone from undermining, her, gradually returning, self esteem. Elise confided, that, compared with former school - fellows, from, the, academically renowned, school - that she had attended - people, who, are now, practising as doctors, and lawyers - she feels a failure. Nonsense! The secret, of success in life, is to find the niche, that suits you! I recommended, that Elise, should seek, existential psychoanalysis, of the kind, that specialises, in self esteem, issues. A poignant story.

We Blossom, And Flourish, As leaves On The Tree
On 13th May 2020, I wrote a letter to *The Wokingham Paper*. The issues, raised, are interesting, because, it does seem to be the case, that, as soon as one, deadly disease, is eradicated, from the earth, another emerges, to replace it. I include part of the letter.

'If, very old people, are fit and healthy, and still able to enjoy life, that is one thing. But, if they are barely, in this world, anyway, could it not be better, to let, wise old, Mother Nature, have her way, and, allow them, to pass away, naturally - instead of compelling her, to resort to drastic measures - such as, the current, coronavirus pandemic? Flowers, start as seeds; then they become buds; they reach full flower; they become over-blown. Then, they start to fade, and, finally, they crumble, away to dust - all, in the course, of a set, time-span. Perhaps, human beings, are meant, to follow, a similar life-cycle.'

We blossom and flourish as leaves on the tree,
And wither and perish, but nought changeth Thee.

We do, indeed, 'blossom and flourish', and then, 'wither and perish'. The debate, is about whether we should, be allowed, to do so, naturally, or whether, the 'withering. and perishing', process, is to be, artificially, and, unhelpfully, prolonged.

Be Fruitful And Multiply

On 6th October, Wes, who appears in the chapter, entitled, 'Bank Holiday at the Crisis House, 2015', from *'Triumph and Tragedy'*, dropped to see us, as he has, on few occasions, during the pandemic. I enquired as to his wellbeing, and to that of his former partner, and three year old, daughter. 'Is she your only child?' I enquired. 'No, I have six children, and I would have seven, if my partner, hadn't miscarried one!' was his reply. 'The eldest is nineteen, then, one is seventeen; the twins are sixteen, one is eleven, and the youngest is three!' Since, Wes, himself, is aged, only thirty-three, you don't need to be, Professor Penrose, to work out that he became, a father, for the first time, at the age of fourteen! Incredible, and he appeared to be, quite proud of it! Needless to say, his children are, by different mothers, and he does not, maintain, them. Wes's saving grace is, that he does, at least, work, on a market stall, in Reading - so, if nothing else, he does, at least, maintain, himself! A poignant story!

Further Funny Stories

Chapter 11

Always look on the bright side of life.
If life seems jolly rotten,
There's something you've forgotten,
And that's to laugh and smile and dance and sing.

This injunction certainly keeps us going at the crisis house, and although we see, both tragedies, and many sad situations, we are always ready for a laugh, and a joke.

Sandie Sacareau: 'The Dying Swan'

One of the most hilarious stories in 'Twenty-five Funny Stories' - from *'Triumph and Tragedy'*, is entitled - 'Sandie Sacareau: Beer Money'. Sandie does not disappoint. In 2018, she still kept us in stitches. The latest incident, was when she walked into the crisis house - howling like a hungry wolf. She then collapsed, into a chair - giving a performance worthy of Covent Garden. Here was Anna Pavlova, the Second - 'the Dying Swan'. 'I only have a fortnight to live!' she wailed. Was she dying of cancer? No! It transpired, that the cause of her distress, was that, the Department of Work and Pensions, had said that she must go back to work! Sandie is strongly built, and is able-bodied. She could easily do a cleaning job, but the mistake that has been made, is in, successive Governments, ALLOWING, fit people, to scrounge off benefits, for decades on end. If you haven't worked, for thirty years, of course the prospect of returning to work, daunts you. Ergophobia, writ large! I have nothing, but admiration, for Iain Duncan-Smith's determination, to end this dependency culture, but, inevitably, as it always does, the band wagon rolled too far, and, disabled people, began to be, unfairly, targeted. This is why Iain Duncan-Smith resigned - since his Christian principles, wouldn't allow him, to see disabled people, being treated unfairly. To get the right balance, as I have proclaimed many times - both to Government Ministers, and in the Press, one has to set up sheltered work schemes. In a scheme, run by people trained in the needs of both the physically, and the mentally, disabled, it would soon become apparent, who could, with a bit of support, return to normal, open market work, who could function, reasonably well, in the Scheme, but would not cope with greater pressure, and who could barely cope - even in the Scheme. The advantage to tax-paying society, would be that everyone, however disabled, would be doing something, and so contributing to this society. Currently, many mentally ill people, do nothing at all - but sit and stare at their four walls. Nothing could be worse for their mental health. Currently, in the summer of 2019, we have Glyn, re-painting the crisis house. He is both, severely mentally ill, and homeless - having relinquished his Housing Association flat, but he is as happy as Larry - doing this voluntary work for us. I keep him going - with a regular supply of coffee and chocolate biscuits - and he is doing an excellent job. So could they all - if provided with sheltered work schemes.

We hadn't seen Sandie, throughout Lockdown, but she suddenly appeared, once again, in the drop-in centre, in August 2020 - looking very much, the worse for wear! Needless to say, she was homeless, AGAIN, penniless, AGAIN, and suffering the physical effects of alcohol and drug abuse, AGAIN. There are times when I consider, that universities, should adopt the Sandies of this world, as walking studies in inadequacy! Could, highly skilled, psychotherapy, have turned them, around, when they were younger? Perhaps! And with it all, I, actually like, Sandie! Now comes the interesting part. Sandie has four children - the youngest, now a teenager, having been adopted away, at the age of three - due to Sandie's heroin addiction. She updated me about the others. Her elder son, is now deputy MANAGER, of a Burger King; her daughter is now deputy MANAGER, of a care home, and her younger son, is now MANAGER, of a British Heart Foundation, charity shop. It is the old, old, story. Have a 'mother' like Sandie, and you know, from a young age, that the only person who is going to make anything of your life, is you - so you do! You go out, and grab life, by the horns. Both sons have stable partners, and children, and Sandie's daughter's partner is a local Police Officer - the quintessence of respectability! Good for them!

Michaela: 'Teach Your Grandmother To Suck Eggs'

Michaela came to us, because she was unable to access, the help that she needed, from the local, statutory, mental health services. Tell me something new!

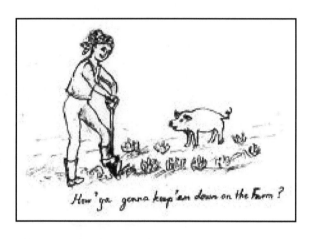

How 'ya gonna keep 'em down on the Farm?

I always think that, ideas, put forward by idealists, would be, nothing short of wonderful - if they worked out, in practice. But they don't! Take the idea of getting rid of private schools! The argument is - that if you have just one type of school - provided by the State - it would have to be good - because it is all that is available! Oh, but it could also - no alternative being available - be free to be tenth rate in peace! I never had children, but had I done so, I would have sent them to the best private schools - where a good education is guaranteed! I would have done so, that is, if they were of normal intelligence. Unlike my, misguided, teacher friend, who features later, in this narrative, I would not have pressurised them through an academic education, if they had special needs! I recall a television programme - in which some parents echoed my views, exactly. They were sending their children to Westminster School - where they KNEW that, a good education, would be provided. In some other schools, it might be, but it might not! Exactly the same, applies to statutory mental health services. They don't want private, or voluntary, alternatives to exist - because these show up their deficiencies. This truth has been illustrated by some most amusing incidents - like this one, in April 2019. The Wokingham Statutory Mental Health Service wouldn't fill in Michaela's Benefit Application Form for her – [Please see: 'Advocacy'] - but they, evidently, very much resented my doing so! They don't want to do it, but they don't want anyone else to do it, either! When Michaela came into the crisis house - to tell us that our application, on her behalf, had been successful, she commented, 'This is the only place where you can get any help!' I wish I had a thousand pounds for every time that I have heard that - in more than forty years of voluntary mental health service! I would be a millionaire! To share the joke with readers, I wrote the following letter to *The Wokingham Paper* (May 2019).

Mental health and the environment
'I refer to my letter - 'Toasting Victory' - (25th April). We have now had a successful Mental Health Awareness Week - with valuable input from Royalty, and other public figures, so I am toasting this, as well. I have always believed mental health education to be of vital importance, so, for many years, I served on the National Schizophrenia Fellowship's National Council, and, as their volunteer, I organised their education programmes. As well as grass-roots work, I ran international research conferences. The research conclusions were not always as people might expect. I recall bringing Dr. Assen Jablensky over from Bulgaria - to speak at my conference at Imperial College. He headed up the World Health Organisation's Pilot Study into schizophrenia - which, perhaps surprisingly - concluded that the incidence and prevalence of the disorder - do not vary - whatever the culture. Remote Indian village, or New York, its incidence remains at one in a hundred, and its prevalence at four in a thousand! I also brought, Father of Biological Psychiatry, Dr. Seymour Kety, over from America. He conducted an exhaustive, longitudinal, study of all the families in Denmark – where identical twins had been separated from birth - one being raised by the natural parents, and the other by adoptive parents. Where, in later life, one such twin developed schizophrenia, so did the second, in a statistically high, number of cases. He thus demonstrated that schizophrenia runs in the biological family, and is not caused by environmental factors - though these can affect its successful management. Such research findings can be invaluable for people seeking genetic counselling. The mentally ill and their families certainly need mental health education, but they also need

grass-roots practical help - so I then went on to set up the Wokingham Crisis House - in order to provide this. I return to the lady in my letter. After the Wokingham Statutory Mental Health Service declined to complete her Application Form for Universal Credit, she told them that I had done so, instead. 'I hope she knows what she is doing; that form requires medical information!' - they replied. Having, for years, organised education for the mentally ill and their families - delivered by the world's authorities on mental illness - I considered myself to be capable of completing a Benefits Application Form, correctly. I was! More champagne! The lady's application for Universal Credit, proved successful!'

Tell me the same old story – when you have cause to fear,
That this world's empty glory, is costing me too dear.

The trouble - or the advantage - of having, as a young teenager, come under the influence of an evangelical Christian church - is that early adolescence is the most impressionable time in life, and what you learn, and take on board, then, never leaves you. I have very good memories, of the days when I ran the National Schizophrenia Fellowship's education programmes. They became renowned throughout the mental health world, and, in particular, my 1985 National Conference on Schizophrenia, was addressed, on the first day, by Professor Sir Martin Roth - who held the Chair of Psychiatry at Cambridge University, by Professor John Wing, Director of the Medical Research Council's Social Psychiatry Unit - at the Institute of Psychiatry, University of London, by Dr. Derek Richter, Secretary General, of the International Brain Research Organisation, by Professor Steven Hirsch, Professor of Psychiatry, at Charing Cross and Westminster Medical School, by Dr, Adrianne Reveley, Honorary Consultant, Genetics Section, the Institute of Psychiatry, and by Dr. Timothy Crow, Director of the Medical Research Council's Clinical Research Centre - at Northwick Park Hospital. On the second day, it was addressed by - Professor G.M. Carstairs, Medical Adviser to the National Schizophrenia Fellowship, by Professor Kathleen Jones, Department of Administration, the University of York, by Professor Anthony Clare, Department of Psychological Medicine, St. Bartholomew's Hospital, University of London, by Professor Robert Bluglass, Department of Forensic Psychiatry, the University of Birmingham, and by Dr. Julian Leff, Deputy Director of the Medical Research Council's Social Psychiatry Unit, and later, Chair of Transcultural Psychiatry at the University of London. Now, more than three decades later, our psychology students, on Placement at the crisis house, are studying these experts' research - now classical - for their degree courses! But let us practise a little Christian humility! It was the speakers, and not I, who had the, world renowned, expertise. I, am hopelessly, unscientific; I am, merely, a good organiser!

My mental health education work, was serious, but also provided some good laughs. Imagine what it is like - if you are used to receiving training by the world's authorities - being 'trained' by 'Gormless Gertie'! Another laugh I remember - when actually running the conferences - was at the 1985 National Conference - which was attended by some eight hundred people. At lunch time, a lady ran up to me, and said that she had omitted to put her name down for lunch - could she still have one? From vast experience, I always provided for such eventualities - so I was able to accommodate her. 'I could help you run your conferences', she said. I thought - 'Lady' - if you are incapable of organising lunch, for yourself, I doubt your competence at organising national mental health events! There were laughs, but also, anger. At the time that I was running these vital education programmes, the National Schizophrenia Fellowship had taken on a new director. 'If you charged a lot more money for attendance at these events', that money could be used to fund a Training Officer', she said. She got a flea in her ear. I, deliberately, gave up a well-paid professional job - in order to provide voluntary services for the mentally ill, and their families. The relatives of the mentally ill - just like the carers of anyone - physically or mentally disabled - are, invariably, impoverished by their situation. Some have to give up paid jobs - if the onus of caring becomes full-time. Joseph, and his wife, Joan, [Please see: 'Our Advocacy Service'], present a cogent example - here in 2019. Very recently, I have advised Joseph - that the best service that I can provide - is to improve their financial circumstances. We have succeeded in getting Enhanced Personal Independence Payment, for Joan, and so, Carer's Allowance, for Joseph. He can now - either reduce his working hours - so that he has more time to complete the household tasks that Joan is too ill to undertake, or - use the extra money, to get some paid help in the house. Now it is established, that there is a severely mentally impaired person in their household, they can also, now, get exemption from Council Tax - all amounting to a significant improvement in their financial circumstances. As a result of the relief of anxiety that this has achieved, Joan is a transformed woman!

I charged the minimum for my events - so that all could afford to attend them. I had no desire to exploit these vulnerable people - in order to fund the employment of a failed social worker - as a Training Officer - when the job was already being done - successfully and voluntarily, by me! I always arranged events - sometimes on weekdays, and sometimes on Saturdays - so that family members had the optimum chance to attend - since some worked on weekdays, and couldn't get time off, and some had their schizophrenic relative home on Saturdays - and so could only attend on weekdays. This director also wanted me to run everything on weekdays - so that professionals, attending events, didn't have to give up their Saturdays! I enlightened her. The National Schizophrenia Fellowship, in its Constitution, was set up, for the welfare of schizophrenia sufferers, and their families - and not to provide soft-option employment - nor the opportunity to skive off work - for failed social workers! So I ran the education programmes, voluntarily, for some fourteen years, and yes, it was extremely successful, but, nevertheless, 'I had cause to fear, that this world's empty glory - was costing me too dear'! Even more vital than education, is the practical, mundane, grassroots, help, that a crisis house can provide - so I set one up - in Wokingham!

I always find parallels in Agatha Christie's books, and I can identify myself with several of her characters. One such, is Lucy Eylesbarrow. Lucy Eylesbarrow, appears in '4.50 from Paddington', Agatha Christie writes:

'Lucy Eylesbarrow was thirty-two. She had taken a First in Mathematics at Oxford, was acknowledged to have a brilliant mind, and was confidently expected to take up a distinguished academic career. [but] To the amazement of her friends, and fellow scholars, Lucy Eylesbarrow entered the field of domestic labour.'

The inevitable happened. As soon as people realise, that you are extremely able at the job you are doing, they want you to do, something else! I don't count Miss Marple - who wanted Lucy to find a body! No one has ever asked that of me! That was a one-off task, and Miss Marple was not intending to take Lucy, away from her chosen field of work. But Harold Crackenthorpe, a character in the book, who recognised her exceptional abilities - wanted her to join his firm in the city. He said:

'I want to tell you how struck I have been by your ability . . . I feel that your talents are wasted here, definitely wasted. Do you?' 'I don't.

The truth is that we could use someone of your outstanding ability in the firm.'

If only people would learn the ancient, oriental, art of leaving well alone. If somebody is doing a good job, and is, obviously happy, in doing so, why try to change anything? - but people always do. These people never see, that if an able person, wanted to be doing something different, they would be doing so! When it comes to statutory services wanting to suck volunteers into their hierarchy - and, I fear, at the bottom of it, then they should pay heed to an old song that my grandfather used to sing.

Howya gonna keep 'em
down on the farm –
After they've seen Paree?

If someone has, 'seen *Paree*', in the shape of international expertise, then they are wise to avoid all contact with statutory bodies, as we do. Assessed as, incapable of filling in a form, I dread to think what role they would devise for us, if we were foolish enough, to get involved with them! My experience of their attempts at 'colonisation' of the voluntary sector, are - that they are - firstly, persuasive. When that fails, they become aggressive. When that fails, they become destructive, and when that fails, they, sometimes literally, give up the ghost! Furthermore, it isn't always, professionals, who want us to run things differently. A service user, who has joined us, recently, has said, 'The Wokingham Crisis House meets my needs, perfectly. I feel completely, at home here, and I can talk, freely, about the things that are distressing me. As a result, my mental health is much better, and I haven't slept so well for years.' This is, very gratifying, to hear. Nevertheless, providing a facility, in which people can talk, freely, about what is distressing them, is the First Law of Mental Health Psychodynamics! [Please see 'Introduction'.] Fail to provide this, and a mental health service, has no *raison d'etre*. It might as well close down. But, it is what new people, including this man, then go on to say, that always, intrigues me. He, astonishingly, said, 'You are wasted here. Why don't you join up with this organisation? Why don't you join up with that organisation? Why don't you serve on this committee? Why don't you serve on that committee? Can't you influence social services? Can't you do more of this, and can't you do more of that?' Harold Crackenthorpe, to the life! My response, echoes Lucy Eylesbarrow's. It is, that I have no desire to join up with any other organisation - nor to serve on any committees. I have, no influence, over social services, and I don't want them to improve, anyway. I want them to be abolished, and replaced by charities. The Wokingham charities, are, incidentally, coping, brilliantly, in the current crisis, and providing a valuable service, for, literally, thousands of people. I have no desire to do any more of this, nor any more of that. I am very happy, sitting in my chair, sipping sherry, and gazing at the beautiful painting, by John Waterhouse, which is entitled, 'Hylas and the Nymphs'. No doubt, irate feminists, would like me to remove, this painting, from display in the crisis house. [Please see: 'Funny Stories – The Bare Necessities'!] But I won't. Not only, is it beautiful, but, like all classic Art, it is not of the twenty-first century, but, reflects the values of the times, in which it was created. But, I do wish, that one day, a new service user would come in, and say, 'The Wokingham Crisis House, meets my needs, perfectly. I feel completely at home here, and I can talk, freely, about the things that are distressing me. As a result, my mental health is much better, and I haven't slept so well for years, so, Stay as sweet as you are. Don't let a thing, ever change you. Stay as sweet as you are. Don't let a soul, rearrange you!' Or, as the more prosaic would say, 'If it ain't broke, don't fix it!' I advise service users, that one could spend one's whole life, complaining, and moaning, about services - or rather, the lack of them. A frequent complaint is, that if one has been discharged from the service, and then needs it once again, one has to go through the 'Common Point of Entry', and be reassessed all over again - even though one's history remained on file. Is it worth complaining? It is not, because nothing will be achieved. It is, indeed, the case, that when I set up the crisis house, and turned, what had been a collection of scruffy little offices, into a state-of–the-art, mental health centre, I did turn, a pumpkin, into a golden coach; talk about the 'Cinderella' services! But this does not mean, that I have a magic wand, similarly, to transform, statutory mental health services. Instead, I advise, groups of mentally ill people, and their informal carers, to look at what is needed, and to set up, their own, self-sufficient, services – which should be, nothing to do with statutory bodies. Such groups of volunteers, could set up - drop-in centres, befriending schemes, work-related activity groups, social activity groups, talking therapy groups, and carers' support groups - thus meeting a wide range of mental health needs - at minimal cost.

Breakfast At Tiffany's

Although my chief aim, in creating the crisis house, was to provide a pleasant environment - where people with mental health issues, could solve their problems, in civilised peace, I have never had - either the money, nor had the desire, to spend a lot of money, in doing so. Most of our eight hundred pictures, and numerous ornaments, have either been purchased for a song, in charity shops, or have been donated. So I was most amused by the following funny interchange. I had bought two Tiffany Lamps, but I had been unable to light them up, because I couldn't get the correct light bulbs. Then, finally, I managed to find the ones that I needed, and the Tiffany Lamps, duly lit up, our main lounge. 'Do you like my Tiffany Lamps?' I asked Chris Hoskin - who has written the Foreword to this book. 'Did you get them from Tiffany's in New York?', he enquired, with surprise in his voice. I did laugh. Original Tiffany Lamps, probably cost thousands of pounds. My copies, had a, more humble, origin. I bought them - very cheaply - at a shop in Bracknell - which was known as 'Past Times'. It specialised in producing cheap copies, of original works of art, and artifacts - Art Nouveau, and Art Deco - being particular lines that they had on sale - hence their name, 'Past Times'! Such cheap, period pieces, are exactly what are needed to enhance the 'retro' environment of the crisis house - which is so therapeutic for people with mental health problems.

Forty-Seven Years

My love unabating
Has been accumulating
Forty-seven years - forty-seven years!

A frequent discussion, in the crisis house, concerns the situation whereby, it was once very easy, to obtain move-on accommodation for people staying with us. If we had the crisis beds nowadays, it would be very difficult - with people having to wait for years. Take young Jerry, for example. We don't see much of him, because, when he can get work, he does painting, and decorating, on a casual basis. He dropped into the crisis house on Tuesday 28th January 2020. He was homeless, would love to be provided with even the, most humble, bedsitter, but explained that, despite numerous efforts to get accommodation, he had been on the Wokingham Borough Council Housing List - for the past ELEVEN years! However, it is an ill wind that blows nobody any good! As a result of the Government's scheme, during Lockdown, to give local Councils money - in order to get the homeless off the streets, and thus less likely to spread the virus, Jerry accepted the temporary accommodation offered, and this, then led, to his being offered, more permanent accommodation. This is in Reading, and not in the most salubrious area, but it is a whole lot better than being in a tent - especially now that the colder weather is here. Jerry dropped in to see us, on Friday 23rd October, and, on his behalf, I contacted Wokingham Borough Council - to see whether he could be considered, for permanent accommodation, in Wokingham itself, his home town. People don't seem to understand, that the roof over one's head, is man's most important, basic security - that, and his food. What was the first thing that Robinson Crusoe did when he landed on the island? - build himself a shelter, of course! I can beat any story of temporary accommodation - turning into permanent accommodation. Jerry's situation reminds me of a funny story of my youth. A neighbour of ours, Doris, who lived, with her parents, in a big house, had got chatting, to a young man, whom she had met in the local park. He explained that he was divorced. His ex-wife and thrown him out, so he was homeless, and was sleeping on the park bench. Being of a kindly disposition, Doris invited him home for tea. 'Ask him to stay with us FOR THE NIGHT', said her father. 'I wouldn't allow my dog to sleep on a park bench!' Forty-seven years later, I happened to be walking down the high street, and who should I encounter but Doris, and the man - no longer so young? Doris's parents had long since passed away, but the man was still 'staying the night' in her big house! Forty-seven years! Forty-seven years!

Stuart Clyde: 'When to Say - 'When'!'

> *Pretty little Sally goes walking down the alley.*
> *Displays her pretty ankles to all of the men.*
> *They could see her garters, but not for free and gratis,*
> *An inch or two, and then, she knows, when to say when.*

Stuart - who was now involved in the Cuckoo's Nest Project, came over from Reading to see the crisis house. Consistent with crisis house tradition, I offered him a lunch-time drink. He opted for Irish Coffee. In Agatha Christie's novel, *'The Clocks'*. Colin is invited to 'Say when' - as the whisky is poured. Agatha Christie writes:

'Hardcastle took his keys from his pocket, and opened the front door. 'Come on in', he said. He led the way into the sitting room, and proceeded to supply liquid refreshment. 'Say when.' I said it, not too soon, and we settled ourselves with our drinks.'

This is the standard, social convention. Not a whisky drinker, myself

- 'little old wine drinker, me' - I followed the convention. 'Say when!' I said to Stuart, as I poured the whisky in. I had to stop pouring - for I feared that the whisky bottle, would be empty, before he said, 'when!' So I learned my lesson. Unlike, 'pretty little Sally, who features in the song, 'Oom Pah Pah' , evidently, everyone DOESN'T know 'When to say when'!

Dan Kent: 'The Bare Necessities'

Look for the bare necessities,
The simple bare necessities,
Forget about your worries and your strife.

Here, in January 2020, Dan Kent is back - progressing along the path to recovery, adjusting to his bereavement. Restoration of libido, is always a reliable indicator, of recovery from depression, and Dan's, current, party piece, is to go around all the eight hundred pictures, and, hundreds more, pieces of sculpture, in the crisis house, and focus upon the 'Nudes'. I decided to join in the fun, and tell him about the artists. 'That picture is The Rokeby Venus', by Velasquez', I explained. 'It hangs in the National Gallery.' In the picture, the Rokeby Venus, is looking into a mirror, and the image seen in such pictures, so the Gallery Tour Guide explains, may not be a reflection of her own face, but may be expressing some specific emotion - such as happiness, grief, and so on.

The Rokeby Venus (also known as The Toilet of Venus, Venus at her Mirror, Venus and Cupid, or *La Venus del espejo*) is a painting by Diego Velázquez, the leading artist of the Spanish Golden Age. Completed between 1647 and 1651, and probably painted during the artist's visit to Italy, the work depicts the goddess Venus in a sensual pose, lying on a bed and looking into a mirror held by the Roman god of physical love, her son Cupid. The painting is in the National Gallery, London.

We come to the next work of art. 'The Birth of Venus', is a particular favourite, of mine - which I have seen, many times, in the Uffizi Gallery, in Florence.

The Birth of Venus (Italian: *Nascita di Venere*) is a painting by the Italian artist Sandro Botticelli, probably made in the mid 1480s. It depicts the goddess Venus arriving at the shore after her birth, when she had emerged from the sea fully-grown (called Venus Anadyomene and often depicted in art). The painting is in the Uffizi Gallery in Florence, Italy.

We move on to the next painting. 'That one is Manet's 'Olympia'.'

Olympia is a painting by Édouard Manet, first exhibited at the 1865 Paris Salon, which shows a nude woman ('Olympia') - lying on a bed - being brought flowers by a servant. Olympia was modelled by Victorine Meurent and Olympia's servant by the art model Laure. Olympia's confrontational gaze caused shock and astonishment when the painting was first exhibited because a number of details in the picture identified her as a prostitute. The French government acquired the painting in 1890 after a public subscription organized by Claude Monet. The painting is on display at the *Musée d'Orsay*, Paris.

Adding to our collection of nudes, I like our two paintings, by, the Pre-Raphaelite style, artist, John Waterhouse. One is of, semi-naked, nymphs, and another of Narcissus - gazing into a pool.

John William Waterhouse RA (6th April 1849 - 10th February 1917) was an English painter, known for working, first, in the Academic style, and, for then, embracing the Pre-Raphaelite Brotherhood's, style, and subject matter. His artworks were known for their depictions of women - from, both, ancient Greek, mythology and Arthurian legend.

Born, in Rome, to English parents, who were both painters, Waterhouse later moved to London, where he enrolled in the Royal Academy of Art. He soon began exhibiting at their annual summer exhibitions, focusing on the creation of large canvas works, depicting scenes from the, daily life, and mythology, of ancient Greece. Many of his paintings, are based on authors such as Homer, Ovid, Shakespeare, Tennyson, or Keats. Waterhouse's work, is currently, displayed at several major British art galleries, and the Royal Academy of Art, organised, a major retrospective, of his work in 2009.

We climb the stairs, and come to a large painting of a scene on a tropical island. 'That, colourful one, is of native girls, with pomegranates. The artist, Paul Gaugin, decided to go and live on a tropical island, and paint pictures of the half-naked, native girls.' He was, evidently, the inspiration for the following song, which was popularised, by the, recently knighted, Tommy Steele!

I'm the only man on the island,
The only man on the island.
It's nice living - in the tropical paradise.
There's a hundred and fifty girls to love -
Underneath the coconut tree.
And the only man on the island is me!

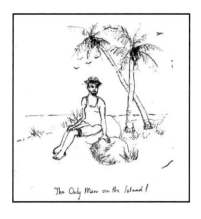

The Only Man on the Island !

Eugène Henri Paul Gauguin, (7th June 1848 - 8th May 1903), was a French, post-Impressionist artist. Unappreciated, until after his death, Gauguin is now recognized, for his experimental use of colour, and Synthetist style, that were distinct from Impressionism. Toward the end of his life, he spent ten years in French Polynesia, and most of his paintings from this time, depict people or landscapes from that region.

We also have several nude sculptures. 'That one is Michelangelo's 'David'. It is on display in the Academia Gallery - in Florence.'

Michelangelo returned to Florence in 1499. The republic was changing after the fall of its leader, anti-Renaissance priest Girolamo Savonarola, who was executed in 1498, and the rise of the gonfaloniere Piero Soderini. Michelangelo was asked by the consuls of the Guild of Wool, to complete an unfinished project, begun 40 years earlier, by Agostino di Duccio: a colossal statue, of Carrara marble, portraying David, as a symbol of Florentine freedom, to be placed on the gable of Florence Cathedral. Michelangelo responded, by completing his most famous work, the statue of David, in 1504. The masterwork, definitively established his prominence, as a sculptor, of extraordinary technical skill, and strength of symbolic imagination. A team of consultants, including Botticelli and Leonardo da Vinci, was called together to decide upon its placement, ultimately the Piazza della Signoria, in front of the Palazzo Vecchio. It now stands in the Academia - while a replica occupies its place in the square.

We move on, again. 'That one is 'The Venus de Milo'.'

The Venus de Milo is an ancient Greek statue, and one of the most famous works of ancient Greek sculpture. Initially it was attributed to the sculptor Praxiteles, but based on an inscription that was on its plinth, the statue is now thought to be the work of Alexandros of Antioch.
Created sometime between 130 and 100 BC, the statue is believed to depict Aphrodite, the Greek goddess of love and beauty. However, some scholars claim it is the sea-goddess Amphitrite, venerated on Milos. It is a marble sculpture, slightly larger than life size, at 203 cm (6ft 8in) high. Part of an arm, and the original plinth, were lost, following the statue's discovery. It is, currently, on permanent display, at the Louvre Museum in Paris. The statue is named after Aphrodite's Roman name, Venus, and the Greek island of Milos, where it was discovered.

Now we come to a particular favourite, of mine. 'That one is 'Discobolus'.'

The Discobolus of Myron, ('discus thrower'), is a Greek sculpture, completed at the start of the Classical Period, figuring a youthful, ancient Greek athlete, throwing discus, about 460-450 BC. The original Greek bronze is lost, but the work is known through numerous Roman copies, both full-scale ones in marble, which was cheaper than bronze, such as the first to be recovered, the Palombara Discobolus, and smaller scaled versions in bronze. A discus thrower, depicted, is about to release his throw: 'by sheer intelligence', Kenneth Clark observed in The Nude, "Myron has created the enduring pattern of athletic energy. He has taken a moment of action, so transitory, that students of athletics, still debate, if it is feasible, and he has given it the completeness of a cameo." The moment, thus captured in the statue, is an example of rhythmos, harmony and balance. Myron is often credited with being the first sculptor to master this style. Naturally, as always in Greek athletics, the Discobolus is completely nude. His pose is said to be unnatural to a human, and today considered a rather inefficient way to throw the discus. Also there is very little emotion shown in the discus thrower's face, and "to a modern eye, it may seem that Myron's desire for perfection, has made him suppress, too rigorously, the sense of strain, in the individual muscles", Clark observes. The other trademark of Myron, embodied in this sculpture, is how well the body is proportioned, the symmetria.

The potential energy, expressed in this sculpture's tightly wound pose, expressing the moment of stasis, just before the release, is an example of the advancement of Classical sculpture from Archaic. The torso shows no muscular strain, however, even though the limbs are outflung.'

Nudes, or beautiful landscapes, paintings or sculptures, it is so important for the mentally ill, to have stimulation around them - focussing on things outside of themselves. We have a regular debate, in the crisis house drop-in centre. Amongst more than a thousand pictures, and *objets d'art*, that grace the crisis house, some are, undoubtedly, valuable. Should we seek a valuation, and put up, for auction, those that would bring us in some, much needed, money? I say, 'No!' By definition, mental illness deprives, its sufferers, of enriching environments. Surely, therefore, our valuable works of art, should stay here, to enrich the lives of our service users! Dan, and his nudes - a funny story, but serious as well! One of the carers, who accompanies, Tommy Warfield, to the drop-in centre, and who has, in the past, experienced her own, mental health, issues, loves all the pictures and *objets d'art*, in the crisis house. You certainly, could, spend many happy hours, walking around the house, and looking, at everything, in detail. Dan is, in background, more of a scientific, than, of an artistic, bent. 'Are those nude paintings, and sculptures, pornography?' he asked me, quite seriously! I replied, 'My dear Dan, most things, in life, are debatable, but, with others, there is no dispute. 'The Rokeby Venus', by the great artist, Velasquez, the beautiful, 'Birth of Venus', by Botticelli, Manet's, 'Olympia', John Waterhouse's, 'Hylas and the Nymphs', and his, 'Echo and Narcissus', and Gaugin's 'Girls with Pomegranates', are, unquestionably, Art! Similarly, Michelangelo's, 'David', 'The Venus de Milo', and, 'The Discobolus', are also, quite certainly, Art!' It is not a question of whether, or not, one approves of the subject. Apparently, in 2018, there was, a Feminist objection, to 'Hylas and the Nymphs', being on public display. But, firstly, one has to remember, that artists belong to their times, and, therefore, to the values of their times, and, secondly, I am willing, to have, in the crisis house, anything that is, culturally, enriching - bearing in mind, the deprived environments, of so many, mental health facilities. A common misconception, is that the mentally ill, are also, mentally subnormal, but this is not the case. They are quite capable of taking in the information that I have provided, about the famous artists, and their classical works of art.

Tommy Warfield: 'We're In The Money!'

Friday 24th January 2020 certainly proved to be a red letter day for donations to the crisis house. I shall start with the funny ones. Tommy Warfield sat, as usual, sipping his drink. Today he had opted for whisky and ginger ale. Then he asked me, firstly, whether I ever watched the television programme - 'Who Wants to be a Millionaire?'. I replied that I, occasionally, looked in on it. 'Then I am going to ask you one of the questions that was, once, asked on it, and, if you reply correctly, I shall donate five pounds to the crisis house.' I agreed to play. Question - 'What is sixty-nine? in French?' I replied that 'sixty-nine' is *soixante-neuf* - but January, is a somewhat chilly time, to think of practising it! Five pounds went into the collection box, and I awaited his next question with some apprehension. I needn't have worried. 'If you can name eleven famous 'Williams', I shall donate a second five pounds to the crisis house.' I duly reeled them off - 'William the Conqueror, William Shakespeare, William Wordsworth, William Wilberforce, William Whitelaw, William Rufus, William of Orange, William the Fourth - the Sailor King, our current, Prince William, William Penn, and William Pitt.' A second fiver went into the box. It occurred to me, that Tommy wanted to make his donations to the crisis house, anyway, but he also wanted to make me earn them! This reminds me of Agatha Christie's short story, 'The Unbreakable Alibi' - [Please see: *Partners in Crime*]. In the story, Una Drake, had agreed to marry Mr. Montgomery-Jones - provided that he could solve the mystery of how she could be - both in London, and in Torquay - at the same time! This is Agatha Christie's narrative.

'I am worrying about the girl', said Tommy. 'She will probably be let in to marry that young man - whether she wants to, or not.' 'Darling, said Tuppence, don't be foolish. Women are never the wild gamblers, they appear. Unless that girl was already perfectly prepared to marry that pleasant, but rather empty-headed, young man, she would never have let herself in, for a wager of this kind.'

I don't believe that men are wild gamblers either - as evidenced by Phil. On the same afternoon that Tommy was making his donations, our service user, Phil, arrived, and explained that he, also, wanted to make a donation to the crisis house. Expecting to receive ten pounds, I said,

'How kind, all donations, large or small, are most welcome!' and I was thinking, that we were having a good day for small donations. Phil then handed me two rolls of bank notes - which amounted to, exactly, two thousand pounds! An absolute windfall, but, to Phil, it was also an investment. He is a very lonely, and isolated, paranoid schizophrenic, and the crisis house is, probably, to him, the most valuable thing in his life! For further explanation, [Please see: 'Benefactors'].

> *We're in the money!*
> *The skies are sunny!*
> *Old Man Depression,*
> *You are through.*

The Political Telephone

I have long maintained, that, if you go on for long enough, in this life, one day, you will have heard everything! On 25th February 2020, it happened. I had heard everything! The crisis house had been without landline telephone, and internet, access, since the beginning of January. Last October, we were told that the network was to be upgraded, that engineers would come out to fix things, and that we could keep our old telephone number. All went ahead, but, at the beginning of January, the line went dead. I made numerous mobile telephone calls, and sent numerous e-mails, but could get no sense out of anyone - even though we were, continuing to pay, for the service! Finally, on 25th February, I got hold of someone in the Technical Department - never doubting, for one moment, that the problem was anything - other than technical. 'Perhaps you should send out an engineer, I said, the problem may be in the house, itself.' It was then, that I heard everything! 'The problem isn't technical, the man replied. It is political'! Those were his very words! 'It is political'! They say that we freak out! How can a telephone line be political? He explained, further. 'It is because you want to keep your old telephone number.' I assured him, that, if this was causing a problem, he should give us a new number, and get our service, re-connected, as soon as possible. For a Communications Organisation, they sure do have a problem, with communicating. If keeping the old telephone number, presented them with a difficulty, why didn't they just say so, give us a new number, and save everybody the hassle? This conversation was followed up, with another e-mail, from them, explaining that our service had been restored, but when I arrived at the crisis house, on Friday 28th February, the line was still as dead as a dodo! *Mirabile Dictu*, at 11am, a telephone engineer turned up - saying that he had come to fix the line.

He proceeded to do so - most efficiently. The faults were technical - after all. Internally, the new socket wasn't working, and the exterior cable had snapped - probably due to the, recent, inclement weather. So communication with the outside world, was restored, at last! A very funny story - well, if you didn't laugh, you'd cry! The tragic aspect is that we don't know whether - in our two months of being incommunicado - desperate people, in mental health crisis, had been trying to contact us, failed to do so, and thus, not able to access the help that they needed, possibly even made suicide attempts - and all through a simple failure to fix a telephone!

There was a sequel to the saga of the political telephone. I received a call at the crisis house - purporting to be from a different telephone company, and explaining that we had been recommended, to be billed by a different company, and to receive our services, at a cheaper rate. In the light of what had happened, at first, I was taken in. It all sounded plausible - until I was asked to provide our Bank details! 'I never give Bank details over the telephone', I replied, and then I hung up. I think that one's wisest stance, is to treat everything as a scam - unless one has proof positive, to the contrary! A final point about the telephone story, is that, I am, greatly relieved, that, at least, the service has been restored - now that we are dealing with the, coronavirus, pandemic. I have never made so many telephone calls - as in recent weeks - to ensure that our self-isolating service users, are being supported, throughout the crisis.

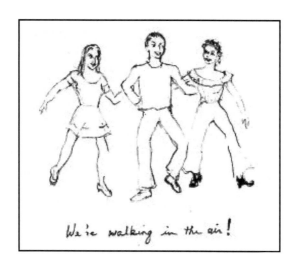

We're walking in the air!

We're Walking In The Air

We're walking in the air.
We're floating in the moonlit sky.

As I explain, in the following letter to *The Wokingham Paper* (5th March), I avoid meetings, unless, like the one, described, they are financially rewarding, and so, on the rare occasions, that I appear, I am always asked the two questions, posed in the letter. A third question, never openly expressed, but, nevertheless, tacitly there, is 'And how can we get our hands on it?' My, tacit, answer is - 'You never will - as long as I am around.' Nevertheless, I answered the question on ownership, with deliberate emphasis. If other people ever tried to evict us from Station House, and obtain occupancy for themselves, they need to realise that they would have no floors to walk on. They would be, literally, 'Walking in the Air!'

'I greatly enjoyed participating in the 'Strictly Charity' Event - which you covered in The Wokingham Paper *(27th February). It was a huge success. Being a burrowing animal, I rarely attend events, but when I do, I am always asked the same two questions - 'Who owns Station House?', and 'Who will take over running it, when you are no longer able to do so? The answer to the first question is that Wokingham Borough Council owns its leaky old roof, and its crumbling old walls, but we own everything else - including some of its floors! Talk about a 'tumbledown shack by an old railroad track', but just like the 'shanty', in the old song, Station House is our 'everything', and is perfect for our purposes. The answer to the second question, is that I am not a bit concerned about who will take over the running of Station House, when I am no longer able to do so. I have quite enough to do - solving the problems of today - without having to spend time, worrying, about those of tomorrow! I am a great admirer of Sir Winston Churchill, who said, 'The churchyards are full of people who thought that they were indispensable!' When the time comes, our younger members, may decide to continue with it. Alternatively, another local charity may find a use for it. Either way, it will be taken over by younger people - as everything always is, eventually. Either way, it will continue to provide a useful service in the local community, - which is the only thing that matters!'*

Boys Will Be Boys

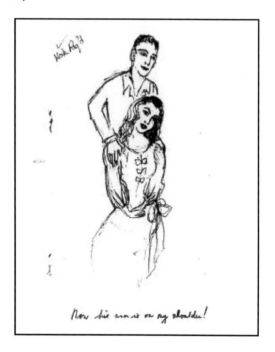

What do you wanna make those eyes at me for,
If they don't mean what they say?

As I have explained, both in *'Triumph and Tragedy'*, and, now, in *'There's A Place For Us'*, I strongly discourage, romantic attachments, between the mentally ill people, who use our services. Such attachments, absolutely guarantee, an exacerbation of existing problems. Is my advice taken? I fear not. A current situation, in March 2020, is an excellent one, for our Psychology Master's students, to observe. As I explain to them, the problem is, so often, the failure to learn by experience. Thus, we have, a current service user, who, in desperation, sought romance, in the mental health drop-in centre. The man whom she targeted, suffers from bi-polar affective disorder, and it was his, entirely suitable, former partner's, inability to cope with his mental health, that had brought about the end of their relationship - some time, previously. This man was not, particularly, looking for a new relationship, and, certainly not, with someone, older, and also mentally ill. But boys will be boys, and if there is the chance of a bit of free sex - with no strings attached - then, I say, that a man will usually take it! In the modern idiom, this is known as,

'Friends with benefits!' The billing and cooing, duly commenced, and we watched it all, with interest, and with great amusement. As I explained to the Master's students - 'If a former relationship has gone, disastrously, wrong, one needs to sit down, reflect upon it, and try to figure out why it went wrong. Indeed, when we had our crisis beds, this was one of their functions. Get the person out of a fraught situation - to come and stay in a sanctuary, where there is no pressure on them, and they can then, take the time to think it all out, and, work out, how to avoid future such disasters'. Was there any, such reflection, undertaken by this lady? There was not, and, although I like the man involved, I cannot convince myself that his intentions are honourable. 'He wants to marry me.' He wants to marry her, my Aunt Fanny!

> *Ma, he wants to marry me,*
> *Be my honey bee.*
> *Every minute he gets bolder,*
> *Now he's leaning on my shoulder,*
> *Ma, he's kissing me!".*

The man, concerned, told us that - when the lady was cosying up to him, and whispering sweet nothings into his ear - he didn't want a relationship with her. Nevertheless, he would sit, close beside her, on the sofa. We have plenty of chairs; he could have sat elsewhere. He said that he didn't find her attractive, but, just like May's little brother, in the full version, of the following song, I saw him kiss her! However, I believe him, implicitly, when he says that he doesn't want a relationship with her. He doesn't - just anything that may be offered, on a plate!

> *Hold your hand out. naughty boy.*
> *Hold your hand out, naughty boy.*

I can advise, till the cows come home! It is no good appealing to common sense; it is no good appealing to one's instinct for self preservation. As the following song declares:

> *They said, 'Someday*
> *you'll find*
> *All who love are blind.*
> *When your heart's on fire,*
> *You must realise,*
> *Smoke gets in your eyes.*

All the service users of the drop-in centre, are in stitches, as this story unfolds, so I cannot, in all conscience, include it in, anything other, than my chapter, entitled, 'More Funny Stories'. However, it could, equally appropriately, be included, with 'More Poignant Stories', or even, with 'More Tragic Stories'. Tragic, that people can be so blind! However, the one chapter in which it, certainly never, could be included, is with 'More Success Stories'! It's an ill wind that blows nobody any good. The coronavirus pandemic, has enforced social distancing, so, during this time, we have, to sit, at least, two metres, apart - and this, for the time being, dampens ardour, and the bubble, is pricked!

I'm forever, blowing, bubbles,
Pretty bubbles, in the air.

President Donald Trump, is, currently, being castigated, for saying, sarcastically, that people should inject themselves, with disinfectant, to protect them from the coronavirus. I tell people, in the drop-in centre, that I would like to have, a large container of common sense, and some syringes, and needles, and so, inject people, with a good dose of common sense! All right, I may, like President Trump, be joking, in order to lighten, the current, sad atmosphere, but, nevertheless, it is a fact, that there is, many a true word, spoken, in jest!

Predictably, despite social distancing, some of the nonsense, persists. In June, 2020, this lady came into the drop-in centre, but the man had not arrived. When he did, she greeted him with, no less, ardour. 'I only came here to see you', she said. 'And, honey, I missed you!' Then, there was further, giggling, flirtation, and lots of banter, with, very explicit, sexual innuendos. You can't win, and, 'being good', they are not!

And honey, I miss you
And I'm being good
And I'd love to be with you
If only I could.

Exactly as anticipated, by November 2020, the disadvantages of two mentally ill people getting together, romantically, have become apparent. Now he is, both literally, and metaphorically, 'leaning on her shoulder', and the strain is beginning to be felt. I have used the situation, to explain to Elise, why we only allow a same-sex Befriending Scheme, and have other strict, but necessary rules, with our Befriending Service.

Making Rosie Laugh
It is such a sad time, for Rosie, at present, with the loss of her son to the coronavirus, so it is good, to see her in fits of laughter, as I explain that human beings, always do what they want to do - however foolish it may be, and they only take notice of any advice, that I may give - if that is what they wanted to do, anyway!

Answer: 'No!'
It is a sad fact of life, that most voluntary organisations, eventually, are colonised by mainstream services. Sometimes, the infiltration, is subtle, sometimes - blatant, but, usually, it happens, at some time. With me, it never has, and it, never, will!

No John, No John, No John, No!

In 2020, I am advising Elise, as to how, to acquire skills, for coping with mental health issues - since she may, eventually, wish to enter the field of counselling, or psychotherapy. She needs to learn when to say, 'No!' We are carrying on, through the coronavirus pandemic, looking towards a brighter future, and to the thirty-year anniversary, of the crisis house, which is due, at the end of March, 2021.

There's a good time coming,
But it's ever so far away.

On Wednesday, 29th April, 2020, I wrote the following letter, to *The Wokingham Paper*, explaining, how I have been able, to keep the crisis house going, for, the full, thirty years.

'When one considers, the heartbreak, that the coronavirus pandemic, is causing some people - bereavement, and their businesses, going to the wall, minor inconvenience - such as not being able to get one's hair cut, is nothing. But, like everyone, I am longing for some easing, of restrictions. I hope, in particular, that we will be able to have, a proper celebration, of the crisis house's thirtieth anniversary - which is due, in March, 2021. So, how have I been able, to keep the crisis house, going, for thirty years? The answer, is that I have put, all my effort, into it, and had nothing to do, with anything, or anyone, outside. As a result, the crisis house has received, no fewer, than eleven top awards - seven of them - local, and four of them - national. I only do, what I do, no more, and no less, and I never change anything - unless it is, clearly, a change

for the better. I have received, plenty of requests, for change, over the years, but I am very well-versed, in the art of saying, 'No.' The requests, may not have been worded, exactly, as I word them, now, but their meaning, was, nevertheless, as I express it. Request, number one: 'Now that you have done all the work, and have set up, a successful, service, can we come swanning in, take over, and have all the say-so, while you continue to do all the work?' Answer, 'No.' Request, number two: 'Now that we have provided some funding, for your crisis beds, can we send you, high-dependency, mental health patients, who need, round-the-clock, nursing, and so, get them off our hands?' Answer - 'No.' Request, number three: 'Now that I am cosy, and comfortable, staying in the crisis house, and doing nothing, to solve my problems, can I continue to stay here, for free, for the rest of my life?' Answer, 'No.' Request, number four: 'We don't like the fact, that you are, an independent, centre of excellence, so can we get away, with pretending, that there is something, wrong, with your service - to justify, closing it down?' Answer, 'No.' Request, number five: 'I have tried, and failed, to destroy the crisis house. But I need your services, so can I, now, come back, and use them?' Answer, 'No.' Request, number six: 'We have stopped, the funding, for your crisis beds, but can you continue, running them, on fresh air, and can we continue to send homeless, mentally ill people, to you, for you to accommodate?' Answer, 'No.' Request, number seven: 'Hasn't the time come, to get rid of the crisis house bar - in case, somebody abuses it?' Answer, 'No.' You don't get rid of the bar; you get rid of the abuser! Request, number eight: 'Now that I am, cosy and comfortable, in the drop-in centre, can you get rid of the people, I don't like, so that I can have it, just for myself, and for those I do like?' Answer, 'No.' Request, number nine: 'If, then, I go away, will you come, running after me?' Answer, 'No.' Anyone who wishes to use our services, is, most warmly welcome, to do so, and, anyone, who doesn't, is, equally welcome, not to! Request, number ten: 'You don't open, on all the days, of the week, so, on the days, that you don't open, can we come, clomping in, use you resources, and facilities, and leave you, to clean up, after us?' Answer, 'No.' I explain, to our young volunteers, that there will always be some people, who, even when offered, the opportunity, do nothing, to resolve, their situation. But equally, there will always be people, who do brilliantly, turning their whole lives, around, for the better. Over the thirty years, we have had people - who came to us - homeless, jobless, penniless, and from, a broken, relationship, and, in due course, left us, with a new home, a new job, money, and a new partner. This is why, I look forward, to taking the crisis house, into its fourth decade!'

With regard to request number nine, my sentiments, are expressed, cogently, in the following song:

> *I got along without you before I met you,*
> *Gonna get along without you now.*

It is evident, that the, forthcoming generation, of charity workers, need to, take a leaf, out of the book, of the nymph, whose, resolute, answer, is expressed in this poem.

Top of Form - Overheard on a Saltmarsh

> *'Nymph, nymph, what are your beads?'*
> *'Green glass, goblin. Why do you stare at them?'*
> *'Give them me.'*
> *'No.'*
> *'Give them me. Give them me.'*
> *'No.'*
> *'Then I will howl all night in the reeds,*
> *Lie in the mud and howl for them.'*
> *'Goblin, why do you love them so?'*
> *'They are better than stars or water.*
> *Give me your beads, I want them.'*
> *'No.'*

Coping With Severe Neurotic Disorders

> *Abe, Abe, Abe, my boy,*
> *What are you waiting for, now?*

Some of these neurotic disorders, really do, take the biscuit, as the following story, illustrates. A good portion, of my life, is, inevitably, devoted to form-filling, so it was, nothing unusual, for me, in January 2020, to complete a form - updating, an insurance company, on an individual's entitlement to, ongoing, Income Protection. In May 2020, the lady concerned, while lamenting, the enormous number of tasks, that she had to undertake, said, 'There is, still, that form, for the insurance company.' It had been, filled in, correctly, in January, but she insisted, upon, altering it, and presented me, with a second version -

which, was also, complete, and so, should have been, put in the post. What was she waiting for? Her Befrienders, have said, that nothing ever gets done, and, no task, is ever completed. She is, always, pursuing, a result, and never, achieves one. This is the, sad reality, of, the severe, neurotic disorders. Years pass, decades pass, and, eventually, life itself, will have passed. I could have included, this story, with my. 'Poignant Stories', but I thought that I would, cheer it up, with the old, music hall, song, 'Abe, Abe, Abe, my boy, what are you waiting for, now?', and place it, with the 'Funny Stories!' On Monday 27th July 2020, a good six months after I had completed the first version of the form, this lady visited the crisis house, and explained that she had still not submitted it. No reason was given; it was simply a case of - 'Abe, Abe, Abe, my boy. What are you waiting for now?'

A new member joined us on Tuesday 21st April 2020. He had experienced very bad treatment, from mainstream services, and having elicited my views of them, asked whether I ever did any campaigning. Although Part Nine, of this book, is entitled - 'Continuing The Campaign For Mental Health Education - Through The Exchange Of Letters', I regard, my stuff, more, as expressing views, and as keeping the mental health debate, alive, than, as actual campaigning. I certainly don't expect to change, or improve, anything in mainstream services, as a result of my letters, and I reiterated, to this new member, the same advice that I have given to people, throughout the entire, thirty-year history, of the crisis house. 'Set up your own service, as we have done, with the Wokingham Crisis House, ensuring, through the Rules and Constitution of your organisation, that you restrict membership, to the mentally ill, and their informal carers. Don't allow, anyone else, either to muscle in, or change anything.'

The lack of social skills that are a feature of severe, mental illness, make life very sad, for sufferers, but, there is no doubt about it, such a lack also causes the most hilarious situations.

Don: 'The Darkness Deepens'

> *At Trinity Church, I met my doom.*
> *Now we live in a top back room.*
> *Up to my eyes in debt for rent.*
> *That's what she's done for me.*

In the crisis house drop-in, Don and I were discussing marriage, and its pitfalls. Don said that he had tried it, twice, and that he was determined, not to be bitten, a third time. He said that his favourite hymn, was 'Abide With Me', and that he had chosen it, for his, first, wedding, but the minister who was conducting the wedding service, wouldn't agree with this. I'm not surprised! We rolled around, laughing. Some hymns - such as - 'The King Of Love, My Shepherd Is', and 'Love Divine, All Loves Excelling', can be sung, equally suitably, at both weddings, and at funerals, but I can't think of any hymn, less suitable, for a wedding, than 'Abide With Me' – unless it were 'Fight The Good Fight'. One wonders, upon which lines, of this hymn, bride, groom, and guests, would focus. Would they be, 'Help of the helpless, oh, abide with me'? - or, possibly, 'Change and decay, in all around, I see'? To top all, the lines, 'I fear no foe, with Thee, at hand, to bless!' completed our session, of rolling around, in stitches. However, if Don's attitude to marriage, is now that of 'meeting his doom', perhaps a funereal touch would be appropriate - hence, the title of this funny story - 'The Darkness Deepens'. For those with a more optimistic outlook, the following hymns are suitable, for a wedding.

The King of love my Shepherd is
Whose goodness faileth never.

Love divine, all loves excelling,
Joy, of heaven, to earth, come down.

The Triumphant Toilet Seat
The hinge of one of our toilet seats had broken. Some of our members tried to fix it - but without success.

In the end, I decided to get a new seat, and have a go at fixing it, myself. I was not very confident - my mechanical skills being about as good as my driving skills! However, I persevered. I was relieved, on reading the instructions for the fitting, that they were, at least, in English. Too often you have to wade through Chinese, Japanese, Russian, Polish, Arabic, French, and German! 'Come on, I said to myself. You may be technically challenged, but you are not mentally retarded.' I toiled, and toiled - struggling to follow those instructions. I must have been at it, for nearly two hours, and then, suddenly, it was done! It was fitted. I had done it! Talk about, 'Have a go, Joe!' Understandably, I was pleased with my success. My driving lessons made it into 'Funny Stories', in *Triumph and Tragedy*, so it is only fair that my triumphant toilet seat, should make it into 'Further Funny Stories', in *'There's A Place For Us'*! After all, I'd 'had a go!'

'Have a go, Joe, come on and have a go.'

How Many Social Workers Does It Take, To Change A light bulb?
How many social workers does it take to change a light bulb. Firstly, you need twenty - to conduct a feasibility study - and then, a further, twenty, to carry out a risk assessment. A further twenty are needed, to set up meetings - to discuss the results of the feasibility study, and the outcome of the risk assessment. Then you need a further twenty - to pursue a longitudinal study - into the science of light bulb changing. Twenty, highly qualified social workers, are then needed, to study the philosophy, and psychology, of light bulb changing - before any actual changing of a light bulb, can be contemplated. So you need at least one hundred social workers - and that is even before the changing of the light bulb, is put into practice! Very funny, but, a true incident, reported by one of our befrienders, casts, a more serious light, on the problem. In March, she visited a mentally ill, resident, of a mental health supported house, in Reading. She was informed that their bathroom had been, without a light, since the previous December. It was an old house, with a high ceiling, so the mentally ill residents had been unable to replace the dud light bulb, and so, had been stumbling around in the dark, for months on end. The serious point is that we should stop paying social workers, to sit around in meetings, and instead, put the money into front line care workers, who will ensure that mentally ill people, have safe, and pleasant, environments, in which to live. One carer, who visits the crisis house, with a client, said that she liked the job, but was only paid the minimum wage, and so struggled, financially. Social care, certainly needs to be looked at - since this situation, is unacceptable.

The Cats Have Gone
In mental health services, communication skills are of the essence, and service users frequently lament the fact that so many care workers in the mental hospital, have an inadequate grasp of the English language. Even when people speak intelligible English, they often assume, incorrectly, that people understand them - which is not always, the case, as the following, funny story, illustrates. I arrived at the crisis house, one morning, and a message had been left for me. 'Could you please let the garage know, that the cats have gone. I can understand one cat going, but not two.' I checked that our two cats - Cuddles and Shayna, were

present, and correct - though I was intrigued as to what the garage could do, if our cats had run away! However, I relayed the message, faithfully, as requested, to the garage. 'I was told to tell you that the cats have gone. It is understood that one cat may go, but not two!' Realising my bewilderment, the garage manager explained, solemnly, 'The cats, are the catalytic converters on the exhaust of your minibus.'

There was also, the occasion, when our doorbell rang, and a lady enquired, 'Have you seen Paul, with a brown princess?' Observing my bewilderment, I was solemnly informed, 'A brown princess, is a car!' Lack of mutual understanding, works the other way, as well. We live in Bracknell, and our telephone number, was only one digit different. 'Can you tell me anything of the wind speeds on the Amazon?' A caller would enquire, without preamble. 'I can tell you nothing of the wind speeds on the Amazon', I would reply, solemnly, 'but I can tell you the correct telephone number, for the Meteorological Office!'

Chapter 12

Further Tragic Stories

Doomed From The Start
In 2016, Alexis died, and his story is told in the section on sadness, and premature death.

Fondly Remembered
In 2016, one of our long-term befrienders, Janet, died after a long battle with cancer. She was seventy-six. Janet used to make cakes for the crisis house, and these were much appreciated by our service users. In the Autumn of 2017, Catriona, another of our long-term befrienders, passed away. She did a lot of befriending for the Association, and was, for five years, our, very efficient, committee secretary. For the hilarious circumstances in which she achieved this position, please read in 'Triumph and Tragedy': 'Twenty-five Funny Stories': 'Angie Higginbottom: The Secretary of the Politburo'.

Catriona also passed away at the age of seventy-six, and our Association received a small donation, in her memory.

A Sad Suicide
Also, in the summer of 2017, Jan, son of our late member, Fenella Bewley, committed suicide. After the death of his mother, in November

2012, Jan often mentioned taking his own life, but, after a period of years had elapsed - since his bereavement - I thought that he had settled well. It therefore came as a shock, when it finally happened, and a shame that he didn't involve himself more with our Association - for the support that he so desperately needed. This story is also, particularly tragic, in that Jan's mother was the best volunteer that our Association ever had, and, more than nine years after her death, is still spoken of, with affection, and respect, by our members, and is still missed, for the enormous amount of good work that she did, in her seventeen years of service with us. She helped so many people back into worthwhile, quality, lives, that it is such a pity that this was not achieved for her son.

Coral Smith: 'No Longer Able To Cope'
It is most unusual for me to get a call for the crisis house, at home, but I did receive one late in 2017. The caller was actually using outdated information, and was looking for a crisis bed. She explained that she had, staying with her in her one-bedroom flat, a friend who was both an alcoholic, and a prescription drug-addict, and that she could no longer cope with her. I explained that we no longer offered crisis beds, but that she should bring her friend to the crisis house next day, anyway, since we were, usually, able to help in such situations. The caller's desperation was illustrated perfectly, next day. She rushed into the crisis house, dumped her friend in a chair, and ran for her life! I asked one of our service users who, though accommodated, by then, had a long history of street homelessness, to take the lady under his wing, and point out to her, all the local help that was available - which included the local Salvation Army - who provide both hot meals, and clothes. Eventually, in 2018, the lady managed to get a room in the house of her former partner, who was also the father of her adult son. She attended our drop-in centre, regularly, and seemed to be benefiting. Then, she just stopped coming. We thought that the reason might be that her former partner's house was in Finchampstead - some miles from Wokingham Town Centre - and necessitating expensive bus journeys. Then, one morning, the friend who had originally contacted us, came in, and said that Coral had been found dead - presumably from an overdose of prescription drugs. Had we got to know her better, and for a longer time, we might have been able to save Coral. A tragic story!

Such A Waste Of A Young Life
Early in 2019, Dora, an occasional user of the crisis house, called in to tell us that Stuart had passed away - probably dying from a dose of

adulterated heroin. This was sad, and a shock, since Stuart, an inveterate heroin addict, had used our services for many years. He was aged only in his early thirties, and it seems such a waste of a young life. Stuart's surname was 'House', but he was always nicknamed - 'Houseless' - because all his accommodations broke down, sooner, or later, and he, invariably, ended up homeless, once again. It is a sad fact, that - over the past five years - more people, in our ranks, have died, prematurely, from drug-related incidents, than from any other cause.

Neville Sandford: 'Hopes Dashed'

Neville came to us in September 2014. [Please see: '*Triumph and Tragedy*'.] We had high hopes for him, at first, and then, largely due to unsatisfactory accommodation, he appeared to be making no progress at all. 2019 saw a change in this. Having, at last, achieved a stable place to live, he started, step by step, to struggle along the Recovery Path. He started to regain organisational skills, and to take on life's responsibilities. In January 2019, he finally cleared, completely, outstanding debts - of ten years duration! He started to budget his money, and spend it, sensibly, on new clothes, and shoes. He regained coping strategies for solving any problems that arose in the, shared, mental health supported house, in which he was now living. It was great to see a person - with our support - progress along the recovery path. Neville celebrated his twenty-ninth birthday in May 2019 - with a determination to have his life back, intact, by his thirtieth. In conversation with him I reiterated my belief - 'Up to the age of thirty, you can get away with almost anything. Your body is young, and can withstand immoderate quantities of drugs and alcohol. You can backpack around the world, and still get back in time to establish a career, and settle down to marriage and a family. After thirty, doors do start to close. Everything can still be achieved, but with every year that goes by, in your fourth decade, it becomes more difficult.' I thought that Neville, who was very intelligent, had taken this advice on board, and was acting accordingly - though with realistic and achievable goals. But, then came the reversal! On Friday afternoon - on 31st May 2019 - Neville came into the drop-in centre, and told us that he was definitely going to commit suicide. He gave us a garbled account of some disagreement that had occurred at his shared house - but this didn't appear to be serious enough to provoke such a reaction, so I told Neville that I thought that he should go to hospital for a while. I went to the telephone to contact a doctor, and arrange his admission. Neville, however, said that he was not willing to go into hospital immediately - because he had an appointment to pay off a drugs dealer the following

Tuesday - when he also had a follow-up appointment with his dentist, and an appointment to see his doctor on the following Thursday. I wasn't happy, but I agreed to delay things until the next week. On Saturday 1st June, he took a massive overdose. He was admitted, as an emergency, to the Royal Berkshire Hospital, and then transferred to King's College Hospital. They considered a liver transplant, but, because of his poor condition, instead resorted to dialysis, and put him in an induced coma - since he was suffering from epileptic fits, and they feared swelling of the brain. He died on Tuesday 18th June. We were, of course, all very sad. Neville had been popular; we all believed him to be making a good recovery, and it is tragic when such a young life is snuffed out. On Thursday 1st August, seven of our own members joined around seventy other mourners at Neville's funeral - which was organised by the local Salvation Army - of which he was a member, and a valued volunteer. His work for them was praised in the Eulogy. We sang 'All Things Bright and Beautiful' - because, bright and beautiful, Neville had indeed been, but it was a very sad occasion for all those who valued him.

The following letter- published by *The Wokingham Paper* in the week that Neville died, highlights, once again, how deficient statutory mental health services are, and how wonderful it would all be - if I ruled the world!

If I ruled the world, every day
Would be the first day of Spring.

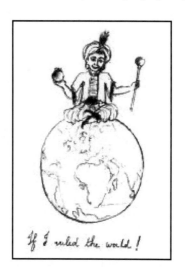

'*Having been presented with two suicide cases in the past week, my best advice is - 'Get the doctor, and get the person admitted to Prospect Park Mental Hospital, without delay.' This is not because I think that Prospect is good; but it has a distinct advantage over other mental health services. It does exist! Section Four - the Emergency Section of the Mental Health Act - is extremely useful - because you only need one doctor to get the person admitted to a Place of Safety. Then, if it is decided that the person needs longer detention - under Section Two, or Section Three - authorisation by a second doctor, can be organised in the hospital, itself.*

In the first instance, the person told me that he was definitely going to commit suicide - so I went to the telephone, to contact the doctor, because I thought it safer if he were admitted to Prospect - straight from the crisis house. But he stopped me. He said that he had an appointment to pay off a drugs dealer - who would inflict awful reprisals if the debt wasn't paid on time. So I agreed, reluctantly, to delay contacting the doctor - until the appointment was kept. Next day, this man took a fatally massive overdose, and so had to be admitted to hospital, anyway!

The second instance concerned a man who had been evicted from his accommodation, and so was homeless, mentally ill, and suicidal. I advised that a doctor should be contacted, and that this man should be admitted to Prospect Park Hospital. In such dire circumstances, there is little that I can do, anyway, since I don't possess a ready supply of homes for homeless mentally ill people - much as I would like to - if I ruled the world! Popular mythology has it that people who talk about committing suicide, never do it, but the Samaritans don't agree with this view - and they should know! I have experience of both situations. I have known people who gave no warning whatsoever, and carried out intentional, and, carefully planned, suicides. But I have also known many - like the two described - who gave every warning, so I wish that we had better mental health services - to respond to these cries for help. In the last week, as well, one of our service users offered to explain to me the sociological model of mental illness - 'It's society that is sick - and not the 'mentally ill' people!' Too cerebral, for me! I have enough of a job - coping with the medical model!'

We have service users - out of their heads on cannabis - who do believe that it is society that is awry, and that there is no such thing as mental illness! In Agatha Christie's short story, 'The Flock of Geryon' - from '*The Labours of Hercules*', Miss Carnaby describes the euphoria - created by cannabis - to Hercule Poirot and Chief Inspector Japp. There is the wonderful dream - followed by prosaic, everyday, responsibility.

'I was thinking', said Miss Carnaby, 'of a marvellous dream I had at the First Festival - hashish, I suppose. I arranged the whole world so beautifully! No wars! No poverty! No ill health! No ugliness!' 'It must have been a fine dream!' said Japp, enviously. Miss Carnaby jumped up. She said, 'I must get home. Emily, [her invalid sister- for whom she was carer], has been so anxious.'

These people - with their Utopian dreams - never explain how things would be - if everyone abandoned daily mundane tasks - in order to embrace wonderful dreams - nor how their ideal world is to be paid for. Furthermore - although mental illness is, indeed, common, there are people who manage to cope in 'sick society' - without succumbing to breakdown. This would suggest that some people are more susceptible to certain mental illnesses - just as some are more susceptible to physical disorders.

Rosie And Carl: 'He Lost The Battle'

Rosie, is a, long-standing, service user, at the crisis house, and she is one, very keen, to keep the crisis house going. Her story is as follows: Her mother was admitted to a mental hospital, diagnosed with schizophrenia, when Rosie, and her sister, were still young teenagers. Mother never returned home; she died, in the mental hospital. Rosie's father was left to bring up the girls, and could not cope. Her sister, who suffered from learning disabilities, went into a home, for the mentally handicapped, and she, also died, some years, ago. Rosie was sent to a special school, in Kent. When, at the age of eighteen, she returned to Berkshire, she worked, briefly, and then, married a businessman, who was much older. She had three children, two girls, and a boy, and the boy, Carl, was born, with defective kidneys. His handicap, among other things, contributed to the breakdown, of Rosie's marriage, and to her, consequent, mental health problems. More recently, Carl was admitted, to a special unit, for yet another, operation. A previous, transplant operation, had failed, and Carl, had resorted back, to dialysis. In order to come under the care of a top specialist, Carl had to be admitted to a hospital, in Manchester. The operation was a success, but he contracted coronavirus, lost the battle, and died, aged, only forty-eight, in April 2020. Rosie, of course, was very distressed, and, particularly, so, in these difficult times. with funeral directors, being overwhelmed, and, funerals, so difficult, to organise. Since she also has financial problems, not least, because transporting a body, through counties, is very costly, I advised, that the best course, might be to choose cremation, locally, in Manchester, without a service, for the immediate situation, and then, hold a memorial service, on Carl's birthday, in 2021. Things, hopefully, will be back to normal, by then, and this will also enable, Gaynor, Carl's sister, to come over, from Canada, for the memorial service. In the end, Rosie opted to have Carl's body transported back to Wokingham, despite the expense, but, due to the current crisis, the funeral could not be held for some weeks. On Friday 5th June 2020, Rosie, still obviously, very distressed, dropped into the crisis house - in order to tell us that Carl's funeral had, at last, taken place. Numbers attending, were restricted, and they sang, only one hymn, 'Dear Lord and Father of Mankind'. What is it, about this particular hymn, that wrenches at the heartstrings, and makes so many people choose it, for a funeral service? Rosie said that, in the light of her tragedy, she was doubting God, as a father, but that, at least, Carl, was now at peace, somewhere.

> *When my time is come,*
> *Let no teardrop fall,*
> *And no darkness hover,*
> *Round me where I lie.*

Rosie's daughter, who lives locally, and was very close to Carl, is experiencing great difficulty, in coping with her bereavement. Her boyfriend has moved in to live with her. Rosie thought that this may not be wise, since her daughter needed time, and space, to grieve, but, on the other hand, I thought that, he might provide good support, at this most tragic time. Sad to relate, when Rosie dropped in to see us, on Friday 22nd July, she said that she and her daughter were not speaking, and that neither Carl, nor Rosie, had liked the boyfriend. It is bad enough, coping with bereavement, but if family relationships, are fractured, as well, life becomes a living nightmare. Rosie has had such an awful time, so I love getting her to laugh. To achieve this, I told her the following two funny stories. The first concerned the vicar of the church that I attended in my youth. He arrived when I was just fourteen years old, and attending his Confirmation Classes. He was aged twenty-eight, and was tall, dark, and handsome. All the young girls were drooling over him! He said that his wife had, prior to marriage, been a domestic science teacher, and was very good at making cakes. He promised that she would bake one for the Youth Club, which we all attended, on Saturday evenings. He duly arrived, accompanied by a dumpy little old woman - whom, we youngsters, assumed to be his mother. Not a bit of it. She was his wife! Vicars, in the Church of England, usually stay for about eight years, in one parish, and are then, moved elsewhere. Many years later, a friend from the church, went to visit this vicar, and his wife, in their new parish. She was greeted by the distressed wife. Apparently, her husband had got friendly with a pretty young nurse, and was leaving her! The Church authorities wanted to save the marriage, so they paid for the vicar, and his wife, to have psychoanalysis. This is what the analysis revealed. When the vicar had married, as a young man, he was looking for a mother. After some years, he no longer needed this, and so sought a woman who would be a wife! All that money, spent on psycho-analysis! We youngsters at the youth club could have told them that! As an adulterer, the vicar could not keep his job in the church, so he and the nurse, duly married, and set up a nursing home together - with the nurse being matron, and the former vicar, dealing with the business side of things. Though unfortunate, for the discarded first wife, so far as I know, the second marriage, was a success. Rosie and I, were not laughing at the people involved; we were laughing at the psychoanalyst's, blinding, but expensive, statement of the obvious!

Clean Clara, the poet sings,
Cleaned a hundred, thousand things.

The second funny story, was one that my mother told me. It concerned a man whose wife was always cleaning, and sweeping up, around him. He dared, not so much, as drop a biscuit crumb, but she would be after him, with the vacuum cleaner! He couldn't stand this, constant, harassment, so he left his wife, for a woman, who was as dirty, as his wife had been clean!

Wash me in the water that you washed
Your dirty daughter in, and I shall be
Whiter than the whitewash on the wall.

Rosie roared with laughter, when she heard these stories, so we had, quite a happy time, together. In September 2020, Rosie reported further, that she missed her son, as, of course, she would, but that her younger daughter, and Andy, were now, working together, running a Landscape Gardening Business. Since her daughter had been made redundant from her former job, due to the pandemic, I thought that this was an excellent venture, and confirmed that these partnership schemes, can work, very successfully, in business, with each partner bringing individual skills to the project. Rosie, herself, also now seemed, more relaxed, about the situation. You have to keep your sunny side up!

Keep your sunny side up, up,
Hide the side that gets blue.

I tell you naught for your comfort,
Yea, naught for your desire.
Save, that the sky grows darker, yet,
And the sea rises higher.

Turning and turning in the widening gyre
The falcon cannot hear the falconer;
Things fall apart; the centre cannot hold;
Mere anarchy is loosed upon the world,
The blood-dimmed tide is loosed, and everywhere
The ceremony of innocence is drowned.

Nightmare In Reading
On Sunday morning, 21st June 2020, news broke that there had been a murderous rampage, in Reading, on the previous evening, and that three victims of stabbing had died. We have a number of service users, who live in Reading, and this news is causing them great distress. All three victims are greatly mourned. One of the three who died, James Furlong, was a, much loved, history master, at the Holt School, in Wokingham, and the whole town is in mourning. The school, itself, held a day of mourning, and the, nearby, St. Paul's Church, opened its doors - for mourners to light candles, and to leave floral tributes. Some of our own members, participated. My own great niece attended The Holt School. James Furlong was a brilliant history teacher - particularly for 'A' Level students - inspiring great enthusiasm for the subject. My great niece actually left the school after GCSEs - preferring horses to academia! She won the Berkshire County Junior Cup, for horse riding, and, on leaving school, commenced the Berkshire College of Agriculture's Course on Animal Welfare - even having to attend to horses, during Lockdown. In fact, it could be said of my great niece, that, like Venetia Kerr, as described by Lady Horbury, who was speaking, scathingly, of her husband's, clear preference, for another woman, '[she's] half a horse herself!' [Please see: Agatha Christie's, *'Death in the Clouds'*]. I don't know what it is about horses, but it is a fact, that they appeal to some

girls - to the exclusion of all else! But, academic, or not, all The Holt School's pupils, past and present, will continue to grieve at the, untimely, death, of their, beloved, history teacher. A tragic story.

Adonais

He has outsoared the shadows of our night.
Envy and calumny, and hate and pain.
And that unrest, which men miscall delight,
Can touch him not, nor torture him again.

Gee Gee: 'A Sad Death'

Gary Gardiner was always known by the nick-name of Gee-Gee - although some, more poignantly, nick-named him, 'Crispy Duck' - because he had, once, sustained serious injuries, in a fire. We were saddened to hear that he had died of a heroin overdose - in July 2020. We had known Gee-Gee for many years, and he was an, inveterate, addict, so, in his case, we did not expect recovery, but it was, nevertheless, sad, to hear of his, premature, death.

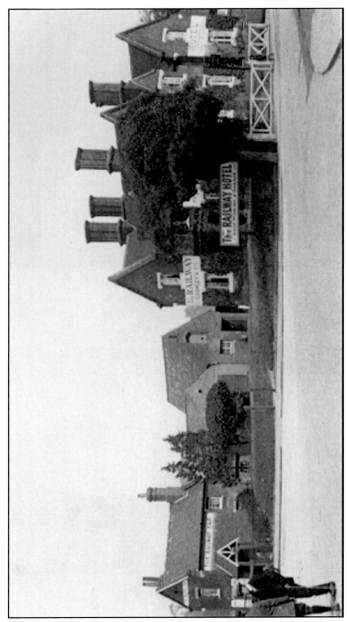

Railway Tap Pub - 1901

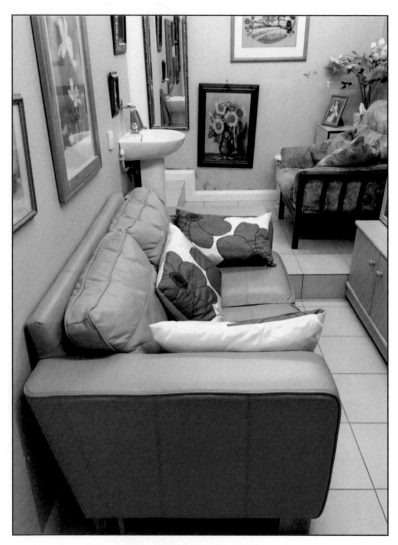

The Crisis House Interior

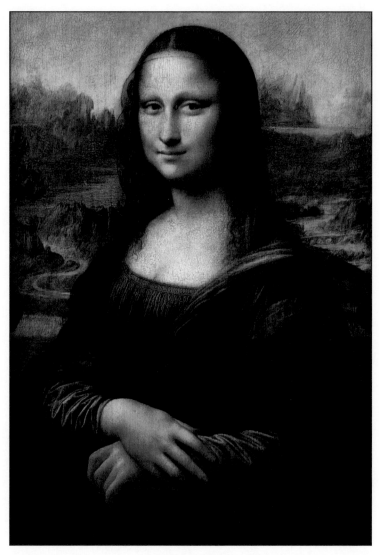

Mona Lisa

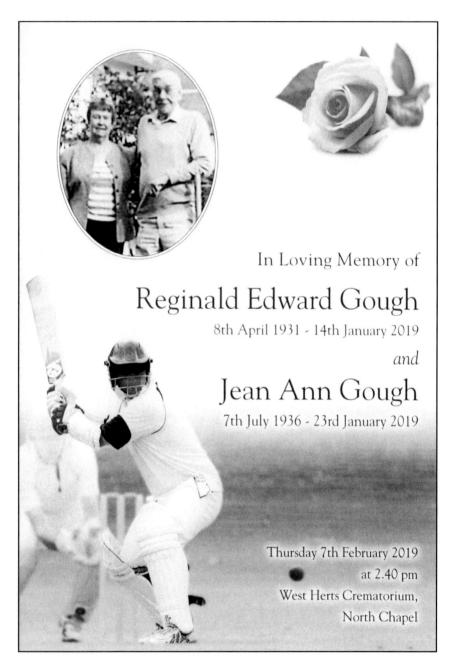

In Loving Memory of

Reginald Edward Gough

8th April 1931 - 14th January 2019

and

Jean Ann Gough

7th July 1936 - 23rd January 2019

Thursday 7th February 2019
at 2.40 pm
West Herts Crematorium,
North Chapel

Reg And Jean's Funeral

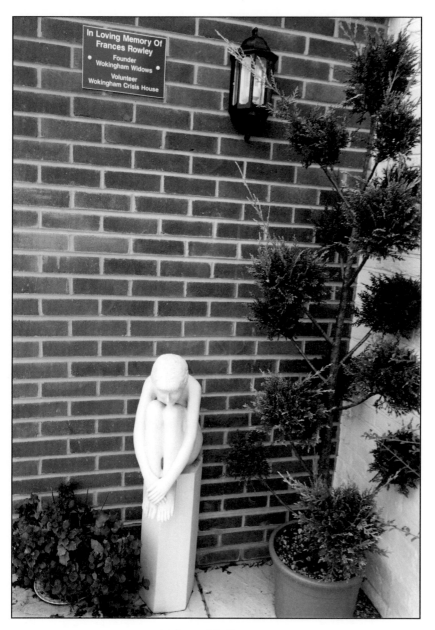

Tribute To Frances

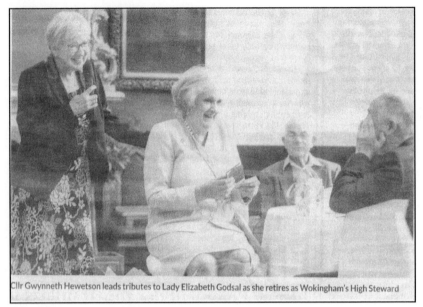

Cllr Gwynneth Hewetson leads tributes to Lady Elizabeth Godsal as she retires as Wokingham's High Steward

Lady Elizabeth Godsal Retirement

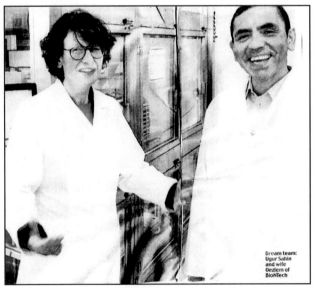

Dream team: Ugur Sahin and wife Oezlem of BioNTech

The World Changers

PART FIVE

Children, Sadness, And Premature Death

Chapter 13

Obituaries

It would be lovely if life were all one glad, sweet song, but it isn't. It is, thus, sad to record that there have been some deaths amongst our ranks since the publication of '*Triumph and Tragedy*', in 2016. In the summer of 2016, Alexis, younger brother of Jim Force died from an overdose of alcohol and heroin. He was aged only thirty-three. I remember Alexis, when he was a youngster, of just fourteen, coming to visit Jim - who was a guest, in the crisis house, at that time. Alexis always had problems in adult life, but it was sad to see that life, cut short, so tragically. You think that you have had it hard? The background, of these brothers, is as follows. Their mother had a mental illness, bi-polar affective disorder, and was also a battered wife. She had five sons - all by different fathers, and all the fathers abandoned the family after, cruelly bullying, both the children, and their mother, whose name was Victoria. Two of the boys, Brendan and Francis, were adopted away - successfully, so far as I know, but I never had any involvement with them. Jim and Alexis were placed in local authority care, and, the youngest, Kieron, suffered from learning disabilities, and was placed in 'Jigsaw', a home for the mentally handicapped. All this was as a result of their mother, dousing herself in petrol, setting light to herself, and going up as a human torch, in front of the children. No wonder they were disturbed! This irony - of the mentally ill and inadequate, having large numbers of children - with whom they can't cope - while lovely, stable, couples, remain infertile - never fails to exercise my mind. I mention the subject in '*Triumph and Tragedy*' - [Please see: 'Tragic Stories: Catherina Lynham: 'I love having children']. More recently, I had the following letter published in '*The Wokingham Paper*':

Parenting Courses

'*As an avid* Wokingham Paper *reader, I saw in the February 22nd 2018 edition, that St. Mary's Church, Wargrave, is offering a Parenting Course, and that free places are available. Decades ago, when taking a postgraduate Montessori Teaching Diploma, I thought it a good idea that the Montessori Society, even then, was also offering courses for people who just wanted to guide their own children. All their courses and schools are excellent - for people who can afford them, but here, at St. Mary's Church, we have a Parenting Course that is open to everybody. Alas, Parenting Courses won't make bad parents, good parents. They will only make good parents even better. There are, basically, four ways of parenting - two good, and two bad. First, high care, low over-protection. The best. This is the ideal world, the happy, adventurous children of Enid Blyton, and E. Nesbit – the Famous Five, and the Railway Children. Sadly, they usually remain in the works of fiction. Second, high care, high over-protection. Most good parents are in this category. Third, low care, low over-protection. Neglect. It would be good if Parenting Courses could turn these people around, but, if they neglect their children, they would probably also neglect to attend, and learn, from the Courses. Fourth, low care, high over-protection. The worst, affectionless control.*

The essential ingredient of parenting, is the ability to put the children's needs before your own. If you can't do that, you can't be a parent. Thus my niece laughed, when, - on returning from the cinema with her two youngest children, her father asked if she had enjoyed the film. 'I haven't been to the cinema, for myself, for years, dad,' she replied. My niece is an excellent parent, and, having four children - aged 15, 13, 8, and 3 - meeting all their varying needs is no mean juggling act! She possesses the essential ingredient. The children come first. Alas, it is my niece who you will find on the Parenting Course - not the socially inadequate heroin addict! So what do you do with people, even quite intelligent people, who think it all right to leave very young children, unattended, in a foreign hotel bedroom, while they go out to dine? Cui bono? Who benefits? What do you do with people who think it all right to allow a seven-year-old to go, unaccompanied, to the fair? I would feel disinclined to take very young children, abroad, at all. To a two-year-old, with his bucket and spade, the nearest seaside resort is every bit as good as a Mediterranean beach. A five-year-old of my acquaintance, claimed that he had been on holiday to America. It transpired that his parents had taken him across the River Thames - from South Woolwich to North Woolwich - in one of their decrepit old ferry boats. In his young eyes, the narrow bit of the Thames was the Atlantic Ocean, and North Woolwich Gardens - were Central Park.

I wouldn't allow a child, of any age, to go to the fair, unaccompanied. But there, I might be making a mistake, and this is where Parenting

Courses become relevant. By failing to allow children to learn to cope with risk, high care, high over-protection, parents, may be failing to provide them with the skills needed, to cope with life. So Parenting Courses can enlighten them. Commonly, you also find parents, who are, generally, considered to be good. Their children are clean, well-fed, and well-dressed. Their physical care is excellent. But these parents don't always realise the importance of emotional support, and its lack can lead to children experiencing mental health problems. So enlightening Parenting Courses, can be positive, in promoting mental health. Finally, we have the great irony of the unfairness of life - the denial of parenthood to those who would have been excellent. The lovely couples - with good jobs, plenty of money, and nice, big houses - who long for a child to complete their happiness, but no child comes. By contrast, you have the, mentally ill, heroin addict, unable to look after herself. Dare breathe on her, and she is pregnant - frequently with twins! Fortunately, Adult Fostering, is available - as an alternative way for childless couples to satisfy their parenting instincts. Take on, and nurture, a mentally ill adult - Cui bono? Who benefits? Everyone benefits!'

*'There's a Friend for little children
above the bright blue sky'*

Fortunately, there are also friends for children, here on earth, and people who will nurture them. On the subject of parenting and mental health, in May 2017, and November 2017, I had two further letters printed in *The Wokingham Paper*.

Nannies can help fix domestic abuse

'I note from the report in The Wokingham Paper, *that the new leadership at Wokingham Borough Council is to focus on the prevention of domestic abuse as its priority. There are also new proposals for a national strategy to tackle this problem - to be adopted, if agreed, in September. Proposals for harsher punishments, and longer prison sentences for abusers, will not help to solve the problem - because people who neglect and abuse their children do so because they were neglected and abused by their parents - who were neglected and abused by theirs! They can't deliver childcare, because they don't know what childcare is! I think that such people should be provided with specially trained resident nannies. This idea is already in operation, to an extent, by the excellent charity, Home Start. They provide trained volunteers - who are, themselves - experienced parents - to help struggling families with at*

least one child under the age of five. I am thinking of full-time resident nannies for those families with the greatest degree of mental illness and inadequacy. The 'Baby P' case would never have happened if Tracey Connelly had been thus supervised all the time. I can already hear the cries of horror at the costs involved. But would it cost more? The aim is not the short-term one of making life easy for inadequate families, but is the long-term one of breaking the cycle of abuse in the next generation. Our current system of having social workers visiting and making reports, of returning mentally ill mothers, to hospital, when they break down under stress, of taking their children into care, and of sending abusers to prison - doesn't work in the best interests of the children, but does cost a lot of money! Trained resident nannies, would demonstrate excellent childcare to those who have never had it, and no doubt, the nannies would find themselves having to nanny the parents, as well as the children! We have an example with our own members - both - ladies who suffered very severe post-natal depression. One had a brilliant nanny - paid for by her husband's employer. Her boys are now, both, hard-working adults - successfully raising families of their own. The other did not get help with her infant son - who now spends his adult life as an unemployable heroin addict! The nannies are not Mary Poppins! There is no magic in mental health, but Wokingham Borough Council should try out this idea. It works!'

Better assessment of prospective adopters is also required, and stimulated me to write the following thought-provoking letter to *The Wokingham Paper*. This was published on 16th November 2017.

Adoption and marriage

'Do your readers detect a homophobic backlash in the excessively harsh sentence given to child-killer, Matthew Scully-Hicks. Life imprisonment - the same as that for mass-murder - and at least eighteen years to serve! Does the media coverage of the case suggest that Matthew Scully-Hicks is a sadist - who deliberately conned the authorities into allowing him to adopt a baby - so that he could, then torture, and kill her? No, because, if so, he could have abducted, and abused, a child - without going through all the complication of rigorous adoption procedures. I get, instead, the impression of an inadequate neurotic - who hadn't a clue about the strain and stress that a constantly screaming baby can impose. He couldn't cope, and flipped. It wasn't necessarily because he is gay, but it certainly was due to mental ill health! He must have had severe mental health issues - because anyone in a

normal state of mind would simply conclude - 'I am not equipped to cope with this child' - and send her back to the Adoption Authorities. Unlike natural parents, prospective adopters are allowed a trial period. We always discourage the mentally ill who use our services, from getting romantically involved with each other, and producing children. If you can barely look after yourself, you will never cope with a screaming baby! I recall that, when having to nurse my screaming infant brother, my solution was a dummy, dipped in sweet condensed milk. This invariably produced a beatific smile, and instant peace - though I am not so sure, in retrospect, that it was the best thing for his emerging teeth! Still, at least it wasn't gin, or laudanum [heroin] - favoured by over-burdened Victorian mothers! They couldn't send the babies back. Matthew Scully-Hicks could have done so - if he had been in his right mind! The Social Services have emerged, yet again, as their usual, useless, selves. Any prospective, adoptive parents should be required to undergo a mental state examination by a Consultant Psychiatrist - to ensure that they have the stability, and the resilience, to cope with a child - who may be damaged, and difficult - due to the circumstances which made them available for adoption. So should gay couples be allowed to adopt? Adam and Eve, Adam and Steve - the Lord God made them all, and He hath done all things well! Gay men and lesbians should have the same civil rights as everybody else. In 1998, before such ceremonies were commonplace, we celebrated a gay wedding at the crisis house - with all the traditions - wedding cake, presents, and a Minister conducting the service, and assuring us that the Christian Church was blessing gay unions as far back as the fifth century. The couple have just celebrated twenty years together, and I send my congratulations through The Wokingham Paper. *No prejudice here! A child needs both a mother, and a father. Can a man be a good mother? Can a woman be a good father? It is all right for rich celebrities - because they can afford both day-nurses, and night-nurses - so they don't have to do the mundane, and demanding, parenting - day and night! When required to do so, Matthew Scully-Hicks proved tragically incapable. This case raises many questions about adoption, and about the need for mental health assessments for prospective adopters.'*

When looking at some of these tragic cases, the following children's hymn, and prayer, would seem to be, particularly, pertinent!

Jesus, Friend of little children,
Be a Friend to me.

PART SIX

Obituaries 2016 - 2021

Chapter 14

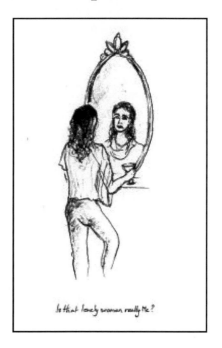

Is that lonely woman really Me?

Not A Bad Innings

In March 2017, my sister, Joan, who had suffered, from mental health problems, all her life, passed away in her seventieth year - not a bad innings - considering her long history of ill health. At her funeral, which was attended by her long-term befriender, Cecilia, as well as by, family members, we sang 'Morning has Broken', 'Those Were the Days', and 'Elusive Butterfly'. 'The bright, elusive, butterfly of love' - brightness, and memories of youth, are the style of modern funerals - rather than the, depressing dirges, that belong to the Victorian age! Celebrate the morning of life! Cecilia, had been, an excellent befriender, for Joan - getting her interested in gardening, and, generally, giving her support. I have chosen, to include, in this book, the song. 'Rose Marie' - in order to mark the beginning of Joan's life, as well, as including, those songs, sung at her funeral, at her life's end. Our mother, had wanted, for me, the names, Pamela Antoinette, but our father, didn't like fancy names. He offered to register my birth, pretended, to forget, that, Antoinette, was the name that our mother had chosen, and registered me as 'Pamela Ann'. When it came to naming, my sister, our mother suggested, first, 'Shirley', and then 'Brenda'. Both names were, 'too fancy', for our father, so our mother settled, for 'Joan', and even our father, couldn't think of any name, plainer, than that. But, on this occasion, our mother registered the birth, and got her own back! She chose 'Rosemary', as a second name, and you won't find any name, fancier, than that. Furthermore, as Agatha Christie writes, in her novel, '*Sparkling Cyanide*', 'Rosemary, is for remembrance'. At the conclusion of the novel, Anthony, and Iris, are looking forward to marriage, and a happy future. Agatha Christie writes:

'He [Anthony], touched a little vase, by Iris's side, in which, was a single sprig, of grey-green, with a mauve flower. 'What's that doing, in flower, at this time of year?' It does, sometimes, just an odd sprig, if it's a mild Autumn.' Anthony took it, out of the glass, and held it, for a moment, against his cheek. He half-closed his eyes, and saw, rich, chestnut, hair, laughing, blue eyes, and a red, passionate, mouth. He said, in a quiet, conversational, tone, 'She's not around, any longer, is she?' 'Who do you mean?' 'You know who I mean. Rosemary.'

Oh Rose Marie, I love you,
I'm always dreaming of you,
No matter what I do, I can't forget you.

Now I include, the songs - sung at her funeral - marking the end of Joan Rosemary's life.

'Morning has broken
like the first morning.
Blackbird has spoken,
like the first bird.

'Those were the days, my friend.
We thought they'd never end.
We'd sing, and dance,
for ever and a day.'

131

When, in Agatha Christie's novel, '*The Do It With Mirrors*', Miss Marple meets up with the friends of her schooldays - Ruth, and Carrie Louise - they laugh over their youthful ambitions and idealism - which included nursing lepers, and becoming a nun. Ruth thought that marriage knocked it all out of people, but Miss Marple, though she never married, was no longer young and idealistic. It is life itself that destroys young elusions - though one can always go on - chasing butterflies!

> '*You might wake up some morning*
> *to the sound of something moving*
> *Past your window in the wind.*
> *I chase the bright, elusive, butterfly of love.*'

I made a donation to our Association - preferring that the mentally ill benefited - rather than having something traditional - like a tombstone - in Joan's memory. My sister's passing was particularly poignant, since - had she and my brother, not developed schizophrenia all those decades ago - I may never have got involved with mental health at all.

Chapter 15

The Passing Of A Wokingham Stalwart

I had known Ellie's mother, Barbara, for many years, and Ellie, herself, stayed in the crisis house from 2002 to 2003. Barbara supported us, with a letter to the Press, at the time that the crisis house was threatened with closure. Barbara was an enthusiastic member of the local History Society, and had published a book on the history of a gravestone - to be found in the, ancient, All Saints Churchyard. Sadly, in 2017, she became ill, with dementia, and died early in 2018 - at the age of seventy. I take the view, as I did with my own sister's death, that, if you reach your seventieth year, you haven't been robbed of life. This is the 'three score years, and ten,' stated in the Bible, as being man's span of life on the earth. If you reach eighty years, you have done well, and any age over eighty, is a bonus from the Grim Reaper! But, as always, it is QUALITY of life, and not just QUANTITY, that is important. One wouldn't want to linger late into one's eighties and nineties - suffering from dementia! Ellie stayed with her stepfather, Rory, to give him support for a while - as he went through his bereavement. In May 2019, I encountered her, by chance. Ellie was now back in her flat, and was on her way to Oxford - to meet up with her Narcotics Anonymous Mentor - she then, having completed, the programme with her Alcoholics Anonymous Mentor. She brought me up to date with the fact that her son, Sam, is now twelve years old, and is in his first year at secondary school. There is no doubt about it - *Tempus fugit*!

Living With Dementia

As I write this, in January 2020, we have, no fewer than three, service users, who are still recovering from mental health problems - exacerbated by the stress of having to nurse parents with dementia. If you have to cope with this, for a few weeks, or maybe, a few months, you might be able to survive, mentally unscathed, but when it goes on for years - mental scarring is inevitable. Thus it is that Keith, Dan Kent, and Jaqui, are all still traumatised from years of this gruelling caring. They had to cope - day and night - with double incontinence, disinhibition, wandering, and constant anxiety. Coping with dementia is, indeed, a major social problem in the twenty-first century. From day one, I have been adamant, that only mentally ill people, and their informal carers, can be involved in our charity. All our Trustees, are one or the other. Who knows what it is like to struggle, year after year, with black, and debilitating, depression? Answer - 'The one suffering from it?' Who knows what it is like, to struggle, often without any help, and twenty-four, seven, with the care of a relative with dementia? Answer - 'The one doing so!' Both mental illness, and caring for the mentally ill, are isolating, positions. Don, when ill with bi-polar affective disorder, said that people would cross the street, if they saw him, coming towards them. They wanted to avoid him, and his mental illness. The full-time carer, hasn't the time, to accept invitations to dinner, nor is he/she in a position to issue them, so, after a while, invitations cease, and the carer becomes, socially isolated. This was, very much, the position of Keith Rode, when he was, for years, caring for a mother with dementia, so it is most rewarding to see him, now restored, to a good social life. [Please see: 'More Success Stories'.] So, 'Who knows if the shoe fits?' Answer - 'The one who is wearing it!' I find it, very interesting, listening to, the scientific advice, that we are being given, during the, current, coronavirus, crisis. In particular, dementia sufferers, are deemed to be, in the 'high risk' group - both, more likely, to contract, and more likely, to die, from the infection. Is there not, in this, an element, of 'nature taking its natural course'? Human beings, are not immortal, and there is, the concept, of 'happy release'! I believe that those, who have actually had to care, for relatives, with dementia, over a period of years, would agree with me.

Chapter 16

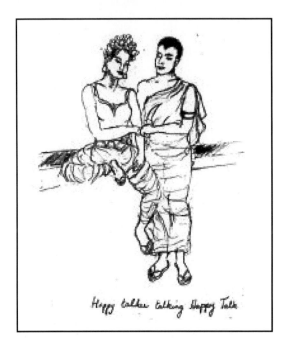

Happy talkee talking Happy Talk

A Very Good Innings

Late in 2018, Jackie Gough telephoned - to say that her mother would like a word. She explained that she was full-time carer for both her parents - who were, now, in their eighties, and suffering from serious health problems. I had a word with her mother, Jean, and followed this up with Christmas greetings - hoping that things were going better. But, sad to report, in January 2019, Jackie telephoned again, to explain that her father, Reg, had passed away, and that her mother, Jean, was also very poorly. Jackie asked me to say a few words at Reg's funeral, and I agreed to do so. I also let, Peter Black, know about Reg's death - since Reg, Jean, and Jackie had all been enthusiastic users, of the holiday caravan. Just nine days later, Jackie telephoned again - to say that Jean - who had been suffering from advanced cancer, had also passed away. Reg died on 14th January 2019, and Jean - on 23rd January 2019. Jackie was worried that the, subsequent snow, would prevent people from attending the funeral, but, fortunately, Thursday 7th February turned out to be a bright, dry, day, with a hint of Spring in the air, and I, like others, travelling across counties, got to the West Herts Crematorium, without difficulty. Some forty mourners attended the service - which was also a cheerful celebration of their lives - as well as a sad marking of their deaths. We listened to 'Happy Talk' - from 'South Pacific, and sang 'All Things Bright and Beautiful'. The Victorian custom of wearing black, and a solemn face, at funerals, is now out-dated so it was good to see people smiling - at 'Happy Talk'.

'Happy talk, keep talkin' happy talk.
Talk about things you'd like to do.

'All things – bright and beautiful –
all creatures, great and small,
All things – wise and wonderful –
the Lord God made them all.'

This is the Eulogy that I read at their funeral:
'I first met Reg and Jean Gough in 1987 - when we worked, as volunteers, in a mental health charity - called The National Schizophrenia Fellowship. This charity supported sufferers from schizophrenia, and their relatives. Reg ran a support group for sufferers - which was called, 'Voices'. I ran a support group for relatives, and I also ran the charity's education programmes. I attended some of Reg's meetings, and so we became friends. Reg, who was born in 1931, had a hard time during the Depression of the nineteen-thirties. He was one of three brothers, and they all had to sleep in one bed! He said that - no sooner had the family got through the poverty of the nineteen-thirties - than the Second World War broke out - so they suffered further privations - with food-rationing. Despite suffering mental health problems, as a young man, Reg did well after the War. He went into the Insurance Business, and he started courting Jean - when she was just seventeen. Attractive, and softly-spoken, Jean was the perfect secretary, and the perfect fiancee. They got married in 1956, and they were very lucky. In 1957, they were able to buy a house, cheaply, because a sitting tenant was living upstairs. But, a few months, after purchase, the old fellow passed away, so they obtained vacant possession of the house. Their lovely daughter, Jackie, was born in the nineteen-sixties, and they continued to flourish. Reg was an expert cricketer, and a member of the prestigious Marylebone Cricket Club. He said that they were determined

to give Jackie as good a childhood as they could, and, latterly, she became their wonderful carer. Reg was hilariously funny - as I said to Jean in our last conversation - days before she, also, died. He would telephone me, and say, 'Sir Reginald here!' Like so many people, we were all very scathing, of the national mental health charity's, failure, to do anything practical to improve life, for the mentally ill, and their families. I served on the charity's National Council, and I showed Reg their Accounts. They had succeeded in spending, a million pounds, on their staff's salaries, cars, and pensions, but we discovered in the Accounts, that, only five pounds, had been spent on the direct welfare of schizophrenia sufferers. Reg asked their National Director whether five hundred sufferers got one penny each! Reg was a great *bon viveur*, and we had some sumptuous meals together! I remember once telling him, that I was going out to dinner with friends, and that I would have lobster - because that was something different, from what I had at home. 'You should try it in the South of France, he said. Lobster thermidor - with cream and mustard.' No doubt, washed down with champagne! I stayed friendly with Reg, Jean, and Jackie, when we left the National Schizophrenia Fellowship. I set up a mental health centre, and Reg and Jean used to come and visit. On one Open Day, I entertained our members by dressing up as the Victorian Music Hall Singer, Marie Lloyd, and regaled them with the full repertoire of her songs. Reg and Jean came to the performance, and I might have been less confident, if I had known that Jean's grandmother had been theatre-dresser to the great Queen of the Music Halls, herself. One of our members, Peter Black, managed to get Lottery Funding for a holiday caravan by the seaside - so that mentally ill people, and their relatives, who often didn't get a holiday, could get away for a break. Reg and Jean became regular caravan holiday-makers, and Peter used to meet up with them for meals. Together for sixty-four years, and married for sixty-two, although their passing is very sad, it is, nevertheless, lovely, that they are, once again, together. Jackie was their splendid carer, and, although she told me, that her parents were her life, she is not alone now, because she has her long-term friend, Steve, to support her. It is the end of an era, but we will continue to keep in touch with Jackie, and I am honoured, that I have been invited to give this eulogy, at the funeral of Reg and Jean Gough.'

National Charities
On the subject of National Charities, and their misuse of funds, there has been some interesting correspondence in the local Press. There were letters, from myself, and others.

The Scandal of Oxfam

'The scandal in Oxfam has brought to a head something that has long been the case - that the Charity Commission should keep a much tighter rein on national charities, and on how they spend public money. I used to make a monthly subscription to Oxfam. Not any more, I don't! I recall going into their shop in Bracknell - asking if they were active in Haiti, and putting extra money in - for the earthquake's victims. They WERE active in Haiti! If I had known that my money would pay for their staff's prostitutes, I would have collapsed, from shock, in their shop! When I was a Trustee on the National Executive of the National Schizophrenia Fellowship, one of my duties was to 'approve' their draft accounts - before they were published. I disapproved, resigned, and complained to the Charity Commission. They had spent one million pounds on salaries, cars, and pensions - for their top-heavy staff - who did nothing but sit around - talking! They had spent, practically nothing, on actual services for schizophrenics and their families - which was their, constitutional, reason for existence. One of the items in the accounts , that was listed under 'Expenditure', was 'Twenty-five thousand pounds - Sundries'! I enquired of them, sarcastically, whether they ran to solid gold paper clips, and diamond encrusted coffee cups? Twenty-five thousand pounds would run the crisis house for years. Their paid staff sat around, talking - while the volunteers did the work! One, handsomely paid, employee, who was leaving after five years 'service', was given a leaving present of two thousand pounds! It should have been a five pound book token! The Charity Commission upheld my complaint, but said that, by Law, they could only interfere in charities, if 'Breach of Trust', [actually stealing the money], could be demonstrated. I consider that paying people to sit around talking, and giving them two thousand pounds as leaving presents, IS stealing the public's money, but this is not the case, in Law. The Charity Commission needs to have wider legal powers. To survive, the National Schizophrenia Fellowship re-invented itself - as RETHINK - and did, at least, then start to provide some tangible services. Now look at National MIND. I have seen their Collection Boxes in shops, and in the Post Office in Bracknell. Where does that money actually go, and what is it spent on? MIND has no services, whatsoever, in Berkshire, and yet it is the people of Berkshire who are putting their money into those boxes! MIND has a charity shop - on the Oxford Road in Reading. The money, raised there, must go to MIND's National Office. It can't be funding MIND's services in Reading. There aren't any! No doubt, it is much easier to keep tabs on little, local, charities - like ours. Any one who *makes a donation to the crisis house, can walk in, at any time, and see how we are spending their money. They can ask the people, directly, 'What do they do, for you?' We never spend the public's money on anything other than the mentally ill - unless it is on our animals - and they are with us, only, because they are therapeutic, and help to relieve mental distress. They earn their keep! The mentally ill love them! One of our volunteers has served with me, faithfully, for forty years! In that time, I have, probably, stood him a couple of drinks! I haven't given him a brass farthing of the charity's money - not even for the petrol he uses when visiting people, for us. By contrast, he makes regular donations to our charity. That is what I call 'dedication'. I don't believe in having paid staff, who are, often, failed social workers, in charities, and, as I told them, I joined the Mental Health Movement because I had a strong vocation to improve life for the mentally ill, and their families, and NOT because I had a strong vocation to pay for your cars!'*

Regarding the controversy over volunteering, and paid work, I do have one strong belief. I am a great Arthur Conan Doyle fan, and I celebrated the one hundred and fifty year anniversary of his birth, in 2009, by visiting the Sherlock Holmes Museum, at 221b, Baker Street, - a museum beautifully set up - in Victorian style. I also celebrated by reading the entire Sherlock Holmes Canon. I love both Basil Rathbone, and Jeremy Brett, as Sherlock Holmes. I love Benedict Cumberbatch - as Alan Turing, but I can't bear him, as Sherlock Holmes! Sherlock Holmes was Victorian! I cannot take to him on a mobile phone! In the Canon, a, particularly favourite, story of mine is, 'The Red Headed League', and I couldn't agree more with its verdict, and the lesson to be learned by the, hapless, pawn-broker, Jabez Wilson. 'Pay the right rate for the job!' I quote from the book:

'Well, it is just as I have been telling you, Mr. Sherlock Holmes', said Jabez Wilson, mopping his forehead. 'I have a small pawnbroker's business at Coburg Square, near the city. It's not a very large affair, and of late years, it hasn't done more than just give me a living. I used to be able to keep two assistants, but now I keep only one; and I would have a job to pay him but that he is willing to come for half wages so as to learn the business.' 'What is the name of this obliging youth?' asked Sherlock Holmes. 'His name is Vincent Spaulding, and he's not such a youth, either. It's hard to say his age. I should not wish a smarter assistant, Mr. Holmes, and I know very well that he could better himself and earn twice what I am able to give him. But after all, if he is satisfied, why should I put ideas into his head?' 'Why indeed? You seem most fortunate in having an employee who comes under the full market price. It is not a common experience among employers in this age.'..... 'Oh, he has his faults too', said Mr. Wilson. 'Never was there such a fellow for photography'.

'Vincent Spaulding' turned out to be the notorious criminal, John Clay. I don't say that all people who accept lower than normal wages, are intent upon something as dramatic as John Clay's plan to rob a leading London bank of its stock of French gold, but, nevertheless, there must always be an ulterior motive!

'Pay the right rate for the job!' Somebody who will accept only half the proper rate of pay for a job, has, inevitably, as in this story, hidden Agenda, or something, scandalous, to hide. Paid work should always be paid, properly. Voluntary work should always be completely, voluntary. And, never the twain, should meet! Voluntary work is not undertaken in order to earn a living; it satisfies other needs! Also pertinent to this debate, is Agatha Christie's short story – 'The Case of the Perfect Maid' - from '*Miss Marple's Final Cases*'.

'Great was the chagrin of the village when it was made known the Misses Skinner had engaged, from an agency, a new maid, who, by all accounts, was a perfect paragon. 'Well really', said Miss Marple, 'it does seem too good to be true'. For ten days longer, St. Mary Mead had to endure hearing of the excellencies of Miss Lavinia's and Miss Emily's treasure. On the eleventh day, the village awoke to its big thrill. Mary, the paragon, was missing! Miss Marple had already warned Miss Lavinia, 'I don't expect she'll leave until she's ready to leave!'

The story turned out to be more complicated than simply that of a missing maid, but the point is cogent. People who appear to be too good to be true, usually ARE too good to be true. It is the same with jobs that appear to be too good to be true. In Agatha Christie's novel, '*The Secret Adversary*', Tuppence was suspicious from the beginning Was it really likely that anyone would pay her a lot of money - simply to make a pleasant trip to Paris, and stay in an exclusive pensionnat for three months? Also, in Agatha Christie's short story - 'Jane in Search of a Job' - from '*The Listerdale Mystery*', Jane - though desperate for a job, and thus accepting the offer of one, nevertheless, pondered:

'So far, I can't see the catch. And yet there must be one. There's no such thing as money for nothing. It must be crime. There's nothing else left.'

Crime, indeed, it was!

These people who expect volunteers to work on the same basis as their paid counterparts share this ridiculous naivete. Anyone who wanted to work for social services would surely be WORKING for social services, and getting the right rate of pay for the job! Volunteers DON'T want to work for social services! The two types of work should be kept, as we have always kept them, completely separate. Voluntary work is, nevertheless, very important for the health of society - as my letter to *The Wokingham Paper*, illustrates.

The Importance of Volunteers

'I sympathise with Francine Twitchett. Please see the letter - entitled - 'The Importance of Voluntary Drivers' - The Wokingham Paper - February 1st. You hear of even worse situations - of people being discharged from hospital in the middle of the night - vulnerable people - with no transport arranged - having to make their own way home. The Wokingham Volunteer Centre is excellent, and recruits hundreds of volunteers - but evidently, the priority need is for more volunteer drivers. Pertinent to this debate, is this question - 'why did hospitals dispense with those most splendid of volunteers - the Almoners?' The Lady Almoner worked, totally voluntarily, and was totally practical. When the patient was ready for discharge, she checked that he had an address to go to, food in the house, the heating on, next of kin and GP informed, medication, and aftercare, arranged, and someone there - to receive, and look after, the patient. In addition, I recall - that when my sister was due for discharge from hospital - having suffered from pneumonia - the Almoner arranged for her to have a fortnight's convalescence - by the sea, at Bognor Regis - in order to recuperate fully - and, of course, arranged transport - there, and back. Marvellous voluntary service! Now, you can't even get the transport home! But what has been done before, can be done again. We need to recreate a culture of voluntary service, and, most important, to value it.'

Chapter 17

Mr. Wokingham

Bob Wyatt, who agreed with my views on the inadequacy of statutory social services, and on the importance of voluntary services, passed away in March 2019. When he first visited the crisis house - on our Open Day in 1992, he had just retired. He was very highly regarded throughout Wokingham - as his Obituary, published in *The Wokingham Paper*, illustrated. One of the hymns sung at Bob's funeral was 'Jerusalem'.

> *And did those feet in ancient time*
> *Walk upon England's mountains green?*
> *And was the Holy Lamb of God*
> *In England's pleasant pastures seen?*

Chapter 18

A Great Campaigner

Joan Penrose

My friend of some thirty-four years, Joan Penrose, passed away in 2019 - at the age of eighty-eight. I first met Joan in 1985 - at, a Housing Conference, that I organised for the National Schizophrenia Fellowship. Joan, herself, was a qualified teacher, but, with such a heavy burden of mental illness in her family, Joan decided, like me, to devote her life to campaigning for better mental health services, and this she did, successfully, right up to the end. It is, a shame, that Joan didn't live, to see Roger Penrose, receive, together with, Professor Reinhard Genzel, and Andrea Ghez, the Nobel Prize, for Physics. Joan regaled me with a story of her courting days. Roger Penrose, who, at the time, was a tutor, at Cambridge University, told her that he thought that he had a genius, in his PhD class. 'Nonsense. Genius, indeed! You're just trying to impress your girlfriend!' Joan replied. His genius student, Stephen Hawking, went on, to collaborate, with Professor Penrose, for many years, and their work, actually rivalled, that of Albert Einstein! To celebrate, both Sir Roger, and Joan, Penrose, I wrote the following letter, to '*Wokingham Today*'. This was published, on Thursday 15th October 2020.

'I was sorry that my friend, the late Joan Penrose, who died in 2019, didn't live to receive the latest news. Joan was a great, mental health campaigner, and we worked, together, for years, in the National Schizophrenia Fellowship. She was an ardent supporter, of, and a regular visitor to, the Wokingham Crisis House. She attended the twenty-five year anniversary celebration, of our Association, with one of her sons, and all three of her sons, visited the crisis house. They are all, formidably intelligent, and they are all, very good, at Maths! Joan also attended our Book Launch, for 'Triumph and Tragedy', in 2016, and thereafter, promoted this book, among the people whom she knew, in the mental health world - as she always had promoted the crisis house, as a model of mental health excellence. She would have been so proud, and her sons must be so proud, of their father. I fear that 'black holes' remain a mystery to me, and are not my scene, at all - any more than they are for any man in the street. There is a story - probably apocryphal - that, on one occasion, Albert Einstein, was so absorbed with his Theory of Relativity, that he forgot to put his trousers on, and someone had to run down the street after him, to make sure that he became fully clothed! They are, rarely practical - these, absent minded, professors! Nevertheless, I take my hat off, to Sir Roger Penrose - the Nobel Prize, for Physics - what a wonderful success!'

Another funny story, of professorial absent-mindedness - tells of the occasion, when, the writer, G.K. Chesterton, wired his wife, as follows: 'I am at Crewe Station. Where should I be?' No doubt, for those of us who lack, scientific aptitude, the only black hole that we are likely to look into, is of, a financial, character. Nevertheless, caught with your pants down, or not even on, or stranded, and bewildered, at Crewe Station, I take my hat off to Nobel Prize winners. Black holes may mean nothing, to most of us, but it must be something, in this life, to know that you are, up there, with Pierre and Marie Curie!

Chapter 19

Played Out With Music

Chris Hoskin's Sister - Mary

In February 2020, Chris attended the funeral of his sister, Mary. She had reached the ripe old age of ninety-five, and had been ailing, for some time. At the funeral, they sang the Quaker Hymn, 'Dear Lord and Father of Mankind' - which, coincidentally, is my favourite hymn, and which I have mentioned, as the most appropriate hymn, for mentally ill people - seeking asylum - in my chapters on 'Benefactors'. His sister was very musical, and, in particular, was a talented violinist - her own, favourite composition, being, 'The Lark Ascending'. To honour her musical accomplishments, Massenet's 'Meditation' - from 'Thais', was played, at the funeral. Chris was, of course, sad, that his sister, had, finally, passed away, but we agreed that a merciful release is accorded to dementia sufferers, when their passing away, ends lives, where they, no longer recognise, loved ones, and that, no longer, provide any quality, or enjoyment. Incidentally, Mary's daughter, Elizabeth, who is a trained psychotherapist, has donated, generously, to our work at the crisis house.

Dear Lord and Father of mankind,
forgive our foolish ways;
reclothe us in our rightful mind,
in purer lives thy service find,
in deeper reverence, praise.

Chapter 20

She Passed Away, Peacefully

On Tuesday morning, 20th October 2020, Tony Heyes's wife, Ethel, passed away, peacefully, after a battle with ovarian cancer. Her family were at her side to the end. From childhood, Ethel Heyes, distinguished herself. She achieved the highest marks for Maths, in the Eleven Plus, Examination, for the entire area, in which she lived, and went on, to study Maths, at Oxford University. Tony had studied Maths, at Cambridge University, so when they met, both in their twenties, and both working in computers, it promised to be a good match. It was. They married, and had two children - Neil, and Jenny - Neil, becoming an accountant, and Jenny, firstly a corporate lawyer, and then, retraining, in psychology. In due course, Ethel and Tony, became grandparents, to Joseph and Erin. Ethel spent many years working, very successfully, in the Citizen's Advice Bureau, and, actually received a national award for this work. In leisure time, Ethel and Tony, were enthusiastic bridge players. They also enjoyed travelling abroad. After fifty-five years, together, as Joyce Grenfell says, 'Parting is hell.' So all our thoughts, and condolences, are with Tony and the family, in their sad bereavement.

If I should go before the rest of you,
Break not a flower, nor inscribe a stone.
Nor, when I am gone, speak in a Sunday voice,
But be the usual selves, that I have known.
Weep if you must, parting is hell,
But life goes on, so sing, as well.

Chapter 21

Denise Grimsdell: 'A Feisty Fighter, and a Good Sport'

Denise passed away on 24th December 2020 - after a long battle with scleroderma. Denise joined us early in 1999, and served as our committee secretary. In due course she progressed on, to work in dementia care. Her illness was very tragic, and her widower, Richard, whom we are supporting in his bereavement, said that, in a way, the end was a happy release. We are also supporting Denise's son, Philip. Our lasting memory of Denise is that of a good sport! She was an enthusiastic skier, skater, badminton and squash player, swimmer, and hiker! We like to think of her, in her days of robust health, and physical prowess.

Alex Bryson: 'Triumph Over Adversity'

Alex passed away on Sunday 27th December 2020. Aged only fifty-seven, he died suddenly, in his sleep, from a heart attack. When Alex joined us, he was battling alcoholism - successfully. My lasting memory of Alex, is of the occasion when he visited us in September 2018. He was beaming with triumph. He had completed, successfully, all his rehabilitation programmes, and had been accepted by the Probation Service, to work - supervising young offenders. His daughter said that his premature death was particularly sad, after such a triumphant recovery, and that his plans, eventually, to retire to his native Scotland, would now, never be realised.

Tony Whitfield: 'Sociable To The End'

Tony Whitfield passed away, very suddenly, on Monday 18th January 2021. It was a sudden heart attack, and I had been speaking with him on the telephone, and playing one of his beloved 'guessing games', with him, literally, hours previously. Our condolences are with his wife and daughter. In earlier life, Tony had had a successful career in Public

Relations. He was with us for nineteen years, and will be greatly missed. Requiescat in Pace.

PART SEVEN

Chapter 22

Further Updates

Updates on the people mentioned in *'Triumph and Tragedy'*, reveal exactly what you would expect - a mixture of great success, average achievement, and, sadly, some who have made no progress at all.

Gabriela Rani

The notorious Gabriela Rani, was for a time, no longer let loose in the community. It had, finally, been decided that she needed high support accommodation - where she could, both get the care that she needed, and cease to be a nuisance, and a danger, to other people. So she was placed into care in Newbury. Now, in June 2019, I gather that she has returned to her former accommodation in Crowthorne. Her ambition was to marry an aristocrat! Nothing changes. She has now placed a photograph of an extremely glamorous young woman - on social media - pretending that this woman is herself! No doubt, the PHOTOGRAPH will attract interest, but what will happen, when it comes to actually meeting up with Gabriela? Past experience provides the answer. When Gabriela spent three hundred pounds - on her mother's credit card - to advertise for meeting prospective partners in *'The Times'* - which then had an introduction service for high class [and, thus, expensive], introductions, she described herself as - 'Attractive, slim, elegantly dressed, cultured, young lady - of Mediterranean origin - wishes to meet young, good looking, well educated, successful, businessman, for a relationship - and possibly - marriage.' The good looking, well educated, successful, businessman, duly arranged a date - and met Gabriela! He said - 'You are not what I expected', turned on his heel, and went! What is so fascinating, is this failure of the mentally ill, to learn anything, by experience! It is always this desire for the magic wand, the crock of gold at the end of the rainbow, and - to be fair to Gabriela - I have to say that my experience of this attitude is, by no means. confined just to her! So what will the future be? She probably lost the secure, supported, accommodation - as was the case with Tommy Warfield [Please see: 'Success Stories, Maintained'] because it was required for a patient with even more urgent needs!

Ewan

Ewan was never going to cope in a flat. We knew that, from his, eighteen-month, stay, in the crisis house. We moved him into, a minimal, bed-sitter, and he couldn't even cope, there, so we were surprised when the Council went on to provide him with a lovely, large flat - in a good area. Of course, he couldn't cope. What a waste of a flat! Needless to say, it quickly became a drugs den - with local dealers going in and out - what I believe is known, in the jargon, as 'cuckooing'. This caused, intense annoyance, to Ewan's respectable neighbours - some of whom, had paid, four to five hundred thousand pounds, for private sector flats, in that complex - where, only a small number, had been put across, for social housing. They complained, and complained, and the Police were constantly involved, but, nevertheless, Ewan stayed there, for some years, his behaviour becoming increasingly bizarre. Things came to a head, with his party piece. He went around Wokingham, breaking into the green boxes, and disabling all the broadband! That did the trick! He was Sectioned, and then placed, in secure accommodation, in Oxfordshire - where he remains. I frequently tell the students, who are, on placement, with us, that you are only, guaranteed services, if you become a nuisance. Unfair though it may be, depressed, but quiet, and well-behaved people, are often just left to suffer. Now, in May 2019, it is quite a time, since we have seen, Ewan, drop in to the crisis house. He did so, more frequently, when he first moved to Oxfordshire. Is it that, like a cat without butter on his paws, for a while, he returns to the place, from which he has moved, or is it, that he no longer needs the drug dealers of Wokingham - because he has found, new dealers, in Oxfordshire? Indeed, on 31st May 2019, a friend of Ewan, visited our drop-in centre, explained that he had been, in touch, with him, and that things were going, OK, in Oxfordshire. OK, in Ewan's world, means that he has secured, a regular supply of heroin! I am a realist. Human beings always do what they want to do. You won't make any difference, if they won't!

Since Elise is thinking of embarking on a career in psychotherapy, I have explained to her, that one achieves much more change, for the better, with those who are young, or with those who had been successful, in life, prior to breakdown, and so are motivated to restore themselves to normality. I am afraid that neither Gabriela, nor Ewan, come into these categories. Furthermore, I have actually mentioned to some of our psychology students - who wish to pursue careers in psychotherapy - that the medical route is the best one. 'But, medicine is hard!' some reply. Of course it is hard; anything worth achieving is hard! But those who genuinely want to be psychotherapists, will strive along the difficult path. As Agatha Christie writes in her novel, '*Death in the Clouds*':

'There are not so many round pegs in square holes as one might think. Most people, in spite of what they tell you, choose the occupations that they secretly desire. You will hear a man say, who works in an office, 'I should like to explore - to rough it in far countries.' But you will find that he likes, reading the fiction, that deals with that subject, but that he himself prefers the safety, and moderate comfort, of an office stool'.

My earlier points about the menial jobs that I undertook - when a young student - confirm Hercule Poirot's statement. I was no more, a hospital skivvy, than was 'the talented' Tuppence Beresford, who worked as a VAD during the First World War, as well as driving a General! Instead, I was to set up, award winning mental health services and to write books about them! Hercule Poirot's points about the 'armchair traveller', ring true. I recall once, having a conversation with a teaching assistant, who claimed that, given the chance, she would have been a linguist! Aged about forty, why did she not, then obtain, the Linguaphone Programmes, and go ahead, and learn the languages? What she actually liked, was dreaming about this achievement - rather than getting down to, the hard work, that, the mastering, of anything worthwhile, involves! However, worse than deceiving oneself, about one's ambitions, is something that one encounters frequently, in mental health. You have failed to achieve a goal, so someone else, has to do it for you. You endeavour to live - through them! This often results in a mental breakdown for the 'someone else'! It is difficult to comprehend how supposedly intelligent people can be so lacking in insight.

I'm following my father's footsteps.
I'm following my dear old dad.

I recall a very distressed lady visiting the crisis house. She said that her mother had come from a humble background, but had succeeded in qualifying as a doctor, and was working as a General Practitioner. The lady explained that, from the age of four, her mother had made it clear, that her daughter, also, was going to be a doctor! Possibly, she feared that if her daughter failed to follow in her mother's footsteps, then the family might go back down the social scale! But her distressed daughter didn't want to do it! To mollify her mother, she took a first class honours degree, in science, at Leeds university, but she was, by then, so mentally disturbed, that she could hardly comprehend what was being said at the ceremony - where she received the university prize - as their top science student. She was capable of being a doctor, but she didn't want to be one. Isn't it better to allow youngsters to find their own preferred path in life? Intelligent youngsters, who want to pursue a particular career, will find out what they have to achieve, to do so, and will then, get the qualifications, necessary. If they don't, it is because they don't want to do it! In some instances, they ARE following father's footsteps - closely, and not being impressed by them. Malcolm Chase - who appears in 'Triumph and Tragedy', his chapter, being entitled - 'Manners Makyth Man' - had a daughter. Unlike her father, who was a Cambridge science graduate, she left formal education on the very first day that she could legally do so, and didn't pursue any informal education, thereafter! To Malcolm's distress, she had numerous tattoos, worked as a barmaid, and was shacked up with a lorry driver! When her father remonstrated about her lack of education, she retorted, 'Much good it all did you, daddy!' Malcolm said to me, ruefully, that there was no answer to this. I simply, take the view, that you can't live, someone else's life, for them! His daughter was happy with her life - otherwise, she would have changed things. If your children are independent, and happy, what more can you want? Intelligent youngsters, supported, but not coerced, will find, the right path, for themselves. But, some youngsters, are, simply, incapable of doing it! I had a teaching colleague, who just would not accept, that her son, who had an IQ, of ninety, would never be, successful, academically, and should have been allowed to attend, non-academic, training - for a practical occupation. He ended up, as an, unemployable, drug-addict. As I explain in my letter, on good parenting, the essential qualification, for this, is the ability, to put the child's needs, before your own! This lady was, constantly complaining, that his, 'good', background, must, surely, enable her son, to achieve something in life. It didn't, because it wasn't a, 'good', background, and it ruined his life. There is an old, and wise, saying - 'You can't put in what God left out!' Hers, was also, a fascinating example of 'Denial' - [Please compare, the chapter, 'Tell Me the Old, Old, Story' - from 'Triumph and Tragedy' -

'Twenty-Five Poignant Stories']. 'Perhaps, a career, in medical photography, would be suitable for him', she would say. She had, by this time, accepted that he was not, with an IQ of ninety, going to qualify, as a brain surgeon! 'All our, educational background, must count for something!' she would add. As she said this, the potential 'medical photographer' - who had, first, been sent to a, very academic, preparatory school - where the masters wore gowns, and then, to an expensive, private, boarding school - which he left - having achieved, no academic qualifications, whatsoever - would sit, slumped there - regarding one, with a bleary eye. He was so out of his head, on cannabis, that he could barely speak - never mind, undertake, the highly skilled, and technical, tasks, required for medical photography! He once, actually said, to me, 'Pam, when I was at school, I used, in a chemistry exam, to get three marks out of a hundred. Do you think that I am stupid?' 'No', I replied. 'I do not think that you are stupid; it is your parents, and your headmaster, who are stupid. If you are getting three marks out of a hundred, for chemistry, you are on the wrong course, for you, and you should be doing woodwork, or, at least, something, practical!' It is 'the old, old, story', once again - both funny, and tragic! Properly, unselfishly, and realistically, supported, her son might have been able, to hold down, an unskilled job. As it was, he achieved no quality of life, at all - neither occupationally, nor in any other way! I am one of those people who genuinely value practical skills, as much as academic achievement. If you have a burst water pipe - it's no good calling up your lawyer, is it? Our member, Chris Hoskin, regales us with the story of a man, to whom he was giving, Maths tuition. This man was completely, and utterly, hopeless at Maths, but he was a highly skilled acrobat! 'Let him abandon Maths, and continue with acrobatics', was Chris's, wise conclusion. Skills are just as valuable as erudition, and Agatha Christie acknowledged this in her '*Autobiography*' - when talking of servants. 'They had skills, rather than education', she wrote. Very useful skills too!

We had this discussion, in the crisis house drop-in centre, on Friday 5th June 2020. Don, who had spent the final seventeen years of his full-time working life, before retirement, as a refuse collector, asserted that all jobs require a skill. So true. I am well aware that all jobs will never have equal status, nor command equal pay, but all jobs, are, nevertheless, necessary.

In contrast, to the teaching colleague - whose, unrealistic ambitions, ruined her son's life, there was the, wholly healthy, attitude. of another teaching assistant - with whom I worked. She explained, that her daughter, was a fourth-year medical student, and that her son, who wasn't academic, was training, successfully, to be a plumber. She added, with wry humour, that, once qualified, and set up in business, her son might actually earn more money, than her daughter! This lady had the, absolutely right, attitude, as a parent. It is also the correct attitude for, professional educationists, to adopt. I recall, my Montessori Tutor, saying, fifty years ago, that pupils who opted for a technical, rather than, for an, academic, secondary education, would probably end up, earning three times as much, as their clever, and more academic, counterparts. And doesn't excellent, and properly valued, technical education, come into its own - during the, current, coronavirus pandemic? Because it values technical education, equally, with academic, education, Germany, has been miles ahead of us, with its testing techniques, for the virus, and for discovering the most promising vaccine, as well.

One, of our newest, service users, Elise, has been the victim, of undue, educational pressure. She explained, that at, the famous, but pressurised, school - which she had attended - everything lower than an 'A' grade, was regarded as a failure, and she had been, in tears, when, on one occasion, she had obtained an 'A' grade in all subjects but one - for which she had achieved a 'B' grade. All other pupils, had achieved, 'A' Grades, for everything, and so, Elise, felt, a failure. This attitude is ridiculous. The whole point of having a 'pass' mark for an examination, is to demonstrate, that you have reached the standard. On occasions, it may be the minimum standard, but it is still reaching the standard. Furthermore, it is no good having strings of qualifications, if you are then, so emotionally damaged, and lacking in confidence, that you fail to cope, in the jobs, for which the qualifications, are intended to prepare you. I regaled Elise with the story of one of our former Placement students - Indiana. She was a happy, party girl, and she passed her final examination by one mark! No feeling, in my opinion, is more satisfying, than that of scraping through, by the skin of your teeth. Just made it, and had a good time, as well! Fortunately, Elise has chummed up with Pamela, and they are meeting, and attending a support group together, when the drop-in centre isn't open. Such natural, and spontaneous, mutual befriending, forms a valuable part of our, overall, befriending scheme. The following, comic, children's song, makes the point that – though you do need arithmetic, and geography, in life, personality, and common sense, also count for a lot

> *I don't like school, don't like work.*
> *I don't like arithmetic.*
> *And, as for rotten geography,*
> *Geography, makes me sick!*
> *In exams, people say,*
> *I will never pass,*
> *But, as for personality,*
> *I've the best one, in the class!*

Then there is the other side of the coin - those who are, over qualified, for the jobs available. Two of our 2018 Master's Psychology students eventually got jobs as teaching assistants. I was relieved that they didn't, like so many graduates, end up stacking shelves in Tesco's - on a permanent basis, but I was, nevertheless, intrigued. If they wanted to work with children, why hadn't they taken professional education degrees? Teachers may not regard themselves as very well-paid, but they are certainly, better-paid, than are teaching assistants - whose pay, just about matches that of cleaners! Furthermore, qualified doctors and teachers can always get jobs - if, not in this country - then, abroad!

A poignant effect of the coronavirus pandemic, is that we won't, at the current commencement of the new academic year, be able to welcome our usual group of psychology students - on placement, at the crisis house. Indeed, today, on 1st October 2020, I have had to decline the offer, of a new psychology graduate, to volunteer in the crisis house. Normally, I would be delighted to welcome her, but, in order to limit the spread of the virus, we are having to limit, attendance at the drop-in centre, to our, regular, 'bubble'.

PART EIGHT

Update On Our Services

Chapter 23

Our Drop-In Service
Our drop-in service has developed significantly over the past five years,

and is always very busy, and well-attended. Having spent fifty thousand pounds - from our 2009 Legacy - on upgrading, and improving, Station House - with a carefully planned five-year programme, we then decided only to spend further, substantial, sums of money on the building - where strictly necessary. In May 2018, we had to spend, six hundred and eighty pounds, on repairing the passage floor - because it was, literally, falling through. In August and September 2019, we were fortunate in having Glyn's voluntary service. He wanted to show his, gratitude, for all the coffee and biscuits, that he consumes, so he painted, and decorated, our Ladies' Cloakroom, our Gentlemen's Cloakroom, our private counselling room, and a outside wall that had been disfigured with graffiti. He did an excellent job. The Ladies' Cloakroom is, of course, pink; the Gentlemen's Cloakroom is, of course, blue, and the counselling room is God's colour - green. Nothing could be more relaxing and therapeutic. Pale green walls, a matching pale green carpet, a dark green settee - with both light, and dark green, cushions, and pictures on the walls - showing country and riverside scenes - in England's green and pleasant land! I decided that the, dark green, velvet curtains, which formerly hung at the window, were too heavy, so I donated some, with a, William Morris, pale green, willow leaf, pattern - perfect! I particularly like seeing Pamela, who suffers from such a severe anxiety disorder, sitting, so relaxed, in our lounge. She is always so elegantly dressed, and sitting there, sipping gin and tonic, from a crystal glass with a fine stem, she positively epitomises civilised, and refined, society. I say it, ad nauseam, but I shall say it, yet again. Anyone who wants to enjoy the best drinks, in the well-furnished, and pleasant, ambience, that is our drop-in centre, is most welcome to join us. But if you prefer to sit on a broken plastic chair, staring at a bare, dirty, wall, drinking the cheapest, and most horrible, tea, that can be bought, and waiting, in vain, for a social worker to sort out your life, then go to social services' facilities - where they exist. We're not stopping you!

Chapter 24

Our Befriending Service

Bev

Bev is one of our long-term befrienders - who has been working for us for, thirteen years. She retired as Headmistress of a school in September 2018, and so then had more time to devote to our service. She has been in touch with one mentally ill lady, Dolly, for the whole of that time. This is fortunate, because Dolly is agoraphobic, rarely gets out of the house, and, in all those years, has only visited the drop-in centre on four occasions. Bev keeps in touch, with her, by telephone, visits Dolly at home, and even manages to get her out for coffee, on occasions. Now that she has retired from teaching, Bev is now in a position to complete a Level Four Counselling Course. Dolly did manage to visit the drop-in on one occasion in 2019. She is still having enormous problems. Her father died, recently, making life ever more difficult, but Bev is always there to provide support. I telephoned Bev, on Monday 23rd March, to explain our policy, of keeping the drop-in centre open, during the coronavirus crisis. She agreed, wholeheartedly, with our stance, and promised to drop in, and see us, on Friday 27th March. Fortunately, she had passed her Counselling Examination, and so, unlike those who hadn't passed, was not subject to all the delays in holding re-sits, that have become, inevitable, because of the coronavirus pandemic Bev, who, in addition to other volunteering, has worked for the Samaritans, shares my view, that our mental health drop-in service, needs to continue, throughout the pandemic - albeit, in a reduced, and socially distanced, way. Bev managed to get in, to see us, in August 2020. She is persevering with her counselling work, but everything has, of course, been made difficult - due to the social restrictions, necessary, because of the coronavirus pandemic.

Johnnie

Johnnie once befriending Delpha, is now befriending her son, Paul. Paul has suffered a lot of mental health problems. He dropped out of Warwick University, but, eventually, he managed to complete an Open University Degree, and he is now doing quite well - working in Johnnie's Gardening Project. He is distressed because his mother is terminally ill, so Johnnie sometimes brings him into the drop-in centre - from Reading - where they both live. I also telephoned Johnnie, on Monday 23rd March - to explain our policy. He gave me the following updates. Delpha, who has for a considerable time, been suffering from scleroderma, remains ill, but is continuing with some activities. Paul is continuing to do well.

Tony

Tony has come up with a useful initiative, during the pandemic crisis. He has set up a Zoom Internet Group - and the Group includes Brendan, whom Tony has befriended, so successfully, for years, Aileen, for whom

Tony has acted as advocate, Keith, for whom Tony, is also advocate, and Julie, Keith's cousin, who first referred him to the crisis house.

We greatly value the service of our long-term befrienders, but we are also very pleased to welcome, new, and younger, people for this service. Thus, Charne, joined us in 2019. She had moved to Wokingham from South Africa, because her husband had taken a post as administrator of an international group of private schools - one of which is the former Bearwood College, in Wokingham. Charne is befriending Elise, and Pamela, and it is particularly useful to have young people, with these modern smart phones - which enable them, to text, the people being befriended, when the drop-in centre isn't open. Charne is very friendly, and personable, and we are delighted that she has joined our befriending service. She has also come up with a new initiative - a Crisis House Newsletter - the first edition, being produced, in January 2020. A pleasant, and diverting, task for us, has been advising Charne, new from South Africa, as to the most beautiful places to visit in the British Isles. There are many who would agree with the view expressed in Agatha Christie's novel - *'The ABC Murders'*. Agatha Christie writes:

'We, [Hercule Poirot and Franklin Clarke], went on down the lane. At the foot of it, a path led between brambles and bracken down to the sea. Suddenly we came out on a grassy ridge overlooking the sea, and a beach of glistening white stones. All round, dark green trees ran down to the sea. It was an enchanting spot - white, deep green, and sapphire blue. 'How beautiful!' I exclaimed. Clarke turned to me, eagerly. 'Isn't it? Why people want to go abroad to the Riviera when they've got this! I've wandered all over the world in my time, and, honest to God, I've never seen anything as beautiful.'

Thus is described, beautiful Churston, in the county of Devon. I don't agree entirely with Franklin Clarke. I think that you would have a job to beat the beauty of the scenery - coming down from Switzerland - to the Italian Lakes – Garda, Como, and Maggiore, or, alternatively, ascending to Fiesole, above the city of Florence, and looking out over the Arno Valley - with the silver river, and the dark green cypress trees - the unrivalled beauty of Tuscany. Our recommendations to Charne, of beautiful places to visit, in the UK, are described in one of our letters to the local Paper - later on in this narrative.

Fortunately, despite all the problems caused by coronavirus, and

Lockdown, Charne and her family, did manage to get away, on holiday, in the summer of 2020. They opted for the pleasant spot, of Poole, in Dorset. Some of my choices of beautiful places, to visit, in the British Isles, have songs, to describe them.

> *If you ever go across the sea to Ireland,*
> *Then maybe at the closing of your day,*
> *You can sit and watch the moon rise over Claddagh,*
> *And see the sun go down on Galway Bay.*

> *The sky is bluer, in Scotland.*
> *The grass, is greener, there, too.*
> *The air smells sweeter.*
> *The rivers are deeper.*
> *The mountain's, a lovelier view.*

> *By yon bonnie banks and by yon bonnie braes,*
> *Where the sun shines bright on Loch Lomond,*

> *High in the misty Highlands,*
> *Out by the purple islands,*
> *Brave are the hearts that beat*
> *Beneath Scottish Skies.*

It was good, on Monday 14th September, to see Charne drop into the crisis house. Elise has been in regular contact, but we, throughout, and since, Lockdown, had seen Charne, only by videolink. Her children are now both back at school, but distancing rules, are very strict, so Charne, for the present, will be able to see us, only occasionally. To celebrate her thirtieth birthday, in November, Charne, together with her family, and Elise, hope to book a break in a log cabin, in the country. Elise was looking at Hastings, as a possible venue, but we advised against. Rundown seaside resorts, are not the most relaxing of places. Charne, coming so recently, from South Africa, is not familiar with the most beautiful places, in the British Isles, but we, just for a long weekend, recommended the Cotswolds. Absolutely idyllic. Visit that lovely little town - Bourton-on-the-Water - with the stream, flowing through its centre. We at the crisis house, have some most enjoyable outings there. In the end, Charne and Elise, settled for a long weekend, at the charming little Surrey town, of Farnham - not very far away, but, far enough, to experience it, as a break from one's normal, routines, strains, and stresses.

As well as the more traditional type of befriending, there is also what I would describe as 'mutual befriending' - thus have Elise and Pamela become chums. In January 2020, Elise moved from a one-bedroom flat, into a two-bedroom flat - and this has proved to be a godsend for Pamela. While Pamela, Elise, - and with Charne coming in to help, as well - are de-cluttering, Pamela's flat, she is able to stay overnight in Elise's spare room. On Friday 31st January 2020, the proud girls brought in - to show me – photographs of the rapidly de-cluttering flat. I was, nothing short, of amazed at the progress. This is where team work kicks in! I took the opportunity of speaking to the person who has been designated to place Pamela under 'Vulnerable Adult Protection' legislation, and I told her, bluntly, that we didn't want a social worker, calling around, waffling, and so taking up Pamela's precious time! What is obviously needed, once the clutter is cleared completely, is a regular cleaning service, so that further cluttering cannot recur. The coronavirus crisis, has, of course, changed everything, and, rapidly, too. Charne's husband had been in touch with an individual who had tested, 'positive', so Charne decided to self-isolate. Then all the schools closed, so she had to stay, at home, with her two children - aged - eight, and three. Though not coming to the drop-in centre - where people are so vulnerable, Charne had been meeting Elise, for a drink in a local pub, but now, all the pubs and cafes, have closed, as well. It is a situation, where things can change, almost by the day. On Friday 3rd April, I was able to catch up, with Charne, by video-link. She certainly is, busy with the children, but she was delighted that our service is able to continue, and is looking forward, to being back with us, once the crisis is over. With a gradual easing of Lockdown, Charne's three year old son, Davian, will be returning, part-time, to pre-school, on Monday 1st June. Since Charne has been home-educating her three year old son, and her eight year old daughter, times, have indeed, been very challenging for her, and we are all longing for September 2020, when, hopefully, she will be able to return to our ranks. It is sad, as well, that her parents have not been able to make, their planned, visit to England, this summer, but, hopefully, this will take place next year. Elise has kept in regular touch with Charne, throughout he absence, due to the coronavirus pandemic, and, since the easing of Lockdown, has even been able to meet up with her, regularly, for drinks, but it will be lovely, once the whole crisis house family, is re-united, under one roof.

Chapter 25

Our Advocacy Service Over Five Years

And when we say 'we've always won',
And when they ask us how it's done?
We'll proudly point to everyone
Of the soldiers of the Queen!

What I admire about our principal Advocate, Tony, is that he always wins!

Advocacy

An area of our work that has increased, and developed, significantly, since the publication of *'Triumph and Tragedy'*, in April 2016, is advocacy. As my letters to *The Wokingham Paper* highlight, the Government's shake-up of the Benefits system has had a significant effect upon mentally ill claimants, and I have raised concerns - both with Health Ministers, and with Ministers for Work and Pensions. We are fortunate in having two excellent, and very well qualified, Advocates - Tony and Bev. They will, not only, prepare all the papers that are required for benefit applications, and Appeal Tribunals, but will accompany the service users to the hearings. Tony has now been working with me for forty years. He appears in *'Triumph and Tragedy'*, as a 'Good male befriender', and is, incidentally, still in touch with Brendan, who has only recently returned to England - after, a very successful, decade of working in Germany. Tony also features. in 'Twenty-five Funny Stories' - please see - *'Cui Bono?'* - 'Who benefits?' You will recall that this is where I threatened him with capital punishment - after he had spent the entire Christmas Party - talking to our blonde, beautiful, psychology student! We won't allow opposite sex befriending, but we do allow opposite sex advocacy - because this work is undertaken in the crisis house, itself. But human nature never changes! Tony had completed sterling work with two female service users. 'I think I can continue to do more with one of them', he said. Which one? The one who is young, and beautiful, of course! Agatha Christie - with her marvellous perception of the frailties of human nature - expresses this truth throughout her works - from the first 'Miss Marple' novel – *'The Murder at the Vicarage'* - to her final 'Hercule Poirot' novel - *'Curtain'*.

In 'Murder at the Vicarage', the vicar, the Rev. Len Clement, goes to visit one of the murder suspects, Mrs. Lestrange. He says,

'She was a curious woman - a woman of very strong magnetic charm. I myself hated the thought of connecting her with the crime in any way. Something in me said, 'It can't be her!' Why? And an imp in my brain replied, 'Because she's a very beautiful and attractive woman. That's why?' There is, as Miss Marple would say, a lot of human nature in all of us.'

In '*The ABC Murders*', there is, an amusing, exchange, between Hercule Poirot, and Captain Hastings. It had been decided, that each of the men in the case, should accompany one of the women, to protect them, when they were attending the races, at Doncaster, the latest town, in which ABC, was due to strike. Poirot says, to Hastings, as Agatha Christie writes:

'I find you, Hastings, singularly, though, transparently, dishonest. All along, you had made up your mind, to spend the day, with your blonde angel'. [Miss Grey]. But Hercule Poirot, goes on to insist, that Captain Hastings, must accompany Mary Drower, because the next victim of the ABC murderer, would, presumably, have a surname that began with 'D'!

Then, in '*Curtain*', Captain Hastings, now elderly and widowed, speaks with Elizabeth.

'Elizabeth told him, 'I'm far more lonely than you are.' 'My dear girl, your life's just beginning. What's thirty-five? I wish I were thirty-five,' I added maliciously. 'I'm not quite blind, you know.' She turned an enquiring glance on me, then blushed. 'You don't think - oh! Stephen Norton and I are only friends. He's, he's just awfully kind.' 'Oh, my dear, I said. Don't believe it's all kindness. We men aren't made that way.'

And that, Agatha, is precisely why I have insisted on same/sex befriending. To fit in with modern political correctness, I have now renamed it 'gender appropriate', befriending. Advocacy is different, because it is usually a matter of taking up a time-limited case, and it is all conducted, openly, but, even then, human nature might feel inclined to extend the process - where a beautiful woman is involved!

Pretty woman,
walking down the street,
Pretty woman
the kind I'd like to meet.
Pretty woman,

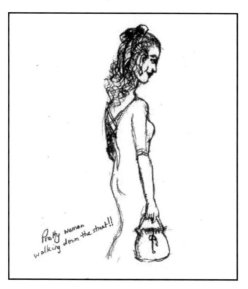

Incidentally, in '*Curtain*', knowing that a romance between Stephen Norton and Elizabeth Cole could never come to fruition, Hercule Poirot enjoins, the lonely, Captain Hastings, to approach the lonely Elizabeth, and make a match of it!

As I have explained, the bulk of our advocacy work is concerned with re-enabling people to access benefits. A major quality required - if one is to do this work, successfully - is assertiveness. The importance of this - if one is to be successful in life - is demonstrated, cogently, by Agatha Christie, in her short story - 'The Manhood of Edward Robinson' - [Please see: '*The Listerdale Mystery*']. Edward had been dominated by his fiancee, Maud, but an exciting adventure changed all that, and he insisted that their marriage should take place next month.

'Will you, said Edward, yes or no?' 'Ye - yes', faltered Maud. 'But, oh Edward, what has happened to you? You're quite different, today.' 'Yes, said Edward. For twenty-four hours, I've been a man, instead of a worm, and, by God, it pays!'

159

The mentally ill are timid, fragile, and easily bullied, so they need strong, assertive, advocates - who will insist upon proper assessments, and won't take 'no' for an answer!

The Benefits Reforms, and the consequent need for advocacy, form a major focus for our Campaign for Mental Health, in the local Press. In response to Paul Farmer's letter on the subject of the Benefits Reforms *The Wokingham Paper* (6th July 2019), I praise brevity, but I also consider detail to be important. Paul's letter follows:

On Universal Credit
'Universal Credit - a total shambles. End of letter.'

I replied with the following:

'I refer to Paul Farmer's letter - [26th July]. Brevity is unrivalled for punching a point home, but the devil is in the detail, and it is our Government's shake-up of the entire Benefits System that is a total shambles - not just Universal Credit. Common sense has been abandoned, and as fast as one learns the new names and rules, they change again. Universal Credit is to be paid, monthly. Traditionally, those on low wages or Benefits, got their money weekly - because it was recognised that it is easier to eke out a small income over a week. Things that are traditional, become so, because they work. One of our members said to me, 'If my Benefits are paid monthly, I'm afraid that I might spend money on cigarettes, and not leave enough over, to pay my rent.' Government Ministers - who have always enjoyed a good income - don't have this temptation. You long for those cigarettes today, the money is there, and your rent is not yet due! Iain Duncan-Smith, architect of the Benefits Revolution, promised a system where people would always be better off working. We all agree with this, but it has to work in practice. Take Housing Benefit - which is to be incorporated in Universal Credit. A person who has suffered a severe mental breakdown, cannot, on recovery, just walk into a well-paid, permanent job. It is a case of taking what you can get - zero hours contracts, part-time, casual, and insecure. As soon as you take any work at all, your Housing Benefit is axed. You might get a month's casual work, and then, a fortnight with no work at all, but Housing Benefit is not re-instated immediately, so you fall into rent arrears. One of our members, who does casual work on building sites, got so fed up with constantly falling into rent arrears, that he relinquished his council flat, asked us to receive his mail, and now lives in his car - space-restricted, but hassle-free! Common sense requires a

system that acknowledges the realities for people getting back into work, and so enables us to achieve Iain Duncan-Smith's vision. When we took a mentally ill heroin addict off the freezing February street, and paid for him to stay in a Wokingham B. & B., it took ten weeks for Housing Benefit to be organised, but, even then, the B.& B. would only accept cash - not direct payments - so I asked the Council to pay the Housing Benefit into our Charity's Account - to enable us to continue paying the addict's rent. Such an arrangement is not within their system, so they paid all the money to him, he spent it all on drugs, and was back on the street. The stone of Sisyphus!'

As with all our other, elderly, members, during the coronavirus crisis, I am keeping, in touch, with Tony, by telephone. He reported, relatively, good news. All face-to-face, assessments, have been suspended, so people, like Aileen, don't have to endure, the anxiety, of attending Tribunals. Furthermore, the Department of Work and Pensions, due to the crisis, is so inundated with Benefit Applications, that it is unlikely to chase up, with checks, on existing claimants, for the, foreseeable, future. His success with Keith's reassessment for Employment Support Allowance, is also described, as follows, in the following, individual examples, of advocacy.

Keith Rode

> *All I want is having you,*
> *And music, music, music.*

Keith contacted us in a distressed state in 2017. He explained that his Employment Support Allowance had been axed peremptorily, without warning. I believe that the renaming of Incapacity Benefit as Employment Support Allowance is a particularly stupid, and confusing, change for the worse! Incapacity Benefit was what it said it was - a benefit for people too incapacitated to work - and this included both mental, and physical, disability. Keith explained that he had been unable to work for the past twenty years, during much of which time, he had been the full-time carer of a mother with dementia. He had now reached the age of fifty-nine, and was perplexed as to what work he would be able to take up - after such a long period of unemployment. He suffered, severely, from anxiety, depression, and irritable bowel syndrome. Our advocate, Tony, took up his case. He made an excellent job of preparing all the papers. Keith said that it was as good as having one's own lawyer, and described Tony as 'marvellous'. Tony was able to drive, and accompany, Keith to the Tribunal - which was fortunate - because Keith, due to overwhelming anxiety - collapsed in the course of the proceedings, and practically had to be carried out, by Tony. But he did win his case. His Employment Support Allowance was restored. With the relief that this engendered, Keith was able to get a better quality of life, and was even able to resume some work, with music and radio, that he had, previously, been too ill to undertake. Keith had been improving in health, and in an ability to take up hobbies, when, in April 2019, he was called up, once again, for an assessment of his capability for work. Tony resumed his advocacy, and they met, at the crisis house, on Friday 26th April 2019. As before, Keith found Tony's support invaluable, and Tony also encouraged him to come to our drop-in centre more frequently - to get out of his four walls, mix with other people, and receive ongoing support. Keith dropped in on Friday 3rd May. Tony had met him, once again, to prepare for his 'Capability for Work' Assessment - due on Tuesday 7th May. Keith reported that his mental and physical health had been improving - until this latest Assessment loomed, but now, it had deteriorated. Tony will, of course, accompany Keith to the Assessment, but his anxiety will not abate, until he hears of a successful outcome. Keith visited us, once again, on Friday 10th May. Tony believed that the Assessment had gone well, but Keith, nevertheless, broke down in tears, three times, during the course of it. His arms and legs are covered with psoriasis - due to the intolerable pressure which is being put upon him. I am sticking to my campaign for sheltered workshops. At present, the severely mentally ill, are either pressured into jobs, that they can't do, or are left staring at their four walls, doing nothing! Surely it would be better, for them, for the economy, and for society, itself, if they worked in sheltered conditions! Since, with Tony's support, Keith's Assessment went well, he has become more confident, and is now able to get to our drop-in centre, regularly. Fortunately, the outcome of Keith's second Tribunal was highly successful. Not only did he remain in the Support Group, but he was also awarded the Severe Disability Premium - this making a huge difference to his financial circumstances. As I write this, on 1st September 2019, Keith is a changed man. With a better income, he is now able to have a better quality of life. He is developing his radio disc jockeying - which our members describe as 'brilliant'. He also now talks to friends on the telephone - where, previously, he had been isolated. So greatly has Keith's social life improved, since, through our advocacy, he has been able to get back into radio disc-jockeying, that, in February

2020, he was able to accept an invitation to spend a holiday at one of his radio colleague's, house in Cornwall. Previously, socially isolated, now, both working, and holidaying, and back into his music, his is a most gratifying success story.

Because he suffers from Type Two Diabetes, Keith made the decision, to self-isolate, during the coronavirus crisis. He was experiencing difficulties in getting his food shopping, and medication, but, fortunately, Elise came to the rescue. She is doing both, for him, and he is, most grateful, for this service. I have been having, regular, telephone conversations, with Keith, ever since he started self-isolating, and, fortunately, he says that he is not, adjusting, too badly, since he has experienced, a lot of social isolation, in the past. It must be much more, difficult, for people, whose lives are usually, packed full, with social activities. He has expressed, once again, how grateful he is, for Tony's advocacy – enabling him to complete his application form for a review of his entitlement, to Employment Support Allowance - which, as I have explained in 'Success Stories', indeed, proved to be, successful. Although, in July 2020, still self isolating - on account of his vulnerability, due to suffering from Type 2 Diabetes, Keith is cheerful, and doing well. He no longer has to take medication for his condition; a strict diet keeps it under control. He is benefiting greatly, from Tony's Zoom meetings, and he even, when I spoke to him on Monday 27th July, thought that he might, before too long, venture back into our drop-in centre - wearing a mask, and practising social distancing, as we all are. Incidentally, support, at the crisis house, is mutual. We have kept in regular touch, with Tony, by telephone and e-mail, during this gruelling time, while he is nursing his wife, with cancer. On 1st October 2020, I received an e-mail, from Tony, to explain that his wife's Consultant Oncologist, had advised against further chemotherapy. So, her condition is terminal, and palliative care, is what is now required. We are all very sorry, and we are supporting Tony and his family, at what is, a very sad time, for them. Our advocacy, and befriending, is never one-sided; it is mutual. Keith nursed his own, late partner, of seventeen years, through terminal cancer - so he is now, able to be, a tower of strength, to Tony, as he goes through a similar, gruelling, experience, and it was, indeed, Keith, who broke the news, to me, on 20th October, that Ethel had passed away. [Please see: 'Obituaries' - 'She Passed Away, Peacefully'.]

Maurice

We have known Maurice for many years. Originally, we got to know him, because he liked to take holidays at our Selsey caravan, and go sea fishing. He still likes visiting our drop-in centre, and, when doing so, on Friday 14th February 2020, Maurice confirmed, that our holiday caravan was, indeed, one of the best services that we ever had. He has become very dissatisfied with local mental health services, and now sees our Advocate, Tony, on a regular basis, to help with the many problems that he now encounters - due to these deficiencies.

Alexander

In December 2017, I was contacted by our Wokingham MP's Assistant - asking if I could help Alexander, who was severely mentally ill, and had stayed in the crisis house in past years. His Employment Support Allowance had been axed, peremptorily, and he had been without an income, since October. This was Christmas time, so all the offices would be closed until the New Year. I was able to supply Alexander with one hundred pounds - to tide him over the holiday period, and then, through representations, got his Benefits restored early in 2018. Further advocacy for Alexander, follows, under the chapter - 'Alexander Hopkins.'

Eliza

Eliza is a severely ill, paranoid schizophrenic, lady. She used to live in Wokingham, but, some years ago, moved to Oxford. Nevertheless, she stays in touch with us, and I have helped her regularly with Benefit Claims. In 2018, her entitlement to Benefit was to be reviewed, yet again, only two years after a previous successful claim. I asked our excellent Advocate, Tony, whether he would help Eliza to prepare the papers for the Tribunal. Fortunately, a former bedroom at the crisis house, is now reserved for private consultations - where such preparatory work can be undertaken - by Advocate and service user - in total peace and privacy. Such preparation is very detailed, and can take some hours to accomplish. Because he has a car, Tony was able to drive to Oxford, and accompany Eliza to the Tribunal - as a result of which, she won her case. These mentally ill people, would never be able to cope with the Appeals Process, without our assistance and Advocacy. This service is one of the most vital that the crisis house offers. Incidentally, Eliza's situation is one that illustrates - sadly, and cogently - how mental illness affects, adversely, not just the sufferer, but close family, as well. Eliza is divorced - still having some, limited, contact with her former husband. She has two sons - one of whom has a partner and a child, and the other who lives with Eliza, and is her carer. When she visits the crisis house, this son accompanies her. We believe that he is very adversely affected by her illness, and his consequent situation is life, and is, himself, depressed, as a result. Some of our members regard him as being more obviously ill, than his mother. There is no doubt that it is no life for a young man in his thirties. Freed from his caring burden, he could, like his brother, be pursuing his own career, having a partner, and family, and, in fact, living what most regard as a normal life. It is a very sad situation, to see the last dregs of his youth draining away. When we first knew Eliza and son, he had completed a science degree, and was due to embark upon studying for a PhD at Reading University, but this was, just at the time, that they were moving to Oxford - so the plan was shelved. Will it ever happen now? There is no doubt about it; the years do roll by. As I quote in *'Triumph and Tragedy'* - 'It's later than you think!'

Aileen

I have described Aileen's situation, in great detail, in the chapter - 'Further Poignant Stories'. She has received both our Befriending and Advocacy Service - with Lucy as Befriender, and Bev, as Advocate. When she came to us, Aileen had been using Reading Mental Health Services for many years, but we felt that she was entitled to a number of Benefits that nobody had accessed for her. Her Employment Support Allowance was due for review - so we completed the paperwork for this. She had been turned down for Personal Independence Payment - so we re-applied, and she is to be called up for another interview - hoped to be successful. As I explained in 'Poignant Stories', we applied for her to receive a Reading Borough Council Personal Budget, and we also applied for her to be transferred to ground floor accommodation - in the light of her physical disabilities. Previously, she had been placed in the lowest category - Band E - for housing transfer priority, but, due to our representations, she was moved to Band C. The Housing Association confirmed that, in Band E, she would have received no priority at all, but, now in Band C, she would get some consideration for a transfer. We considered that a bungalow would be ideal - since - with a garden, Aileen would be able to grow her own vegetables, and herbs, and since cookery is one of her interests, this would result in an improvement in her quality of life. I disagreed, strongly, with the Reading Borough Council officer's suggestion that Aileen should resort to internet shopping, and delivery of food - directly to her home. For the busy, and healthy, person, internet shopping is, indeed, a convenience. By contrast, for the severely physically, or mentally, disabled, person, a weekly shopping trip with a carer, enhances daily living, and gives them something to look forward to. They can get the shopping, go for a coffee, and make a pleasant day of it all - which is precisely what disabled people need - in order to improve their quality of life.

Our veteran advocate, Tony, also extended his advocacy services to Aileen - with excellent results. He met her several times at the crisis house, and this is where our quiet counselling room, comes in useful. He was able to give her undivided attention - [All to herself, alone!], whilst preparing all the papers for her 'Capability for Work', Assessment. He attended the Assessment with her, and Aileen described his advocacy on this occasion as 'very good'. On Friday 19th April 2019 - [Good Friday]. We celebrated with champagne. It was indeed a good Friday for Aileen. Tony had pulled it off, and succeeded in getting her assessed as 'unlikely to find work.' This means that she is now placed in the 'Support Group', rather than in the 'Work Related Activities Group' - in order to qualify for Employment Support Allowance. Aileen, as a recent psychiatric report - from a distinguished private psychiatrist - has confirmed, is extremely ill. She suffers from severe and chronic post traumatic stress disorder - as a result of childhood abuse. She also suffers from depression and anxiety, and the psychiatrist also considered a diagnosis of 'personality disorder' - which is what we had anticipated. However, in the end, he plumped for 'a complex post traumatic stress disorder'. Whatever, it all adds up to a very ill lady - who is very dysfunctional in daily life. Aileen is so neurotic, that she is unemployable in open market employment, so it is pointless steering her towards this. Now, due to Tony's successful advocacy. she will not have the constant stress of being pressured into something that she can't do! Relieved of the anxiety, occasioned, by the pressure of being forced into a job that she wouldn't be able to do, Aileen became more relaxed. We have a good eight hundred pictures - decorating the walls of the crisis house, and one is the 'Mona Lisa' - which I bought in a charity shop - for fifty pence! Aileen has long dark hair, pale skin, and always wears dark clothes - very much *décolleté*, and she is very beautiful. On Friday 3rd May 2019, she just happened to be sitting, relaxed, and with hands folded, below this picture. There she was, the Mona Lisa in the flesh!

> *Are you warm, are you real,*
> *Mona Lisa?*
> *Or just a cold and lonely,*
> *lovely work of art?*

In August 2019, Tony was taking a well-earned holiday, so I took over his advocacy role with Aileen, temporarily, and so sent this letter on her behalf - having to travel so far to get to a Tribunal - being completely unacceptable.

As her mental health support worker, I am writing to you on behalf of Miss Aileen E. Brown - address - Flat 50, Acacia Avenue, Reading. Berkshire. National Insurance Number - AB 12 C. Reference Number - AB 123/34/00567. [All details changed in order to ensure confidential - ity]. I refer to your letter to her - dated 25th July 2019 - entitled - About your Personal Independence Payment [New Claim Appeals], appeal.

Miss Brown suffers from a very severe, and long standing, neurotic disorder - with anxiety, depression, and sleep problems. She also suffers from nerve damage in her leg - the result of a road traffic accident. She has bouts of vertigo, and suffers from falls. It is for these reasons that she should qualify for Personal Independence Payment. We therefore fail to understand why her Appeal is being handled by the Liverpool Service Centre, and that, in your letter, you ask for her to attend a Hearing at your Preston Mags Venue. I spoke to your colleague about this matter on Friday 9th August, and he also, could not understand why Miss Brown's Appeal was being handled from Liverpool. He said that Sutton is the nearest Appeals Centre for the South-East, so he suggested that I write to you, and copy this letter to the Sutton Appeals Service.

Miss Brown is unable to drive; she has difficulty coping - even with local public transport, and we are perplexed as to why her Appeal cannot be heard in Reading - as all our other local Appeals have been. I should therefore be grateful if you would kindly look into this matter, and arrange for Miss Brown's Appeal to be heard locally. I look forward to your reply in due course. Thank you for your kind attention to this matter.'

Greg

Greg is Sadie Minton's partner of many years [Please see: '*Triumph and Tragedy*' - 'Twenty-Five Success Stories']. He has always been stalwart and hard-working, but, unfortunately, in 2018, he suffered a heart attack, and so was no longer able to continue with heavy work on building sites. Treatment proved successful, and medical examination proved that the tear in his heart valve had healed, spontaneously, so his Employment Support Allowance was axed, peremptorily. Our Advocate appealed, and Greg was able to resume entitlement to Benefit. We also applied for him to receive Personal Independence Payment. Greg is an example of a person who has worked hard all his life, has, through taxes, contributed hugely, to the Welfare System, and is, more than entitled, to claim Benefits, when his own health breaks down. Eventually, Greg recovered his health sufficiently, to be able to transfer from Employment Support Allowance, to Job Seekers' Allowance. He still manages to do his work as Steward - at Chelsea Football Club, and is also now considering taking work as a Security Officer - this being light - as compared with his former work on building sites, and so more suitable for a person with a history of heart problems.

On Friday 26th April, Greg visited us - with Sadie. He is now experiencing further health problems, and is having to undergo hospital tests, and treatment. Fortunately, Sadie is always there to give him her support. In May 2019, he underwent investigative surgery. Further investigative surgery became necessary in November 2020 - fortunately, with good results.

Lucy

Lucy had been in receipt of the High Rate of Disability Living Allowance - ever since she was discharged, from hospital, in 2007. Then, this was axed, and she was told to apply for Personal Independence Payment. This was refused - both on Application, and on Appeal. Lucy complained. The Assessor was a paramedic - with grossly inadequate training to assess mental health. In my representations to Parliament, I have called for a separate Application Process for mental health - since the current Application Process for Personal Independence Payment, is weighed heavily towards physical disabilities. Lucy, with our encouragement, applied a second time, and, this time, she was assessed by a physiotherapist. Because Lucy's arthritis has got worse, she succeeded in receiving the Standard Rate of Personal Independence Payment, but this was still only half the amount of money that she got with Disability Living Allowance, and was awarded, chiefly, for her physical, and not her, mental, disability.

Mary

Mary is another, Reading Service User, who has started coming to the crisis house drop-in centre, for support. When I completed her Employment Support Allowance Application Form, I was amazed, that, at the age of sixty-two, her entitlement was still being reviewed regularly. It is inconceivable that a person of that age, with a mental illness, and who hasn't worked in open market employment, for years, should still have to go through the stressful process of Review.

Sue and Vera

I have known Sue's mother, Vera, for a number of years, but since they live in Henley, they are not frequent visitors to the crisis house drop-in centre. However, Vera contacted me in October 2018 - to help her daughter, Sue, apply for Personal Independence Payment. Sue has a young daughter, and, now, a nice partner - who acts as her carer. They live in Didcot, but were able to get to the crisis house - where I competed all the paperwork for the Claim.

Incidentally, in December 2019, a most startling incident occurred at the crisis house. Vera telephoned me. She explained that she had been visited by a social worker, and by a psychiatrist - presumably with a view to Sectioning her - under the Mental Health Act. I had only met Vera a couple of times, and spoken to her, two or three times, on the telephone, but she had never struck me as being, anywhere near, being Sectionable. She told me that the psychiatrist, a top, distinguished, one, had been nice, but the social worker, horrible! Tell me something new! I suggested that Vera visit us at the crisis house. When she arrived, she was obviously as mad as a hatter - probably one of the most disturbed people whom I have seen on the premises. She had been told that she was suffering from cocaine psychosis, and, there was no doubt about it, she was Sectionable! I introduced her to everybody - including one of, this year's, little psychology students, Nerisha. 'You're the expert What is your opinion of me?' Vera enquired of Nerisha. Afterwards, I told Nerisha that it was excellent experience for her. I have always maintained that the crisis house is the light end of mental health - with most of our people, stabilised on medication, and well behaved. It is, therefore, unusual, here, for students to get experience of acute, and untreated, serious mental illness.

Tessa

Tessa is one of the group known, affectionately, as 'The Reading Invasion' - though she actually lives in Earley - which - though close to Reading, is in fact, within the, vast Wokingham District. She has suffered a severe breakdown, and is very timid, and fragile. In October 2018, she was called up for a review of her Employment and Support Allowance, and she never would have been able to cope with the stress of the interview - without the support of our Advocacy Service. Our Advocate followed the usual procedure of meeting up with her, to prepare for the Hearing, and then, accompanying her to the Interview, itself. She was in a very anxious state, throughout, but, fortunately, all went well. However, although the Tribunal went well, Tessa, with her fragile mental health, succumbed to the stress of the situation, had another breakdown, and had to be Sectioned into Prospect Park Mental Hospital for six weeks. Why put these, mentally fragile, people through all this unnecessary stress, one asks?

Joseph and Joan

Joseph's sister contacted me in 2018. She explained that the family were experiencing great difficulties. She and Joseph were in the process of organising care for their mother, with dementia, but that Joseph had the additional, problem, of also having to look after a mentally ill wife. He was having to work, full-time, as a lorry driver, and could not cope with having to be a full-time carer, as well - having, when he got home from work, to do all the cleaning, shopping, and cooking as well. A fellow feeling makes us wondrous kind! This story resonated with me, because Joseph was a lorry driver. My elder sister - who left school at the age of fifteen - with no qualifications, and, through sheer graft, achieved the position of Legal Secretary to the Queen's Solicitor - [Please see: 'Triumph and Tragedy'], has, for some twenty years, had a partner/companion, who was, in working life, a lorry driver, and he confided his problems, to me. His marriage ended acrimoniously, and he was very bitter about losing the house. Apparently, his wife was one of those women who always has to have a baby! So, as one child reached the age of five, she became pregnant again. They ended up with five children, and one had abnormally large feet. You couldn't buy shoes to fit her in ordinary shops - so they had to be made specially for her - price one hundred and fifty pounds a pair, and that was decades ago! What might they cost now? He said that he simply could not earn enough money as a lorry driver - to support them all. As a result of the divorce, he lost the house, and was relegated to occupying a council flat! Joseph is in a similar quandary. He has to earn money to keep the household going, but he can't cope with both, full time work, and full time caring, as well. I arranged for Joseph and Joan to come to the crisis house, and to meet our Advocate, Tony. Tony was able to spend a lot of time with them - arranging for Joan to re-apply for Personal Independence Payment. Joseph should also be entitled to Carer's Allowance, and if the applications for this extra income are successful, he will be able to reduce his working hours, and thus to cope better with caring for Joan.

We also arranged for Joan to have an updated Mental Health Assessment. I advised Joseph to write down all the important points for this Assessment - since, in the stress of the meeting itself, one can forget to mention crucial concerns.

Joan was assessed for her eligibility to claim Personal Independence Payment on Wednesday 24th April 2019. The Assessment was carried out at home - since Joan may have found difficulty in getting to an Assessment Centre. Fortunately, our advocate, Tony, was able to be present at the Assessment, and was described to me afterwards, by Joseph, as being 'marvellous'. This is what they all say, and it is, indeed, marvellous for our Association to have such an excellent, voluntary, advocate.

In late May 2019, Joseph's sister telephoned once again - to explain that she was bringing Joan to the drop-in centre - in order to do further work with advocate, Tony. She explained some of the difficulties - saying that they would make appointments for Joan to see the doctor - and then she wouldn't attend. 'Is that not, in itself, evidence of mental illness?' I replied. People with normal mental health, are only too anxious to get to a doctor - in order to receive the treatment that will improve their condition. It seemed to us, that it was taking a long time, for us to achieve benefits for Joseph and Joan - bearing in mind that they had first approached us in December 2018. But finally, in August 2019, we received the good news! Joan had been awarded the Enhanced Rate of Personal Independence Payment. She came into the drop-in centre - a transformed woman. All the anxiety had slipped from her shoulders. She could now afford to get out and about, and had, for instance, taken up swimming - excellent, for both, her physical, and her mental, health. Joseph would now be eligible to receive Carer's Allowance - taking away the financial insecurity of just one, precarious income, from his lorry driving. Excellent outcome, and most rewarding, for our Advocate, to see the fruits of all his hard work.

I telephoned Joseph, to find out whether he and Joan, needed any help, during the coronavirus crisis. He duly confirmed, that it would be a great help, if Elise could collect, and deliver, their shopping, and medication, so this was arranged, as well - making life, decidedly easier, for the couple. So Elise has been, providing, this service, for Joseph, and Joan, for some weeks, now - and it is proving, to be, excellent experience, for her, as well as, being, a godsend, for them.

Michaela West

Michaela was referred to us, in March 2019, by the local Talking Therapies Service. She required advocacy. Michaela came to see us - accompanied by her ex-husband - with whom she still has amicable contact. She explained that - as well as having mental health problems, herself, she had been in a relationship with a man who was severely ill with bi-polar affective disorder. They had, four months previously, moved from Wokingham to Glastonbury - to be near his mother - ostensibly for extra support - but his mother proved to be interfering, and domineering, and had driven, a wedge, between Michaela and her husband. Michaela had been acting as full-time carer - supervising medication - but this had broken down, with the breakdown of their relationship. Various incidents had occurred - and, through the Courts, Michaela had been placed under a Non Molestation Order - not to enter Glastonbury. Currently, she was staying with an aunt - in the village of Finchampstead - in Wokingham District, but she was concerned that her possessions - including pets, and private papers, were still in the bungalow at Glastonbury. She had a solicitor - to defend her joint-tenancy of the bungalow, but felt that this solicitor had little understanding of mental health, and was trying to rush the case, which was being funded by Legal Aid - through the Court - without sufficient attention being paid to Michaela's side of the story - hence her need for advocacy. There are times, when I truly believe, that the only service, that actually exists, is our own! I explained to Michaela, that I knew of a local solicitor, who had conducted other cases for our members, and that I would contact him. I duly telephoned his Firm - to be told that he only took criminal cases - with mental health features. I was then transferred to their Mental Health Section - only to be told, that they only dealt with cases of Mental Health Treatment [or the lack of it!], and not with Housing issues. Had I tried Housing Solicitors, no doubt they would have said that they didn't deal with mental health. Michaela's case included mental health, housing, and – if she breached the Non Molestation Order – criminality. I explained to Michaela, that our own advocates were not trained lawyers, so I would try other local advocacy services. I tried to telephone two, and, in each case, their telephone numbers were out of service! So I telephoned our own advocate, Bev. Bev is a retired headmistress, and is quite capable of going over the papers with Michaela - to get what she wants to say, down - in preparation for the Court Hearing. But this will still, of course, have to be presented by a solicitor. Good old Bev said that, of course, she would act as advocate, and made an immediate arrangement to meet Michaela at the crisis house. Bev, duly arrived, on Tuesday 12th March 2019, and spent some hours, in the private counselling room, with Michaela, and her former husband. Michaela - through having this support - is greatly reassured, and Bev will accompany her to any meetings or Hearings that may be necessary.

Putting these people, under pressure, is counter-productive, and is pointless. Michaela reported that the staff member at the Forge - the one who refused to fill in her Capability for Work Assessment Form - usually has her in tears! Fortunately, Bev will be able to accompany Michaela to the Assessment, itself, which is due to take place on Tuesday 30th April 2019 at Fitzwilliam House, Bracknell - the local Job Centre! Such environments can be experienced as being very intimidating - especially if the person has to attend, alone. What the mentally ill need, are environments that relax them - not ones that exacerbate their stress. Have places like the crisis house - with comfortable chairs, soft lights, cups of tea, and sympathetic listeners - then you will achieve improvement in their mental health, and who knows, you might even get them, well enough, to return to work! On Friday 3rd May, Michaela, and her former husband, dropped into the crisis house. She had mistaken the date for her Assessment at Fitzwilliam House, but it had, nevertheless, gone off reasonably well. Michaela complained bitterly about the misrepresentations that were being made about her situation - both by her estranged husband, and his parents, and by some of the officials involved. We advised her, strongly, not to waste any further energy on 'He said, she said'. 'Get shot, as soon as you can, of everything in Glastonbury, and concentrate on rebuilding your life in Wokingham!'

It is always good to drive a wedge through the extraneous, and get to the kernel of the vital. What is vital in Michaela's case, is establishing her tenancy rights. She and her ex-husband were joint tenants of a council house in Wokingham. Their divorce was amicable. He went to live with his mother, and Michaela's new partner moved into the council house. They then exchanged, for another house in Fareham, but his name was only, added to the Tenancy, in the last year of their occupation there. Then they moved to Glastonbury! The ploy, has been to remove, Michaela's name, from the joint tenancy there - and thus render her homeless. Michaela's case resonates with that of Janey and Mick - [Please see, the chapter, 'Sauce for the Gander' from *Triumph and Tragedy*]. If it is genuinely believed, that a vulnerable adult, risks abuse, by another adult living with him, then the duty of the authorities, is to remove the vulnerable adult, from the shared premises, and to a place of safety. It is quite illegal to evict the joint tenant. This is what happened with Janey and Mick, and what has now happened to Michaela. We have advised, if a sole tenancy is awarded to her partner, that we should complain, as we did in the previous case, to the Local Authority Ombudsman. They upheld our case then, and should do so, once again.

On reflecting on Michaela's situation, I am reminded of Agatha

Christie's short story, 'Wasps' Nest' – Please see: *'Poirot's Early Cases'*, Poirot says to his friend, John Harrison, who was engaged to be married to Molly Deane:

'I had seen Claude Langton and Molly Deane together when they thought no-one saw them. I do not know what lovers' quarrel it was that originally parted them, and drove her into your arms, but I realised that misunderstandings were over, and that Miss Deane was drifting back to her love.'

In the case of Michaela, and her former husband, it was his long working hours that parted them, but we all observe, the phenomenon, that Hercule Poirot, observed with Claude Langton and Molly Deane. Michaela and her first husband are, obviously, very much, back together. This being the case, the sooner she establishes Tenancy rights, obtains accommodation back in Wokingham, retrieves her property, and her pets, from Glastonbury, divorces her second husband, and draws a firm line - under this, unfortunate mid-life crisis, the better! In 'Wasps' Nest', Hercule Poirot successfully prevents a murder. Our case may not be that dramatic, but swift action, can prevent further pain and distress, for all concerned. To this end, I sent the following e-mail to Jenny Crossley - at Mendip Housing Services. This was sent on Wednesday 15th May. Michaela's Court Hearing - with regard to her Tenancy Rights - was scheduled for Friday 17th May. On the previous Tuesday, I spoke to Mendip Housing Services; they were reasonably helpful - especially when they heard about our proposed 'safety net'! I also spoke to Michaela's solicitor - requesting a contact for her barrister. Bev had described this solicitor as 'rubbish'. My conversation confirmed this view. I said that Michaela's mental health had not received sufficient consideration, but she was adamant that I could not speak to her barrister before the hearing.

My e-mail to Mendip Housing Services.
'As promised, I am writing to you - following my conversation with your colleague on Tuesday 14th May. It was left that you would contact me by telephone on Friday 17th May. This concerns your client, Mrs Michaela West, address, c/o, number of road supplied, Finchampstead, Wokingham. Former address in Glastonbury, house number and road, supplied. Our Mental Health Association has been involved with Mrs. West since March of this year - when she was referred by the local 'Talking Therapies' Service - requesting our Advocacy Service - which

we have been providing. Our Advocate has, accompanied her, to meetings with her solicitor. We are disregarding all the marital ins and outs of the case. Our aims are twofold - one - was to obtain Universal Credit for Mrs. West. This we have achieved - so she now has her own income - separate from that of her estranged husband, John. Two - to secure her Tenancy Rights. The Court Hearing - with regard to the joint Tenancy of the bungalow - which John still inhabits, is to be heard, at Yeovil, on Friday 17th May. Mrs. West will attend - accompanied by her aunt - with whom she has stayed, since January of this year. This Hearing, should establish Mrs. West's right, to a Tenancy in Social Housing, with yourselves. Mrs. West has held, a Social Housing Tenancy, for the past twenty-five years. Firstly, she shared a Tenancy with her first husband - in Wokingham. When their marriage broke down, he moved in with his mother, and she kept the Tenancy of the council house. John moved in with her, but his name was not added to a Joint Tenancy, until the final year of their living, in another property in Fareham. When they then moved to Glastonbury, their Tenancy was, once again, a Joint Tenancy - so if the Court, on Friday, decided that Mrs. West's name should be removed from the Tenancy, and that John should get sole occupation of the bungalow, then Mrs West will clearly, have had her social housing rights, stolen from her, and we will have to appeal to the Local Authority Ombudsman - as we once did with another, similar case. However, we have serious concerns - even if the Court establishes Mrs. West's right to continued social housing, because we believe that she needs to stay in Wokingham, and not return to Somerset. She needs to draw a firm line under - what has been a most unfortunate relationship - and to concentrate on re-building her life in Wokingham Mrs. West's doctor has confirmed that she is suicidal, and she did, on one occasion, return to Somerset - with the intention of committing suicide there. She is certain to try this again - if she returns to live there - even on a temporary basis. What I need to discuss with you on Friday, is therefore, whether some kind of exchange scheme, can by arranged, between yourselves and Wokingham Borough Council - so that Mrs. West can re-establish her right to social housing in Wokingham. I have spoken to Wokingham Borough Council. Mrs. West is not currently eligible for their Advance Rent and Deposit Scheme - whereby they will lend the deposit, and one month's rent in advance - if the person can find a private sector rentable property. The criteria are - having lived in Wokingham for the past year, or a family connection, or a work connection. Mrs. West does not qualify - because the aunt with whom she is staying, is not considered to be, a close enough, family connection. We are clear that her current living situation, with her aunt, is already starting to break down. People are very kind, and don't mind someone staying for a few weeks, but when the weeks become months, or longer, the arrangement doesn't continue to work so well. Mrs. West's mental health is very fragile, and she has physical health problems, as well. It is therefore vital that she stays in Wokingham - where she has the support of our Mental Health Service, of our Advocate, and the support of her former husband, of her aunt, and other friends. To return to Somerset - which has only unpleasant connotations, and where she would be completely isolated, would, in our opinion, be - literally fatal! So we have arranged a safety net. If the Court decides in John's favour, or if you are unable to exchange social housing rights with Wokingham Borough Council - then we will help Mrs. West to find a private sector, one bedroom flat, or bedsitter flat, in Wokingham - making sure that she is within easy travelling distance of her former husband, her aunt, and our mental health centre. Our charity will pay the deposit for this, and the first month's advance rent. Unlike the Borough Council Scheme, we never lend money. We pay for what the person needs, and if, at a later, and more favourable, financial time, they wish to make a donation to our charity, they are welcome, but not obliged, to do so. Now that we have secured Mrs. West's entitlement to Universal Credit, her application for Housing Benefit, to pay her subsequent rent payments, after the first month, should go ahead, smoothly. I look forward to discussing this with you, further, on Friday. Thank you for your kind attention to this matter.'

At the Court Hearing, the Occupation Order went in John's favour - although the Judge said that it was a very evenly-balanced case. The Somerset Housing Authority agreed to provide Michaela with the Tenancy of a bungalow - but this would still be in Somerset. Michaela thus opted for Cheddar - as far away from Glastonbury, as possible. We all doubted the wisdom of this decision. Michaela has suffered from suicidal ideation, and indeed, her attempt at suicide, took place in a beautiful field in Glastonbury. Cheddar may be a, similarly charming, place, but she would be totally isolated there - and - although she could try house-swapping with someone in Wokingham, this may not be achieved for months, or longer. Thus did we advise her. Nevertheless, Michaela decided to move back to Somerset. She dropped in to see us in August 2019 - temporarily back in Wokingham - looking after her aunt's dog - while aunt and uncle were away on holiday. Things not going too badly in Somerset. The bungalow in Yeovil, where she now resided, was part of a supported housing scheme - so she was not suffering the isolation that we had feared. Her former husband had visited her in Somerset, and continued to be supportive, but she was also engaged in internet dating - and so, evidently, was looking forward, and not backward! I mentioned Michaela's situation to one of our 2019/2020 Master's Psychology students, and we agreed that it is not always wise to be on with the new love, before you are off with the old! Sometimes it is better to take some time to reflect upon why the previous relationship broke down, and then set out to avoid similar pitfalls in any future relationship.

Peter Yates

Peter Yates, had attended the crisis house drop-in centre, a couple of times, but not recently. John Redwood's Parliamentary Assistant put me in touch with him, since he had approached them with regard to the lack of local mental health services. I contacted Peter by telephone, and suggested that he came to our drop-in centre. I kept them informed, as follows.

'I am writing with an update on Peter Yates's situation. As promised, I contacted him by telephone, and then kept in touch. He, eventually, came to the crisis house drop-in centre, on Friday 31st May. He said that he was still very depressed, and suicidal, but, fortunately, one of my service users - whom he remembered - and with whom he clicked - happened to be in, and so was able to give Peter some good support. This service user is also, currently, doing some painting and decorating, for us, so he roped Peter in for this as well - and nothing could be better for his mental health! I said to Peter - that the worst thing for anybody's mental health - is to stay indoors - staring at the wall, and thinking about yourself! Apparently, he is getting some other local support. A lady from Optalis - which is a local employment support service - takes him out on Tuesdays and Thursdays. This is good - as far as it goes - but it will be better still, if Peter comes to us regularly - so that he is participating in a group of people. Peter is interested in sport, so I also mentioned, that people on benefits, can get membership of the St. Crispin's Sports Centre, at a reduced rate. St, Crispin's is very near to where he lives, and so will be ideal. His difficulty is still with the local Mental Health Team - since he believes that he needs an updated diagnosis. His original diagnosis was one of anxiety, and depression, but he is experiencing paranoid symptoms - which - as I explained to him - are always made worse if one isolates oneself. Thus, I hope that we will *achieve regular attendance, and then I will be able to chase up the mental health team - to arrange a current Consultant Psychiatric Opinion. As always, we are only too delighted to help, and do refer other mental health clients to us - if they approach you with problems.'*

Shona

Shona contacted the crisis house for help with a Court Case. She explained that a Judge had ruled that she was unfit to have contact with her grandchildren, on grounds of her poor mental health. Shona explained that she had a very poor relationship with her daughter, and had suffered from reactive depression when they lived in the same house. Her son-in-law was very controlling, and made the situation worse. But, for the past eighteen months, Shona had been living, alone, in her own rented flat, and away from the friction, had recovered her mental health. She had always given both her daughters a lot of help - including very practical help - such as cleaning, and baby-sitting, but now she was being denied access to the grand children, and her elder daughter had even turned her younger daughter - with whom the relationship had been much better - against her. We thought that a letter to the Court - with a request that their decision be reviewed would be helpful. We duly produced a letter - stating that Shona was now recovered from depression, was stable and sensible, and should renew contact with her grandchildren - since this would be mutually beneficial.

Janice

Janice's current crisis illustrates, perfectly, the fact that mental illness is inherent, and genetic. Depending upon what is happening in the sufferer's life, they are at times, relatively well, and, at other times, relatively ill, but the fundamental condition is always there, and I am convinced, inherited. I remember that, some twenty years ago, Janice was very depressed. Then, it was the break-up of a relationship that triggered the illness. When she changed careers - from accountancy to physiotherapy, she also experienced problems, and said, herself, that the physiotherapy turned out to be 'a disaster.' Being dismissed from her job at the hospital, she returned to simple office work, and, from that, took on the care of her aged parents. To most people, losing your mother, at the age of eighty-two, after a five-year battle with cancer, and losing your father at the age of just under eighty-eight, would be regarded as, yes, sad, but surely, inevitable - since people are not immortal! To people with underlying mental health vulnerability, such life events trigger mental breakdown, and this is what has happened with Janice. Her great need is to talk, and to unload, and I am thus hopeful that - by putting her in touch with Anna, a therapeutic outcome will be achieved.

Pamela

On Thursday 26th September 2019, I accompanied Pamela to a Personal Independence Payment Review Assessment. This was held out at Theale, in West Berkshire - even though Pamela lives in Wokingham. I had to laugh when we arrived. Talk about having everything that you say about statutory services, vindicated! We sat in the waiting room - which was furnished with a dozen identical chairs - all with metal legs, and all exactly alike - ordered from a catalogue. A really fat person, could not have fitted into one. I thought, fondly, of the crisis house - with its huge, comfortable chairs and settees - provision for both the fat and the thin - some soft, and some hard - to suit preference, and some - both comfortable, but high - to meet the needs of the arthritic. For twenty minutes, we sat gazing at a bare wall! Pictures? You must be joking! There wasn't even a clock, or a calendar! At the crisis house, we know our social Greenwich Mean Time. Visitors are offered sherry, a gin and tonic, or a whiskey and soda. Are you having a laugh? All right, perhaps that would be a bit much to expect of services funded by the Tax-Payer. But, we weren't even offered a cup of tea - and yet these Tribunals are for people with both physical, and mental, disabilities, and some people have to travel quite a way to get to them. Eventually, we were shown into the interrogation room! The interviewer was something of a dragon, and Pamela, certainly, would not have survived the interview - had she been unaccompanied. She would have run out, in tears. I noted, to my glee, that the interviewer did not like having me there. 'Who are you?' she asked, with acerbity. 'I am the President of the Wokingham and West Berkshire Mental Health Association', I replied, firmly, but resisted adding, 'And with some Trump-like characteristics - not easily intimidated!' The interrogation went on for one hour. At the end, even I was exhausted. God knows what, a mentally, or physically, disabled person, feels like - after such an ordeal! Pamela suffers from a severe obsessional disorder - with symptoms of hoarding, so we took photographs of her flat, to the Hearing - so that the Assessor would get a realistic picture of her problems with daily living - which are, after all, the reason for applying, for Personal Independence Payment. The Assessor was reluctant to look at these pictures, but we insisted. A person, with a physical disability, needs help with preparing meals, because they can't stand at the cooker. Pamela needs such help - because she can't get to her cooker! There is so much clutter in her kitchen, that the cooker is impossible to reach! We thought it very important that the Assessor should see this! At the end of the exhaustive, and, exhausting, assessment, I asked, the Assessor, whether she was a trained nurse - since the interview did include a small amount of physical examination. She replied that all the Assessors had a professional background - which did not, in fact, answer my question. 'A professional background', covers a very wide range of qualifications - which need not be medical at all! Pamela had been extremely anxious throughout, but I insisted on putting in a lot of input - though resisted, and I reassured Pamela that the outcome of this review would be favourable.

Imagine, then, my chagrin, when we received a letter from the Department of Work and Pensions - stating that Pamela was not being awarded Personal Independence Payment. I could hardly believe it! Pamela's, neurotic anxiety, is so severe, that she is incapable of opening her own mail; she has to bring it to me to be opened - so that I can assist, if there is, anything adverse, to be dealt with in her letters. We are, of course, asking for a Mandatory Reconsideration of this decision not to award disability benefit, so, on Pamela's behalf, I duly submitted the following letter to the Department of Work and Pensions.

'*Personal Independence Payment Claimant, Miss Pamela McEllen - Reference Number - AB 123456 YZ - Address - 100, Acacia Avenue, Wokingham, Berkshire. - has authorised me to write to you on her behalf. I refer to your letter of 15th October 2019 - regarding your dis - continuance of her Personal Independence Payment. I accompanied Miss McEllen to her Assessment for this Benefit, and I disagree strongly with your decision to discontinue it. Miss McEllen has been attending our Mental Health Centre, and receiving our Advocacy Service, for some ten years, and your statement that her needs have changed - presumably for the better - is patently untrue. Two years ago, in October 2017, she suffered a severe trauma - which had a deleterious effect upon her mental health. We see Miss McEllen on a regular basis, and both her mental health, and her physical health, have changed for the worse, since a previous Assessment - when it was determined that she DID qualify for a Disability Benefit!*

In your Assessment, you have awarded no points for preparing food - even though we made it clear to the Assessor that Miss McEllen cannot prepare simple meals, unaided, because - due to the unacceptable clutter in her kitchen, she cannot reach her cooker. We were careful to supply photographs of the current state of clutter in her flat, and insisted that the Assessor examined these - though she appeared to be somewhat reluctant to do so - evidently regarding them as irrelevant - though they provided factual, and tangible, evidence of Miss McEllen's mental disorder. I am highly critical of this, since - when assessing mental health clients - evidence of their living conditions - and thus of their daily coping abilities - is crucial for an accurate assessment of their needs. I cannot emphasise, strongly enough, that this Assessor was, inadequately qualified, to make an accurate appraisal of Miss McEllen's needs. Her Consultant Psychiatrist, with his superior training and experience, is easily able to penetrate her superficial appearance of normality, and to assess, how ill, his patient actually is. You identify eating snacks, and putting on weight, as evidence that Miss McEllen has adequate nutrition. They are the opposite. Reliance on junk food, because she is unable to cook and eat healthily, inevitably leads to greater ill health!

I explain to people, ad nauseam, that these Assessments should be carried our by people with a proper mental health training, and I am not satisfied that Miss McEllen's Assessment was. The applicant with multiple sclerosis, for instance, qualifies for Personal Independence Payment, because he/she can't stand at a cooker, and so needs help with preparing meals. Obsessive/compulsive disorder - with which Miss McEllen is diagnosed - is a well-authenticated psychiatric disorder - which results in the sufferer living in such chaos and clutter that he/she is unable to carry out the daily functions of life. Qualification for Personal Independence Payment should disregard the particular diagnosis - whether mental, or physical - and focus upon the person's actual daily living capability. A conclusion as to entitlement to Benefit should be reached - not according to whether the disorder is, mental or physical, psychotic or neurotic - but upon how the disorder inhibits normal daily living activities. Miss McEllen exhibits quite definite neurotic symptoms - including self-sabotage, and poor self care - which affect adversely, all activities of daily living.

Coming to Daily Living Activity - number 2 - you have awarded Miss McEllen no points for eating and drinking, unaided. Certainly, Miss McEllen can hold a spoon to her mouth, but this is not the point, when it comes to mental disorders. She needs reminding to eat and drink, and so can still suffer malnutrition - though not for the same reason, as with an individual who is, physically unable, to hold a spoon! I come now to Daily Living Activity, Number 3 - Managing Treatments. Recently, to her Consultant Psychiatrist's consternation, Miss McEllen had not been taking her medication. Due to her mental state, which includes cognitive deficits, she forgets to take her medication, and, due to loss of Benefit - she could not, in any case, afford expensive Prescription Charges. Our obtaining for her, an annual Prepayment Prescription Certificate Ticket, has helped in this situation. She has now resumed taking medication, but she should never have been deprived, of the Benefit, that enabled her to receive regular treatment.

You have, for Daily Living Activity Number 4, correctly, awarded points for help needed for washing and bathing. Miss McEllen has told me that, when at her most ill, she doesn't wash or bathe, but puts clean clothes on - over an unwashed body! Dressing and undressing, presents its own difficulties. So extreme is the clutter, and chaos, in Miss McEllen's flat, that she is, frequently unable, to find, daywear, in the morning, and nightwear, at night. She needs to have sufficient income, to employ a hoarding specialist - appropriately trained - to de-clutter her flat in a sensitive manner, and then to be able to employ a cleaner, on a regular basis - to keep things up to an acceptable standard.

Coming to Daily Living Activities Number 5 - Managing your toilet needs - Miss McEllen does suffer from, some degree, of stress incontinence, and so should receive points in this category. I cannot understand why her needs in this category have been disregarded - since her problem, with stress incontinence was, quite definitely, emphasised at her Assessment. Daily Living Activity Number 6, Dressing and Undressing, is relevant to the whole picture - because Miss McEllen - like numerous mentally ill people - puts up a front to the world. She is always neatly, and presentably dressed, and this masks her underlying, serious, mental illness. As I have mentioned, she has difficulty in organising her clothes, and it is only through the most extreme, and time-consuming, effort, that she is able to present herself as being normal. This brings me back to my point, that these Assessments, should be conducted by qualified, and experienced mental health professionals, who are capable of penetrating the veneer, and seeing the degree of disability, that underlines it. So severe, did her anxiety state, and consequent exhaustion, become - as a result of her trauma - that, in the Autumn of 2018, her Consultant Psychiatrist, recommended respite care, in the, private, Cardinal Clinic - a service which is not available in the NHS. Fortunately, at the time, I was able to contact the Health Insurance Company on her behalf, to establish that she had cover for this, and to arrange her admission to the Cardinal Clinic. But equally unfortunately, her Health Insurance entitlement has now expired.

Daily Living Activities - Numbers 7 and 8 - Communicating, and Reading, are largely irrelevant, for an applicant, who is claiming Benefit on mental health, and, to a lesser extent, on physical health grounds - because they are more applicable to people with severe cognitive, and sensory impairments. Even so, contrary to your statement, Miss McEllen does not invariably understand signs, symbols, and words - because extreme anxiety disorder does affect, adversely, cognitive functions. Miss McEllen is currently suffering from suicidal ideation, and this must surely affect normal communication, and the processing of basic and complex written information. I also aver that having suicidal thoughts would inhibit her, from engaging in Daily Living Activity Number 9 - Mixing with other people. Miss McEllen's assertions at the Assessment - that she is able to attend various groups, and talk to people within groups - comes into the same category as her neat and tidy appearance - that of, putting up a good front, to the world! She makes every effort to participate socially, but she certainly won't be attending groups, and talking to people in groups, on the occasion that she is attempting suicide! This is a solitary, but preventable, tragedy - provided that the mentally ill receive the right kind of support!

Daily Living Activity - Number 10 - Making Budgeting Decisions - is one of your most inaccurate conclusions. Miss McEllen has great difficulty in budgeting and managing money. So distressing is her anxiety in this area, that she brings official letters - unopened - for me to open and read to her - so greatly, does she fear bills and debt! This disability is of a long-standing nature. Before I took over this service, which was quite recently, it had, for many years, been undertaken by another carer. Miss McEllen's psychiatric diagnosis - of emotionally unstable personality disorder - is very much an anxiety disorder - coming under the umbrella of the severe neurotic disorders. Financial worries make her condition much worse.

I come now to the mobility categories. By definition, mental health problems fluctuate. Miss McEllen will have days when she can plan and follow a journey, and days when she can't get out of bed. Your score of nought for the category - 'Moving Around' - is also inaccurate. At the Assessment, Miss McEllen explained, that she has pain in her right hip, and also suffers from severe sciatica - which does cause constant pain, and for which she does take pain-killing medication. Furthermore, these physical problems are exacerbated by her current state of extreme mental stress. The Assessor states, that there was no evidence of overwhelming psychological distress, at the Assessment. This was because I was with Miss McEllen - to ensure that extreme distress was not caused. Even so, I could detect that she was in an extremely anxious state, and any competent Assessor should have been able to see this. Had Miss McEllen been alone, she would have fled, crying, from the Assessment. Since this is invariably the case with people facing this ordeal alone, our Association now always ensures that people attending Assessments are accompanied by our Advocates.

Your statement that Miss McEllen is receiving private therapy, but has been discharged from the statutory mental health team, is irrelevant to her assessment for Personal Independence Payment. The implication is that only those patients under statutory care and treatment, are genuinely ill, and that, presumably, the ailments of people in private therapy, are largely imaginary. This is nonsense. Miss McEllen has, for many years, been receiving, private treatment, through Health Insurance - indicating the chronicity of her mental ill health. She has now arranged with her General Practitioner, to resume care and treatment from the statutory Mental Health Team - because her, Health Insurance Entitlement, has now expired. She was, until quite recently, under the aegis of the Statutory Mental Health Team, but the NHS Consultant Psychiatrist, didn't think that the NHS mental hospital, Prospect Park was an appropriate, place of respite, for Miss McEllen - hence the resort to the private, Cardinal Clinic - which proved to be efficacious, and was financed from private Health Insurance. Patients in the private Cardinal Clinic are every bit as ill as those in NHS facilities! As a result of the severe trauma of 2017, Miss McEllen is receiving gruelling grief therapy. The trauma increased her exhaustion, and made her, obsessive/ compulsive symptoms, much worse - hence the importance, of the photographs, which were submitted for the scrutiny of her PIP Assessor. Both her Consultant Psychiatrist, and her Psychotherapist, can confirm that this deterioration, in health, has taken place. Furthermore, with advancing age, physical problems have been added to mental problems. Miss McEllen suffers from an arthritic, hip, shoulder, and neck, and these physical problems are made worse by the stress that she is currently suffering.

In all these years, there has never been a time when Miss McEllen was fully recovered, and so ceased to need treatment. Mental Health is a chronic condition - often needing lifetime treatment, and, consequently, lifetime entitlement to Disability Benefits. Her ninety-one year-old mother has been in contact with me - very concerned that her daughter was not getting support - nor the financial help that she needs for daily living. With regard to your Report, she commented adversely on your statement - 'I realise that this decision isn't the news that you were hoping for.' She thought that this was, a most unprofessional, way of expressing things, and I would suggest that if a ninety-one year old, is aware of this, then your Department needs to look, very seriously, at how PIP applications are handled, and at how, consequent decisions, are expressed. Miss McEllen's mother commented that it read as though Assessments were being made on a personal, and so, prejudicial, basis. They should be completely objective. I come back to my most essential point. Doctors are used to making objective judgements. Other 'professionals', quite frequently, are not! So it should be doctors, with a specialism in psychiatric medicine, who conduct the PIP Assessments for mentally ill applicants.

On her behalf, I am, therefore, asking for a reconsideration, of Miss McEllen's assessment for Personal Independence Payment, and I add my own assessment - based on long-standing knowledge of the patient, and of her needs in daily living activities.

Preparing food - six points
Eating and Drinking - four points.
Managing your treatments - six points.
Washing and Bathing - Four points.
Managing your toilet needs - two points.
Dressing and undressing - two points.
Communicating - six points.
Mixing with other people - six points.
Making Budgeting Decisions - six points.
Planning and following a journey - six points.
Moving around - six points.

On the basis of these scores - with the reasons, that I have given, for awarding them - Miss McEllen scores fifty-four points, and so should be entitled to the Enhanced Rate of Personal Independence Payment. I should therefore be grateful if you would look at her claim again.

I would also draw your attention to the section of your letter - entitled 'Other Benefits, support, and advice - Council Tax or Housing Benefit help, and help with Health Costs'. Wokingham Borough Council, have now assessed Miss McEllen, as not being eligible for Housing Benefit, on Low Income Grounds - though she was eligible, previously. An official from her Housing Association, thought that the discontinuance of Personal Independence Payment, was the reason for their axing her Housing Benefit. Since PIP isn't means tested, if this is the case, then this decision is quite illegal. Their Statement gave no reason for the change, so I am appealing against this decision, as well. Also, I arranged for Miss McEllen, earlier in the year, to receive Exemption from paying Council Tax. She had been unaware of her entitlement to this Exemption. But this Exemption, on grounds of Mental Impairment, is dependent upon her receiving at least Standard Rate Personal Independence Payment - so, unless reassessed successfully, she will also lose this Exemption. Nor is she eligible for help with Health Costs - and this was the reason for her ceasing to take prescribed, and very necessary medication. So you are looking at an individual who - having lost Benefit - now has to pay full rent, and Council Tax, and who will, shortly, have to relinquish contact with her long-standing, and trusted, private Consultant Psychiatrist. Were it not for our assistance, she would not even have been able to afford, prescribed medication - which is absolutely essential to the maintenance of her mental health. I think, that in such circumstances, suicide, would be a, highly likely, outcome, but, as I have stated, this is preventable - provided that the mentally ill are given proper support. I look forward to receiving your response in due course. Thank you for your kind attention to this matter.'

In due course, I received the following reply.

HM Courts & Tribunals Service

Dear Pamela Jenkinson
You've been registered by Pamela McEllen as the representative on their PIP benefit appeal.
You will receive all the updates about their appeal by email. You will also be able to contact the tribunal on their behalf and submit information. You can provide them with as much support as you want.

I duly submitted evidence - including my own assessment of Pamela's eligibility, for PIP, and all the medical evidence, available, together with the following, covering, letter.

'*In response to your letter, asking, for evidence, to support Ms. McEllen's Appeal, I have pleasure in enclosing my own assessment of her needs - together with medical evidence, as requested. Since our charity was paying for her final appointment with her Consultant Psychiatrist, on 12th December 2019, I was invited to be present, and I can confirm that he said that her mental health was worse, and that she needed, firstly, continued treatment, from the NHS Consultant Psychiatrist, secondly, a community psychiatric nurse - to monitor her mental health, and, thirdly, a community support worker - to give practical help, with her hoarding problems. Since Ms. McEllen, qualified for PIP when her mental health problems were less severe, she must qualify, now that they are worse. Thank you for your kind attention to this matter.*

As well as appealing the PIP eligibility decision, I have also taken up the cudgels, locally - this being with regard to the hoarding in Pamela's flat. I wrote the following letter to the officer concerned.

'*I understand, from Miss Pamela McEllen, that you visited her at her flat in Acacia Avenue, Wokingham. She suffers from a severe obsessive/compulsive disorder, anxiety, and depression - which are manifested, principally, in hoarding. Since your visit, Miss McEllen has attended a Support Group for people with hoarding problems. This was held at the community centre at Jealotts Park on Wednesday 11th December. Miss McEllen attended with a volunteer from our Mental Health Association, and found the fellowship, experienced there, to be beneficial. However, the practical problems of de-cluttering, and regularly cleaning, her flat, remain - not least, as you pointed out, to eliminate fire risk. Miss McEllen is, herself, very anxious about the situation, but is helpless, until the practical problems are resolved. I, personally, accompanied Miss McEllen, to her final appointment with her Consultant Psychiatrist, at the Cardinal Clinic, Windsor, on Thursday 12th December. Her Health Insurance has now expired, and I believed that she needed me to accompany her, in order to ensure that her care was transferred to an NHS Consultant Psychiatrist, and that she would not fall through gaps in the service. Fortunately, her private Consultant assured me that he would be in touch with her GP, obtain a referral to her NHS Consultant, recommend a medication review, and suggest that a community psychiatric nurse be allocated to her case. He suggested that, for the de-cluttering and regular cleaning of her flat, a community support worker should be allocated to her. Provided that all this happens, many of her problems will be addressed, and managed. At the Appointment, her Consultant said - that we were looking at management - rather than cure. I shall be monitoring her situation, carefully, to see that Miss McEllen gets all the care and support that her private Consultant Psychiatrist recommends. Thank you for your kind attention to this matter.'*

Elise and Charne's heroic efforts to sort out Pamela's clutter, are lauded in this comic song.

> *We've all been doing a bit, a bit.*
> *We've all been doing a bit.*

A most welcome, and significant, development in our history, is how, in late 2019, and now in early 2020, we are attracting some younger people into our ranks. They have proved a godsend to Pamela. Charne and Elise have got together, and helped to declutter Pamela's flat. It is proving to be an arduous, and uphill, task, but they are getting there! Incidentally, as they, being sensitive to mental health, realise, it is no good rampaging in with black sacks, and cleaning materials. Hoarding is connected with depression, insecurity, anxiety, and nostalgia, and they are marvellously sensitive to Pamela's situation. I compare this, ruefully, to the 'professional' service received by Hank. Apparently, the 'support worker' stormed into Hank's house, shouted and screamed at him to clear it up, and left Hank - no further forward, traumatised, and expressing a wish to give the 'support worker' a good smack in the mouth!

Pamela's psychotherapist, Allison, is delighted with the progress that is being made in clearing Pamela's flat - due to the good offices of our befrienders. Elise has come, further to the rescue, by allowing Pamela to sleep in the spare bedroom of her new flat - while the clutter is being cleared. Unfortunately, Pamela's private Health Insurance, for psychotherapy, has now, in January 2020, run out, but we have agreed to pay for her to have six final sessions - spread over a three-month period, so that the therapy is tapered out - gradually, and with appropriate preparation - rather than with Pamela having to find herself, suddenly abandoned. This paying, where necessary, for therapy, is our 'crisis service' - for which we are seeking funding.

Although the de-cluttering is going splendidly, Pamela is finding it all stressful, and exhausting. On Friday 7th February, she came to see me, at the crisis house, in a very anxious state. I promised to write the following letter, on her behalf, which I did, and I then encouraged her to spend the rest of the day, relaxing, at 'Nirvana' - the upmarket health club, that features, so hilariously, in the section entitled, 'Funny Stories', in *'Triumph and Tragedy.'* I suggested that the officers, concerned, met Pamela, at the crisis house, but, unsurprisingly, they insisted upon seeing her flat!

'Miss Pamela McEllen has requested that I write to you, She is in an extremely distressed state. When Miss McEllen came to see me, at the crisis house, on Friday 7th February, I got the impression that she is, currently, having to deal with so many people, and so many issues, that her mental illness - diagnosed as emotionally unstable personality disorder, is getting worse. She is in, an extremely anxious, state - and this, at a time - when her Private Health Insurance has run out - and she is having to transfer to NHS Consultants. With the help of friends from the crisis house, Miss McEllen is making good progress in de-cluttering her flat. Her private psychotherapist, whom, fortunately, we are able to pay, until the course of treatment is finished, is very pleased with the progress, but, at the same time, Miss McEllen finds this mammoth task, of de-cluttering - quite exhausting. She is finding it, particularly distressing, having people visiting her at the flat, while it is still in a state of disorder, and while there is still so much to be done. I, therefore, consider it to be better, at present, for you all to visit Miss McEllen, at the crisis house, for any meetings with her, that are necessary. In our atmosphere of ordered tranquility, she is less likely to be anxious, and so to experience, further breakdown. The crisis house has a, completely private, counselling room - where things can be discussed, with total confidentiality, but there are also, always people here, to give advice, and support, if required. The crisis house is always open from 10.30am to 4.30pm, on Mondays, Tuesdays, and Fridays - with the exception of the morning of Monday 24th February - when I have to attend a Funding Event. I look forward to hearing from you. Thank you for your kind attention to this matter.'

This was the reply.
'Thank you for your email. Unfortunately, we do need to visit Pamela at the property, but you are more than welcome to support her, or she can have someone else there if she would feel happier about our visit. We

do need to discuss the issues she is experiencing with her neighbour, but we also need to monitor the progress of the clearance of the property because it poses a serious fire risk, to Pamela, and to others living in the block.'

I discussed the situation with Pamela, and we agreed that the visit could go ahead - at least, provisionally - provided that nothing else cropped up on that date, and also, on condition that, only Julia, conducted the assessment. Pamela is unable to cope with more than one person at a time. The visit went ahead, and was a success! Julia, and a colleague, attended, but Pamela had, with her, the support of her sister, and of our, excellent, befriender, Charne. Julia and her colleague were most impressed with the huge improvement - in de-cluttering - that had been achieved since a former visit. Now, the next step, will be to obtain regular domestic help, for Pamela, so that a de-cluttered flat, can be maintained - thus giving her a good living environment, and a better quality of life. The coronavirus pandemic has, of course, put a lot of routine things, on hold. I am only too delighted, that our crisis house cleaners, have been able to continue. Charne is now, fully occupied, home-educating her two young children, and Elise, as well as providing essential services, for our members, is doing telephone befriending, and has also registered, as an NHS Volunteer.

As Agatha Christie says, in *'Murder at the Vicarage'* so cogently, there is a huge difference, between theory, and practice! If all had gone as Pamela's, private Consultant Psychiatrist, suggested, Pamela would, by now, have been transferred to the care of her NHS Consultant Psychiatrist, and would be ready to take up NHS psychological treatment - as her sessions with her private psychotherapist, taper to a close. Alas, as the following letter, sent on 21st April 2020, indicates, it hasn't happened! Pamela duly wrote to her, former Consultant's, secretary.

'I'm writing to express my concerns about what has happened since I was discharged from the care of my private Consultant Psychiatrist, on 12th December 2019. Please could you kindly forward this email onto him.

At the final clinic which was attended by myself and Pam Jenkinson from the Wokingham Crisis House, he decided upon 3 steps forward.

1. Firstly he promised he would contact my former, NHS Consultant

Psychiatrist, at Wokingham Community Mental Health Team, that day, in order to see that I had a seamless mental health treatment because my private health insurance had run out.

2. He said to Pam and myself that my mental health was worse, and so I should also be provided with a Community Psychiatric Nurse, in order to monitor medication, and mental health.

3. That I should be provided with a, community support worker, to help with practicalities in my flat.'

My world is a world, free of bureaucracy. This is how I would imagine a service being conducted. On Friday 12th December, the private Consultant Psychiatrist, has his final appointment with his patient. In the course of this, he telephones the NHS Consultant. 'I should be glad if you would kindly see a patient of mine, and a former one of yours,' he requests. 'Her Health Insurance has now run out, but she is suffering from severe anxiety, and needs a seamless transition to your care.' 'Certainly', replies the NHS Consultant. 'Please give me the patient's details, so that I can look up the history, today, and I can see her in my clinic, at 11am, tomorrow!' My world is the world of dream ideals, but then, so is Pamela's world!

On Friday 24th April, I discussed Pamela's situation, with her befriender, Elise. In the letter, as well as the frantic seeking for help, I detect, a naïve, hope, that all would be well, if Pamela, could re-engage, with NHS services. But, I fear not. This, just like Aileen, is the person, suffering from an, extreme, emotionally unstable, personality disorder, seeking the, imaginary, crock of gold, at the end of the rainbow! It doesn't exist. There is no magic, in mental health. On Friday 1st May, 2020, Pamela did, finally, receive, a telephone call, from her GP - which she described as being, 'helpful'. Our stance is, that even if this leads to, a re-engagement, with the NHS Consultant Psychiatrist, it will not prove to be, a magic wand, that waves, all the problems, away!

> *I'm always chasing rainbows,*
> *Watching clouds drifting by,*
> *My schemes are just*
> *like all my dreams,*
> *Ending in the sky.*

Further evidence that Pamela is always chasing rainbows, emerged in July 2020. The Court of Appeal had been in touch - to explain that her Hearing had been allocated, and that it would be conducted, by telephone. Face-to face interviews are not being conducted - because of the coronavirus pandemic. Pamela declared that she was not willing to be assessed, by telephone, and so would wait, until face-to-face, assessments are resumed. This is the 'chasing rainbows' phenomenon, that goes with narcissistic personality disorder. Public bodies have to deal with thousands, and now, with the economic crisis, resulting from the pandemic, sometimes, with millions, of cases. In such circumstances, it is hardly surprising, that an applicant, is a number, and not a person. Pamela could find herself in a position, where she loses her current allocation, and has to go through the whole process, of appealing, a second time. Should we advise her thus? No, because she won't take any notice. So I have simply informed the Tribunal Judge of Pamela's position, and await his response. On Monday 27th July, Pamela visited the drop-in centre, and I was surprised, but pleased, to hear that things had taken a turn for the better. Her complaint to PALS had resulted in her being placed under the NHS Consultant Psychiatrist of her choice. Quite a victory - this! Pamela also, showed me letters, that her sister, her general practitioner, her psychotherapist, and her physiotherapist, had submitted to the Tribunal. All backed up my comments - though there had been no collaboration between us. It was good to see, that we were all singing from the same hymn sheet, and this made me feel much more confident, that Pamela's appeal to the PIP Tribunal, will be successful. Sure enough, now that it looks as though one problem is to be solved, satisfactorily, Pamela is, immediately, off, chasing another rainbow. There always has to be, something, on the, problem, agenda, so now, in August 2020, we are re-focussing, on Pamela's problem neighbours – with a view to the Housing Association placing an ASBO on them!

On the subject of getting a cleaning service, I cannot deny that I was greatly relieved when our, regular, crisis house cleaners, confirmed that they would be happy to continue with our service, during Lockdown - using the appropriate personal protective equipment. Apart from everything else, the crisis house has eight hundred pictures, to be dusted! I shared, perfectly, the anxiety, and then, the relief, of Mrs. Easterbrook – described by Agatha Christie, in her novel, '*A Murder is Announced*'. Colonel and Mrs. Easterbrook, feared that their cleaning lady had taken Colonel Easterbrook's gun, which was missing, may be implicated in the murder, and for which he held no licence. Agatha Christie writes:

'Perhaps Mrs. Butt [the cleaning lady], took it. She always seemed quite honest, but perhaps she felt nervous, after the hold-up, and thought she'd like to - to have a revolver in the house. Of course, she'd never admit doing that. I shan't even ask her. She might get offended. And what should we do then? This is such a big house - I simply couldn't.'

'My sentiments, precisely, Mrs, Easterbrook!' Fortunately, Colonel Easterbrook replied,

'Quite so. Better not say anything.' Just what I say. Keep everybody sweet, and leave well alone!

Pamela visited the crisis house on Tuesday 1st September 2020, and was able to report that, at last, after nearly nine months of waiting, all the professionals appeared to be working together, and consulting with each other, on her behalf. She had, finally, received treatment from an NHS Consultant Psychiatrist, who had treated her before, and so knew her case history, and she had also been allocated a Community Support Worker. Mirabile Dictu, her private psychotherapist, and her, newly allocated, NHS Psychologist, were, finally, talking together. All things come to those who wait! Pamela reported, further, on Tuesday 15th September. Her assessment, for a Personal Budget, had taken place, and she had been assessed as needing personal care, and a de-cluttering, and, regular, cleaning service. The only thing that was not, now, going ahead, was NHS Psychotherapy. When a patient has had a lot of psychotherapy, as Pamela has, the view is taken, that, for one year, the individual should work on the areas which the therapy has explored, before undertaking further sessions. Pamela did not agree, but I saw the logic of this, and explained, that, in any case, a further letter, from me, which she was requesting, would make no difference, if such was their policy. We were chasing rainbows, once again, looking for the, elusive, bluebird, in vain. On Monday 21st September, Pamela telephoned, to explain that she was submitting the questionnaire, that we had completed, together, to the local mental health team, and that, then, she was going away, to Glastonbury, for the weekend - because she needed some respite - after having so much to do! 'There's nothing at Glastonbury; it is empty countryside,' commented one of our members. This is, probably just the point! Were not the old, Victorian, mental hospitals, placed out in the heart of the countryside, for this very reason? Agatha Christie, in her novel, '*By The Pricking Of My Thumbs*'; writes about the work of a very popular, artist, Boscowan. One of his works, was at the heart, of the murder mystery. He painted:

'Quiet, peaceful dwellings, with no human occupancy. He didn't often paint people, you know. Sometimes, there's a figure, or two, in the landscape, but, more often, not. In a way, I think that gives them, their special charm. A sort of isolationist feeling. It was as though he removed all the human beings, and the peace of the countryside, was all the better, without them. Come to think of it, that's maybe why the general taste, has swung round to him. Too many people nowadays, too many cars, too many noises on the road, too much noise, and bustle. Peace, perfect peace. Leave it all to nature.'

'I explained to our members that Pamela's illness, is the most severe form of neurotic disorder. Everyday life exhausts its sufferers, and, as with Pamela now, their need for asylum, becomes acute. Pamela returned from Glastonbury - duly refreshed - just as she had been, when she was discharged from the Cardinal Clinic! Asylum - this is what is needed, in our mental health services. With regard to the practical services, for which she had been assessed, I opened, for her, a letter, which she had received from Wokingham Borough Council - detailing their charges, for these. I suggested that she discuss this with her Assessor - to see whether she would receive, a Personal Budget, since Pamela, already has, financial problems, enough, and can't afford to pay, for social care. With regard to Pamela's PIP Appeal, there was a step, further forward, when, in October, we received confirmation, from the Department of Work and Pensions, that they now had all the information, from us, that was needed, for a decision, to be made. On Tuesday 13th October, Pamela and I, together, discussed her social care finances, with the relevant Council Officer, who promised to look at the situation, sympathetically. Our exchange produced, yet another joke, for my readers. Pamela explained, to the officer, that I was 'her adversary'. 'No, I said, your adversary is your enemy! I am your 'advocate.' Talk about a malapropism! On Friday 16th October, Pamela received, the following letter, from the Department of Work and Pensions, and I, as her advocate, not her adversary, received a copy.

'You appealed against the Personal Independence Payment [PIP] decision, we made on 15th October 2019. Since we made that decision, we have received further evidence. This means I can change our decision. We can now award you Standard Rate Daily Living, from 15th October

2019.'

I explained to my colleagues, that I never waste any time, and energy - 'Chasing Rainbows'. I will only put the effort in, if I think that I shall succeed. With Pamela, I wrote a report, that wasn't much short, of a thesis - because I knew that we had a good chance, of succeeding. Nevertheless, I also pointed out to my colleagues, that the medical evidence, will always carry more weight than the layman's. Fortunately, with Pamela's Appeal, we submitted copious amounts of both - hence our victory!

> *Victory! Victory!*
> *He has given us, victory.*
> *Trust in His almighty arm,*
> *And you will wave,*
> *The victor's palm.*

Elise
Elise joined us in 2019. She had a long history of mental health problems, and had not worked for the past five years. She had seen a private psychiatrist, was due to be discharged by her NHS Consultant, but was still having psychotherapy. I have described in my narrative, 'The Path of Recovery' how Elise needs, firstly, to achieve a greater degree of recovery, and then, to have counselling - with a view to a change of career - since work in the pressured world of business, evidently made her more ill. In January 2020, Elise moved into a new flat, owned, but rented out to her, by her mother. I explained that she was bound to be very stressed, when moving home, since moving is recognised as being one of the most stressful of life events. It went off, quite successfully, but Elise expressed doubts about what, was now, even greater dependence upon her mother. She felt that reducing such dependence was a goal to be pursued, and explained that their relationship was very complex. On Friday 24th January 2020, Elise had to keep an appointment with her NHS Consultant - who insisted upon discharging her - even though Elise explained that her medication still needed monitoring, and that she was not ready for discharge. A further complication emerged. Crowthorne, where Elise lives, is one of those towns which does not have coterminous boundaries. Half its residents are under the Wokingham MP, the Wokingham Borough Council, and the West Berkshire Health Authority, and the other half are under the Bracknell MP, Bracknell Forest Council, and the East Berkshire Health

Authority - with the boundaries, not always, matching, exactly. Elise was, in addition to all the other stresses, having, as a result of her move, to change doctors and services. The, decided, assets of our crisis house services, for our users, are stability, and continuity. We have been in the same place, and with a number of the same volunteers, for thirty years. We know people. They don't have to go through the whole story, again, and, again. Elise's strategy of getting away for Christmas - to visit Iceland, with her brother - was a very successful ploy. Although suffering from a, severe, neurotic disorder, Elise retains an ability, which, unfortunately, many mentally ill people, lack - the ability to think forward, and thus, to avoid, potentially damaging, situations. Christmas 2018, had been a disaster - making Elise's illness, worse, so she determined that this would not happen at Christmas, 2019. This ability, to learn from experience, is vital, in crisis resolution, but sadly, is, so often, absent! Elise, exhausted by her house move, and by de-cluttering Pamela's flat, decided to follow up her Christmas success, by having a long weekend in Spain - both to relax, and to get away, albeit, briefly, from our cold, February, weather. By March 2020, Elise was undertaking the Training Programme for Home Start. Of course, with the coronavirus pandemic, all face-to-face, contact, with elderly people, and with, vulnerable, families, has discontinued, but Elise has found a, most useful. role for herself, in other ways, and I maintain that this is being therapeutic for her, and is helping her to regain self-esteem. Furthermore, with the recent easing of Lockdown, Elise has been able to resume some of her weekends away - visiting friends in other parts of the UK, as well as resuming contact, locally, with Charne, and this is also proving to be therapeutic.

On Monday 6th July 2020, Elise reported that she had taken a further step forward. She had researched, on line, counselling training programmes. These are composed of levels - going up to Level Four - which our long-term befriender, Bev, has recently completed. Elise discovered that a local college offers a short, ten week, introductory programme, and since she is reliant on benefits, I suggested that our charity paid for her to embark upon this programme - in order to establish - whether this was to be a step in the right direction, and would lead to training for a future career. This is a good move - because Elise thought that she could work, part-time, when progressing onto further levels of the counselling training. So, since coming to us, late in 2019, she has progressed through the, necessary, stages. She has got herself out of her walls, and into the drop-in centre. She has done a lot of voluntary work. She is about to embark upon part-time, paid, work and training, and this, hopefully, and in due course, will lead to a full time, paid, and professional, career, in mental health.

In July 2020, Elise received the good news that she has been accepted for the Preliminary Counselling Training Course, at the local, Farnborough College; this starts in September. As promised, in July 2020, our charity paid the fee for this preliminary course, and I assured Elise, that we were only too delighted, to do so. We are keen to do anything that will help people further along the path of recovery. Elise confided more information about the complexity, and dysfunction, of some of her family relationships. This is what I advised. 'It would be lovely if things were the way that we want them; but, often they are not. You can't cut yourself off, completely, from your family, because, therein, are your biological roots. Whatever they are like, you have come from them. But you can make an adjustment to the situation - in order to make life, liveable. You can accept that they are, the way that they are, and then go on to make the best of your life, with its disadvantages.' Elise has a friend who works for British Airways, and who has, as a result, managed to get them, a cheap flight, to a Greek Island, Santorini. This will give Elise, a much needed Summer holiday - before embarking on her training course, in September. Although there have been further peaks of coronavirus in Spain, and both France, and Germany, are at high risk, Greece, at present, appears to be at low risk. Elise and her friend, fly out, on Monday 3rd August, staying until the Friday, so I hope that they are able to have a happy, and hassle-free, time. Since returning from Santorini, Elise has, further, visited family, in Tenby, in Wales, and in Cromer, in Norfolk. Then, with a friend whom she met, in Group Therapy, she visited Nottingham, and Bakewell, in Derbyshire. This need, to be constantly on the move, is, in fact, agitated depression. One has to fill every minute with activity - in order to stave off the, underlying, depression, from which one is suffering. Although Elise, is well on the path of recovery, she has not reached the end of it, yet. With relative youth [aged thirty-three], on her side, I have every hope for a successful recovery, for Elise, but, there is no doubt about it, it is a hard, hard, climb!

> *My buddies and me, are getting real well known.*
> *I get around, round, round, round, I get around.*
> *We always take my car 'cause it's never been beat.*
> *I get around, round, round, round, I get around.*

Throughout September, Elise continued to get around - to West

Wickham, with one friend, back to Tenby, to see others, and, to Oxford, to see others. In October, she visited, a friend, in Bristol, visited Southampton, with a friend, introduced Charne, to the lovely old town, of Windsor. Elise is also, of course, awaiting her stay, in the country log cabin, in November. As in the song, she always takes her car, and, as in the song, Elise has lots of 'buddies', and this, certainly, helps her situation. Prior to her starting her Counselling Course, on Thursday 17th September, we helped her to fill in their Questionnaire. She had to describe the qualities that would make her a good counsellor - so we suggested, 'Empathy, good listening skills, a pleasant manner, understanding of mental health issues, and of, complex, family problems.' I added, 'High intelligence.' I consider this to be important, because a counsellor has to analyse things, as they really are, and not just as they may be presented, or appear to be. I cover this point in my chapters on 'The Path of Recovery'. To be effective, one must deal with reality - however, painful. Now half way through, Elise is doing well on the course, and is considering, once this basic course is complete, progressing, in January 2021, to the next stage. This is, to a part-time, but, intensive course, which will take her to the next level up. We are delighted with her progress. As well as pursuing her counselling training, Elise and Charne, have come up with the idea, of setting up a little 'Room Refurbishing' business - to be advertised, on line. I always claim that the individual will take the step back into paid work, when ready, and this is proving to be the case, with Elise.

Chas

In January 2020, it was so good to see Chas back with us. He had been one of the 'Reading Invasion', but had been obliged to stop visiting the crisis house, early in 2019, because his Employment Support Allowance had been axed, and so his free bus pass was withdrawn, by West Berkshire Council. Social isolation brought about further breakdown, and he had to spend two months in Prospect Park Mental Hospital - which he described as being 'awful!'

These are some of the criticisms, which I hear regularly, about this hospital. 'It is run like a prison. Patients have no freedom. You have plastic knives, forks, and plates, and drink from plastic cups.' This last criticism amuses me. To bring things down to the lowest common denominator, you can, just as easily, poke out an eye, with a plastic knife, as you can, with a stainless steel one! Therefore, why not have Viners cutlery, fine bone chinawear, and all the accoutrements of civilised living, that we have at the crisis house? Further criticisms. 'All the staff are temporary, agency staff, and cannot speak English. Patients are not allowed to smoke - even outside in the grounds, and are only allowed, decaffeinated tea, and coffee.' Such a draconian regime is both, ridiculous, and indefensible. I noticed, recently, with the criticisms, of the Feltham, Young Offenders, Institution, that the inspectors, were maintaining, absolutely correctly, that the young people were there, to learn how to turn their lives around, and this should be fostered, by the environment, and regime, provided there. The same is true, of patients, in Prospect Park Mental Hospital. Once discharged into the community, they will have access to, and need to cope with, all the ordinary things of life - where individuals encounter choice, decision making, and personal responsibility. Chas, appears to be, somewhat depressed, by his recent experiences, but now that his Employment Support Allowance, and so, his bus pass, have been restored to him, we are hopeful that our, therapeutic environment, will enable him, to pick up, and be restored, to mental health.

Des

We'll build a sweet little nest,
Somewhere, out in the West,
And let the rest of the world, go by.

Des, first, telephoned, and then, started attending, the drop-in centre, in May 2020. As with all, distressed, new service users, we give them time, to reveal their problems, at their own pace. If one seeks information from them, severely mentally ill people, can experience this, as interrogation. They clam up, don't tell you what is really distressing them, but instead, tell you what they think you want to hear. Thus, the situation, ceases to be therapeutic. Ironically, one gets a much clearer picture of the actual situation, if one just sits quietly, and listens. In her novel, '*Sparkling Cyanide*', Agatha Christie shows how much she is aware of this truth. Colonel Race, and Chief Inspector Kemp, are investigating the murder of George Barton. The Chief Inspector thinks that Colonel Race, should go and see Iris Marle - younger sister of Rosemary Barton, who had been murdered, the year previously, but Colonel Race says that he wants, first, to see Lucilla Drake. In an earlier chapter, Agatha Christie writes:

'Lucilla Drake was twittering. That was the term, always used in the family, and it was really, a very apt, description, of the sounds, that issued, from Lucilla's kindly lips.'

Now, Colonel Race says to Chief Inspector Kemp,

'I'm going to see her, [Iris Marle], but I'd rather go to the house first, when she isn't there. Do you know why, Kemp? 'I couldn't say.' 'Because there is someone there, who twitters - twitters, like a little bird . . . A little bird told me, was a saying of my youth. It's very true, Kemp - these twitterers can tell one, a lot, if one, just lets them, twitter.'

Des, was extremely lonely, very isolated, and very distressed, about the way that he had been treated, by social services. Bit, by bit, Des explained, that, for some forty years, he had looked after a lady, June, and her daughter, Jenny, who suffered from learning disabilities. As the, by then, old, lady's health deteriorated, the care needs of both, increased, so Des expressed his concern to the social services. Apparently, because he was a friend, and not family, June's niece was brought in, to supervise the care. Eventually, June went into hospital, and died. A full-time carer, was brought in, to look after Jenny, and Des felt that he had been pushed out, and that his long years, of caring, had been ignored. In particular, he had always kept the garden, neat and trim, and now, it was a wilderness. Des was very bitter about the way that social services had treated him, and complained. He showed me, a very negative, and insulting letter, from them. This intimated, that they would not deal with his complaint, that they would put the phone down, if he telephoned, and they advised him, to contact his GP, if he thought that his mental health, was adversely affected. I advised Des, not to pursue his complaint, against the social services, any further - because he would be, hitting his head, against a brick wall. His stance, is, that if nobody ever does anything about them, they will never improve. My stance, is that they will never improve, anyway! In the past, I have, taken up the cudgels, on a few occasions. For instance, I took, a complaint, about a care home, to the Social Services Inspectorate. 'The Social Services Inspectorate, doesn't inspect, the social services', was the Social Services Inspectorate's reply! Then, on behalf of a client, I once sought, emergency accommodation, from the Reading Emergency Accommodation Project. 'The Reading Emergency Accommodation Project, doesn't provide, emergency accommodation', the Reading Emergency Accommodation Project, replied. If one responded to these people in the way that one felt inclined, the Third World War would break out. As it is, I can only quote, to myself, from the hymn, 'Abide

With Me' - 'What, but Thy grace, can foil, the Tempter's Power?' In one instance, that of a Sectioned patient, who, due to negligence, committed, suicide, I did nail, the authority, but, only after a year, of persisting, and after, a detour, from the Health Authority, to the, [then], Mental Health Act Commission, to the Health Ombudsman, to the Secretary of State for Health, and then, back to the Mental Health Act Commission. In this instance, I only succeeded, because the patient, had been under Section, and so, there were, clear, legal issues, involved. I have advised Des, to take a, step back, from the whole, sorry, situation, to get the service that he needs from us, and to have, nothing further to do, with the social services. Since the full-time carer, is struggling, to cope with Jenny, and the niece, is apparently, incompetent, and also, elderly, herself, it is only a matter, of time, before the house, has to be sold, and Jenny, has to be moved into residential care. Welfare, is so much better, delivered, by charities. Just look at the wonderful work, that the Wokingham Charities are doing, in the current coronavirus crisis. The Citizen's Advice Bureau, as reported in *The Wokingham Paper*, on 14th May, has been able to assist, 1,700, households, to access the help that they need, during this pandemic. If anyone doubts, that younger people, are able to take over services, successfully, as older people retire, they need look, no further, than at the new, young, Chief Executive, of the Wokingham Citizen's Advice Bureau. Then, look at the Wokingham Volunteer Centre with 55 volunteers, across the Borough, enabling, vulnerable, self-isolating, individuals, to receive their medication.

All local charities, are providing a wonderful service. The Wokingham Link, is actually providing, 2,000 vulnerable people, with, a fortnightly, phone call, and, over 300, of the most vulnerable, with a weekly, phone call. It is, clearly, best then, not to waste energy, in complaining, about statutory, services, but simply, to put all one's effort, into one's charity, and, let the rest of the world, go by! One of my poignant stories is entitled - 'Talking to the Wall'. On Tuesday 28th July, I thought that I was doing so, once again, when in conversation, with Des. 'Aren't the Social Services accountable to anybody?' he asked, once again. Answer, 'No!' 'But they should be.' 'Answer - They should be, but, in practice, they are not!' It will indeed, be a wonderful day, when society abolishes them, for once, and for all, but until that day comes, it is better to have, nothing whatsoever, to do with them. In the Wokingham Crisis House, Des has found a home - where seldom is heard, a discouraging word, so he is, best advised, to stick with us, and to let the rest of the world go by. Furthermore, he and Don, have chummed up. As well as just talking, non-stop, they have now got into using the, crisis house, table games room, and it is good to see them getting down, to playing draughts, and dominoes. Des reports, great improvement, in his mental health, as a result.

> *Oh, give me a home, where the buffalo roam,*
> *Where the deer, and the antelope play,*
> *Where, seldom, is heard, a discouraging word,*
> *And the skies are not cloudy all day.*

Alexander Hopkins

In September 2020, Alexander's mother contacted me - desperate for help with her son's problems. I wrote the following letter, immediately, to a local Councillor - copying in, Alexander's parents. They had been in touch with this Councillor, since May, but the problems - between Alexander, and his abusive neighbour, remained, unresolved. The main thrust of my response is that it would be no good, going out of the frying pan, and into the fire. Supported accommodation, for Alexander, is necessary.

'I am writing to you at the request of William and Marie-Antoinette Curtis - with regard to the health, and wellbeing of their son, Alexander Hopkins. They have copied me in with the correspondence already exchanged between you. I have been involved with Alexander, and with his parents, for over twenty years, and I can confirm that he is severely, and chronically, mentally ill, and so in need of specialist housing. Alexander's mother referred him to the Wokingham Crisis House in 1999. He had been playing the drums with a band, in France, but had suffered a psychotic episode, so his fellow musicians thought that it would be better for him, to return home. We had mental health crisis beds at Station House, in those days, and Alexander stayed with us from July 1999, until June 2001. We found him to be, invariably, charming, and perfectly behaved, and we experienced no trouble with him, whatsoever. He was, nevertheless, severely mentally ill. He suffered from depression, was prescribed medication, and a diagnosis of Aspergers Syndrome, was also considered. He suffered acutely from obsessive/compulsive disorder - which manifested itself in hoarding, and he had also reversed the biological clock - sleeping throughout the day, and being wakeful, at night.

We never allowed guests to stay in the crisis house for more than two years - since, after that length of time, we had identified their long-term needs, and their situation had ceased to be one of crisis. So, in June

2001, Alexander moved into a flat on the Norreys Estate - which we decorated, carpeted, and furnished, for him. Even then, there was a problem between Alexander, and the resident of the flat above his. This was occupied by a baker - who, due to the demands of his work, had to rise very early, and Alexander's sleep was disturbed by the neighbour, moving about above him. After he moved out of the crisis house, we kept in, limited, touch - both with Alexander, and with his parents. In due course, he moved to another flat, in Crowthorne, and then, I believe, back to a flat on the Norreys Estate - experiencing problems, throughout. After his short prison sentence, Alexander's Probation Officer contacted me - to see whether he could come back to the crisis house. I had no objection, but my fellow Trustees, though they had nothing against Alexander himself, thought that, because of the nature of his offence, the crisis house might be targeted with violent attacks. He moved to a flat in Shinfield, and then to the flat above it.

Alexander's parents are now elderly, and suffering from their own health problems. I always advise the middle-aged parents of a mentally ill son or daughter, to get them settled into supported accommodation, before they, themselves, become too old, and ill to cope. Unfortunately, this is the situation in which, William and Marie-Antoinette, now find themselves. Over the years, Alexander has become, increasingly, reclusive. We have, on occasions, helped him with benefit claims, and helped out, financially, when his benefits were axed, but the social contact has been minimal. In my view, just moving Alexander into, yet another, ordinary flat, when one becomes available, would just be going out of the frying pan into the fire. He is now fifty years old, and it is unlikely that there will now be much change, or improvement, in his mental condition. I have two suggestions for a, possibly, more suitable placement. Firstly, at the age he now is, he could be offered a flat in sheltered accommodation for the elderly. We had a number of elderly people attending the drop-in centre, when Alexander was in residence with us, and he always got on well with them, and was liked by them. Furthermore, sheltered accommodation would, at least, have a Warden, to deal with any problems that arose. My second suggestion, is that of supported mental health accommodation. We may no longer have the mental health hostels, in Wokingham, but schemes do still, exist, in other Berkshire towns. Incidentally, Alexander is always welcome to attend our drop-in centre, as he always has been. Furthermore, we have a lady volunteer, who accompanies another of our hoarders, to a Hoarders Support Group, and I am sure, would be willing to accompany Alexander - once the Group re-convenes, after the *coronavirus pandemic has abated. I hope that my suggestions are helpful, and you are most welcome to discuss things further, with me, if you think that this would be useful. Thank you for your kind attention to this matter.'*

The Councillor duly contacted the officers who were dealing with Alexander's case, and their response - which I sent on, to Alexander's parents, was completely negative!

As always, I didn't expect to get any satisfaction from the statutory authorities, so their response was no surprise. I am not very keen on The Rolling Stones' grammar, but I share their sentiments, wholeheartedly! One is always palmed off, with 'some useless information', and, invariably, one stays, firmly, on square one!

I can't get no satisfaction, I can't get no satisfaction.

Marie-Antoinette, wrote to me, again, in October. I include part of her letter, and my reply, with this narrative.

'I am wondering if you have heard from the Councillor, by now, as William wrote to the W.B.C and they said they would contact all concerned. It was crucial that they saw your correspondence, because they have actually not responded to any of our concerns, and have washed their hands of everything - no compassion, nothing. So we are left, bereft and worrying, about what is happening to Alexander, his cut in benefits - to pay arrears to the rent and council tax etc... As you say, your suggestion of giving him a place at an elderly people's home was such a good idea .He should be left enough to live on; as it is, he is struggling. Do we go to Ombudsman, do we have a case?!
Could C.A.B help, I wonder?'

'The only response that I have received from the Councillor, is this one - which I am forwarding again. I don't agree, that sixty, is the lowest age for eligibility, for sheltered housing for the elderly. In the past, I have actually achieved this for a man of fifty-five, and for a lady of fifty-two. The threshold, depends upon the individual scheme. I think that this route is the best one to follow - since, unlike other accommodation, Wokingham Borough Council has plenty of sheltered accommodation, for the elderly. I shall continue to keep in touch, if I hear any more. The CAB in Wokingham are very good, and I am sure that they would be

able to help. Their Chief Executive is Jake Morrison, and he has a team of experts - in housing, legal issues, and financial problems. I am sure that we can get suitable accommodation organised, for Alexander.'

Don

Some advocacy cases are very complex, but, fortunately, Don's was straightforward. He simply, having reached the required age, wanted to apply for a Concessionary Travel Pass. I filled in the application form for him, and this was submitted to the local Council! Don, as a side effect of medication, suffers from severe parkinsonism. His hands shake, and he has difficulty in grasping a coffee cup, so, although he still holds a Driving Licence, driving is out of the question, and a Travel Pass, is vital, so that he can get about. Incidentally, according to the application form, even before he reached the required age, he could have applied for a Concessionary Pass, on grounds of disability - since 'inability to drive a car', is one criterion, for qualifying.

Mirabile Dictu, everything was straightforward, and Don received his Concessionary Travel Pass, almost immediately, and without complication.

Three New Members

Due to the coronavirus pandemic, we have had few new people, joining us, during 2020, but a lady, who had just moved to Wokingham, from Wiltshire, joined us, on Friday 16th October. She met my fellow-trustee, Patrick, and myself. She explained that she had multiple, and long-standing, mental health problems, and enquired, about all three of our services. We were delighted to welcome her, and it seems likely that she will need, our drop-in service, our befriending service, and, our advocacy service! Then, on Monday 26th October, another new lady joined us. Dan Kent had met her, working as a volunteer in a local charity shop, and introduced her to our service. She, also, has a long history of mental health problems. Both ladies described us, in our Visitors Book, as 'welcoming, warm, and homely'. [Please see the 2020 chapter on 'Comments from visitors to the crisis house'.] On Friday 6th November, a man in mental health crisis, telephoned. A former service user of ours, who had benefited, greatly, from our services, had suggested that he contact us. He explained that he had been suffering from severe anxiety and depression, for some time, and so was having to take, a less stressful, job. Fortunately, his employers were sympathetic, and were arranging for him to access counselling. He said that he had to support a wife, and four children, and that his wife was, also, suffering from mental health problems - exacerbated by Lockdown, and their, consequent, limited contact with, and so, reduced support, from, their, wider family. I made, immediate, arrangements for both to access our services. It is good, then, to report that all, of these, are continuing, and continue to be needed, and used, and are, greatly, valued.

PART NINE

The Ongoing Campaign, For Mental Health Education - Through Letters To The Press

As will now be apparent to my readers, I have become a 'woman of letters' in my old age. This part of the book, describes our campaign, for the mental health education of the public - through the medium of these numerous letters - which have been published in the last five years - after the 2016 publication of *'Triumph and Tragedy'*. It struck me, that, having written so many letters - most of them published in the local Press, and some as part of our Advocacy Service, it would make a better writing of a History - to include them exactly as, and when, they were written, and when they were published - rather than extracting parts of them, to incorporate in my general narrative.

Chapter 26

Exchange Of Letters: 2016 - 2017

These are some of the letters that have been published by *The Wokingham Paper*: 2016 - 2017

Looking out for the mentally ill
'I read, with sympathy, the letter 'Cost of Social Care is going up six hundred percent' - The Wokingham Paper: April 13th. The shake-up of the Disability Benefits System is causing a nightmare for the disabled, and in the case of the mentally ill - whose illnesses are stress-related - is causing further breakdown. Through John Redwood, I have taken these concerns to Parliament. The Ministers claimed that Disability Living Allowance was an out-dated Benefit. Nonsense! While disabilities continue, the need for Disability Living Allowance continues. This

Allowance has been replaced with Personal Independence Payment [PIP], and the 'Low' rate has been abolished - to which I have objected, strongly. Now one can only claim 'Standard' [formerly 'Middle Rate'], or 'Enhanced', [formerly, 'High Rate']. That small amount of help - provided by the low rate of Benefit, often made the difference between a mentally ill person just about coping, or breaking down again, and returning to hospital - at much greater expense to tax-payers! I have also recommended to the Ministers, that there should be a separate application process, for mentally ill applicants - since the PIP process is weighed heavily towards physical disabilities. Furthermore, I have asked for the mentally ill to be assessed by qualified mental health professionals - a useful job for psychologists! Not all mental disorders are immediately obvious, and can, go undetected, by those inadequately trained - though such disorders are just as disabling as physical disabilities. One individual, who approached me for help, recently, because his Disability Benefit had been axed, appears in your feature - 'From the Courts' - [The Wokingham Paper - April 13th] - charged with stealing food. Is this what the disabled are being driven to? Of course we agree with our Government - that we want to get everyone back to work. Nothing is worse for mental health, than idleness, but, the severely mentally ill, cannot cope with open-market employment. They need sheltered work - such as that once provided by the former REMPLOY factories. They were excellent. Why close them down?'

Paul Farmer wrote this letter to *The Wokingham Paper* on 7th September 2017.

Puzzled over mental health care

'Although obviously in awe of what Pam Jenkinson and the Wokingham Crisis House provides, and the variety of folk they help - the homeless and the mentally ill - I am however slightly puzzled. In several earlier letters, Ms. Jenkinson has proposed the abolition of all NHS services/ treatments for the mentally ill, many of whom do find themselves homeless. Instead she appears to favour voluntary services and yet admits to 'scraping the pot' - to find enough money to pay privately when a mentally ill person can't get immediate NHS treatment. If Wokingham Crisis House is 'scraping the pot' while NHS mental health services and treatments, are, however inadequate, available [crisis treatments or less critical treatments]. These cannot provide the crisis care that is needed now, hence having to pay for individuals' immediate private crisis care, as her latest letter admitted. How will/can the

Wokingham Crisis House and its peers provide what would be needed if no NHS mental health care was on offer? There is also the ethical question of - should groups like the Wokingham Crisis House spend their limited financial resources on providing private and very expensive crisis mental health care, or should it use its limited resources to provide crisis care until NHS mental health care is provided, when it is not provided immediately, or for whatever reason?'

I responded with a letter published on 14th September 2017 - part of which, follows.

Puzzled no more
'I refer to the letter - 'Puzzled over mental health care' - [The Wokingham Paper: 7th September]. I don't think that I have ever proposed the abolition of the NHS. It is generally the case - not that our people don't WANT NHS services, but the difficulty in getting them, and the length of time that people have to wait on lists.

The next letter focuses on problems with local medical services.

'In response to your request for readers' experiences of the Rose Street Medical Centre, [30th August], the feedback that I get from its mental health patients, is not damningly bad, but is not good either - with a strong preference, being expressed, for the former Tudor House, and Rectory Road, surgeries. The doctors at Rose Street are generally good - though some are better with physical, rather than with mental, illnesses. But the overwhelming impression I receive - as is the case with all Berkshire's NHS services - is that of OVERBURDEN. They can't cope with the volume of work that they are required to undertake. This is particularly the case with what is left of our mental health services. It is difficult to get very ill patients into Reading's Prospect Park Mental Hospital, and when you do, they can't discharge them fast enough - freeing up the bed, as soon as possible, for the next incoming patient! This hospital's service has deteriorated since it was required to take over the former mental health beds in Ascot, Slough, and Maidenhead. Overburden! They don't have enough trained staff to deliver a high quality service. A nursing sister, of my acquaintance, once commented - 'I don't care about my staff. I care only about my patients.' A most blinkered attitude! If you train, pay, and support your staff, properly, they will then deliver a better service to patients. A greater contrast could not be made between this, and private medical practice. When I

need to get a mentally ill person into the Cardinal Clinic - a private mental hospital in Windsor - I can always get them seen immediately - with the Consultant of their choice, and this hospital has such wonderful facilities, that I am green with envy!

The answer to the problem, lies in a cultural shift - whereby it becomes the convention, the norm - as is already the case in some countries - for people, generally, to take out private health insurance. Keep the NHS as well, of course, but don't be totally dependent upon it. Some people may argue that the NHS IS an insurance scheme. You pay your contributions, and treatment is then provided - free at the point of delivery - as it is with private schemes. Agreed, but the NHS is overburdened. Not all of our members agree with me. Some don't resort to private health insurance, but prefer to pay, directly, for any private treatment - physical or mental - that they need. But to do this, you have to be loaded! Some NHS services - such as their screening for the early detection of cancer, and other preventive initiatives - such as their 'flu and shingles vaccinations' - are excellent. But when it comes to mental health, the last thing that you need, is an environment which is overburdened, frantic, and frenzied. What users comment upon, as the assets of the crisis house - unhurried tranquility, peace and quiet, and the time to talk, and to be listened to - are the essentials that a mental health service requires.'

On the subject of the loss of our beds, and the paucity of services for the homeless mentally ill, I wrote the following letter to *The Wokingham Paper:* 31st August 2017. Unfortunately, our members have told me, that Broadway House never did materialise, solely, as provision for homeless families. Instead, like most properties in Wokingham, it is now high-rent accommodation in the private sector - though I gather that it does have some units which are described as 'social housing'.

Catering for mentally ill

'Pleased though I was, to read in The Wokingham Paper *that the old Nights Inn B. and B. is to be turned into a hostel for the homeless, [August 17th], if it is, as indicated, to cater for families, then that is yet another facility now closed to the single, homeless, mentally ill. They have lost the London Road Hostels, the Hornbeam Flats, the Reading Road Day Centre, and now, the Nights Inn B. and B. How good Wokingham Borough Council's services are, depends on your client group. Schools - brilliant - the best in the UK. Services for the elderly - marvellous! I have taken vulnerable, elderly, mentally ill people, to Shute*

End, and had them accommodated, there and then, on the same day! Wokingham has a lot of accommodation for the elderly - so they get choice, as well. But of services for single people - between the ages of twenty-five, and sixty-five, not so good. No doubt this age group are expected to be working, and providing everything for themselves. I agree that they should be working, but, if mentally ill, in sheltered work, and their housing should be staffed - just as the new Broadway Hostel is to be. Mentally ill people - who were formerly residents of the London Road Hostels, or of the Hornbeam staffed flats - are lucky not to be homeless. They report that the ordinary flats in the community - into which they have moved - are perfectly all right - just as flats. What they miss, is the support from staff. Our charity's finances always remind me of that old Bible story - 'Elijah and the widow's cruse'. Your young readers may not know what a cruse is - like the schoolboy who wrote - 'Elijah took a widow on a cruise!' It is a pot! We scrape around in the bottom of the pot, and always find enough money to pay for what the mentally ill person, in crisis, needs. God knows how we do it, but we do! If the person can't get immediate NHS treatment, we send them to the private, and expensive, Cardinal Clinic, in Windsor. I had just posted the cheque for one, earlier this week, and, crossing the road back to the crisis house, found that a large donation had just arrived in the post - more than covering the Clinic's fee. Elijah and the widow have got nothing on us! We have paid for people to stay in all the Wokingham B. and B.s, but the one that we used, most frequently, was the old Nights Inn. Mayfair, it wasn't, and 'breakfast' existed only in its name, but as well as being close to all the services, including ours, it was cheap! When you are freezing to death on the streets in January, and February, it was a case of 'Any port in a storm!' The other B. and B. s are infinitely better, but are, also, infinitely more expensive. It is good news that the local community is accepting the new Broadway House Hostel for the Homeless, and not seeing it as a stigma. I shall hail the day when the same can be said for services for the mentally ill!'

By contrast, some of my letters look at ideas that have germinated in other parts of the country, but could be replicated, successfully, here in Wokingham. The 'Care Rooms Initiative' was one such idea. It is good, though unusual, in this day and age, to see people coming up with creative ideas. The idea of 'Care Rooms Initiative' stimulated me to write the following letter to *The Wokingham Paper* (2nd November 2017).

Care Rooms Initiative

'I don't agree with the concerns raised about the Care Rooms Initiative - pioneered by Dr. Harry Thirkettle, and which was due to be implemented, in Essex. Berkshire would benefit from such a scheme - and it could be extended to mental health patients - as well as to those recovering from surgery. Prospect Park, now our only Berkshire mental hospital, is always short of beds, and is always reported to be understaffed. Yet there must be patients who no longer need twenty-four hour medical attention, but are not sufficiently recovered, to cope, alone, in the community. A Care Room, with a bit of support, and meals provided, would meet their needs admirably - until they achieve full recovery - and would free up acute mental health beds for those who need this. I frequently advocate long-term Adult Fostering. The Care Rooms initiative would provide the, equally valuable, short-term Adult Fostering. Furthermore, patients frequently complain that Prospect Park's staff don't speak English. Most ordinary Berkshire residents, who could provide Care Rooms, would be able to speak intelligible English! The idea is not so different from that adopted by the crisis house - except that our beds were in a building owned by the local community - La Maison Pour Tous - as the French would have it - rather than in private dwellings. Quite often, Consultants would refer patients to us - and they would stay for a few weeks - while they got used to normal life again, and sorted out permanent future living arrangements. Such schemes work very well, but only if the power remains firmly in the hands of the providers of the service, and not in those of the referrers. We only ever accepted patients for whom we could provide the appropriate level of support, and firmly resisted ever becoming a dumping ground. As a result, we had a very good success rate - as the Care Rooms scheme would if thus run with proper safeguards. I think that it should be tried.'

Chapter 27

Exchange Of Letters 2018

With the dawn of 2018, there was no diminution in both Paul Farmer's, and my, efforts to highlight the lack in services for the mentally ill.

On 18th January 2018, the following was published.

Bring back the asylums

'*Health Secretary, Jeremy Hunt, was quite right to stay in his job. He is a good person, and the problems in the NHS and social care, will only be resolved by cutting out bureaucracy, and putting the resources into front-line staff - not by re-shuffling ministers. When he says that the community system for mental health, is better than the old asylum system, he must demonstrate that this is the case. There is a current drive to get people off disability benefits and back to work, and this is causing a major problem for the mentally ill. The old asylums were very good at providing sheltered work. They all had farms, market gardens, and workshops. Patients had an occupation, and so, in a limited way, earned a living. Now in the community, the mentally ill are either idling their lives away, or being forced into open market jobs - which they can't do! First, look at the common run of mental illnesses, and the disabilities with which they leave sufferers. Now, look at the whole alphabet of available jobs - from Accountancy - through to Zoo Keeping. The one disability that all mental disorders cause - is the inability to cope with environmental stress! So, to replicate the services of the old mental asylums, in the community, the Government must set up sheltered work schemes for the mentally ill, and benefits should be paid - only on condition that sufferers engage with them. Such schemes need not cost much money - if they are run by volunteers.*'

Then, in February 2018, Paul Farmer submitted a letter, and I supported him with this, very forthright, additional letter.

Mental Health

'*I agree one hundred percent with Paul Farmer - [Assessing mental health - The Wokingham Paper - Letters - February 8th]. Mental health services are in crisis, but the crisis is not in what is left of the mental hospitals. It is in the community. If Health Secretary, Jeremy Hunt, can stand up there, and say that community care is better than the old asylum system, then he must put his money where his mouth is! The 'Short' Report, of the nineteen-eighties, said that any fool can close a mental hospital. Equally, today, any idiot can save money by simply not providing services. The clever way is to get rid of all the gobbledygook, and provide simple, basic services - at minimal cost. Healthwatch Wokingham, would have a job to solicit service-users' views of local mental health services. There aren't any! On the only occasion, that I have asked Healthwatch, to investigate the local failure, to provide a mentally ill man with supported accommodation, they replied that he was assessed as not needing the service - because Wokingham hadn't got one - in which case, you might as well get rid of the assessors! We HAD local, community mental health beds, in Slough, and in Ascot. They closed down! We HAD mental health hostels on the London Road, in Wokingham. They closed down! We HAD a mental health day centre on the Reading Road. It closed down! Last Friday, a lady who was moving, from Hertfordshire, to Berkshire, telephoned me - to enquire about Berkshire's MIND services. There are none. They have all closed down! One of our own service-users found to be quite valuable, a mental health support service, called 'Reading Your Way' - which had been working in Wokingham. It has closed down! They would have closed down the crisis house - if I had let them, but wars are won by those with the strongest will. 'Have I not commanded you, be strong?' says the Bible. I don't take commands from Wokingham Borough Council, but I do take commands from God! However, the nation can't be expected to rely upon old women, of iron will, to stand guard over services, nor on ones who will pay for private treatment for people who can't get it in the NHS. Mr. Hunt needs to go back to the drawing board. One of the very few services available - these 'talking therapies' - that he is so keen on - are fine for neurotic disorders. They are no good, whatsoever, for paranoid schizophrenia - which requires supported housing, with supervision of medication, and sheltered work. Patients are less overwhelmed by paranoid thoughts, and, consequently, less dangerous, if they have something to do! This is where the old asylums kicked in. Mr. Hunt needs to look at what they actually provided. Until these services - sheltered accommodation, care routines established by nurses, supervised medication, and sheltered work, are replicated in the community, then mental health will remain in crisis. When I was a child in the nineteen-fifties, we were much poorer than we are now. We were skint from the war. But you never saw anybody homeless - unless it was a solitary tramp - if you went into the country. The mentally ill were in asylums. Old Aunt Fanny had been 'put away'. As a child, you didn't understand where they had put her, but she wasn't freezing to death, in a shop doorway, as she is today. I have been battling to get a paranoid schizophrenic, into care, for over three years, and I have been trying, over a year, even to get a cleaner, for a mentally ill person who can't cope. So my message to Jeremy Hunt, is, 'Let us get rid of the bureaucracy, and get back to the basics!'*

There's a fight to be fought.
There's a race to be run.

On 1st March 2018, Nicola Strudeley, Healthwatch, Wokingham, Locality Manager, joined in the debate. The following is her letter to *The Wokingham Paper*.

'I enjoy reading Pam Jenkinson's and Paul Farmer's frequent letters about the crisis in mental health community services. I am pleased that the town has passionate, dedicated, and committed people speaking up for individuals who are either too ill, or too exhausted, to fight for themselves. Healthwatch, as consumer champion for health and social care, listens to what people have to say about local services, spots trends and themes, and amplifies these to the powers that be. Healthwatch cannot look into individual cases; however, the Citizen's Advice Bureau undertakes case work. Healthwatch engages with all residents of the Borough. We recently spent a week at Prospect Park Psychiatric Hospital - talking to inpatients about their care, hearing from them, what was good, and what could be improved. Last year, we held a focus group of women who had used the crisis team, and produced a Report called 'Voices in the Darkness' - highlighting how the service was not working for the users. This has resulted in the Council exploring alternative ways of supporting people in mental health crisis - such as the Recovery College model. Last week, I had the privilege of attending one of the inaugural get-togethers of a new group - Wellbeing in Wokingham Action Group (WIWAG) a gathering of people who are concerned at the lack of community mental health services, and have the desire to support positive change. The aspiration for WIWAG is to raise awareness of mental health, locally, reduce the stigma, and support people to live the best possible lives they can. I hope that everybody passionate about mental health and well-being, will support the aspirations of this newly formed Action Group.'

On 17th May 2018, I had the following letter published in *The Wokingham Paper*.

Mental health treatments

'I think that schizophrenia is the most neglected area in the whole, neglected, field of mental health. This struck me, forcibly, the other morning - when three chronic schizophrenia sufferers - all happened to be in our drop-in centre, together. One has used our services for thirty-one years, the second for twenty-five, and the third - for twenty-three years. During those decades, numerous people have passed through our hands, have recovered from mental breakdown, returned to work, and

so have gone back to completely normal lives. By contrast, the chronic schizophrenics remain - just as ill - as on the day we first encountered them. They should be in sheltered work, and I have campaigned for this, but Government policy is to work with employers – to get people, with mental health problems, back into ordinary employment. This is a realistic ambition for those recovering from nervous breakdown, but is totally unrealistic for chronic schizophrenia. Our Association has the most marvellous volunteers. Recently, one moved in to stay with a very ill, paranoid schizophrenic, lady - in order to look after her, day and night, until our befriender, could persuade the authorities, to Section this lady into Prospect Park Mental Hospital; literally, care in the community, by the community! But it remains a shame, that our own crisis house beds had to close - because their funding was axed. We only got two thousand pounds a year, from the local Mental Health Budget, [joint Local Authority and NHS funding], but we scraped by, for years, and there is all the difference in the world between getting a small amount of money, and getting no money at all! How, unutterably useful, those beds were - not just for the mentally ill people, but for those who encountered them - the Council, the Police, the Samaritans, the Mental Hospital. Here was a place to which you could come - just like that, and virtually no questions asked! No one had to pay anything, and there was no, lengthy, assessment process. A bed was here, waiting for you, and everything for your immediate needs was here - in a chest of drawers. Here you could stay - for days, weeks, months - up to two years - sorting everything out, in a place devoid of pressure, and of critical emotion - in fact - an asylum! Asylum - by far the most ancient, and the best-proven idea, in the entire history of mental health services. How foolish we are - to have abandoned it!'

Chapter 28

Exchange Of Letters 2019

NHS Mental Health

Paul Farmer submitted a letter - highlighting the deficiencies in our only mental hospital.

It had been my hope, when I set up the crisis house in March 1991, that once it had been accepted as a model of excellence - as it went on to be - then crisis houses, on this model, would proliferate throughout the United Kingdom - just as Women's Refuges have - using the

Chiswick model - established by Erin Pizzey - in the nineteen-seventies. It hasn't happened! It is the old, old, story. People just cannot believe that effective services can be run by volunteers, and believe that anything, outside of statutory control, is bound to be dangerous, and a failure - despite all the evidence to the contrary! I recall attending a Mental Health Conference in 1994 - and that is now a quarter of a century ago! At the conference, I described my crisis house project. Some managers from a Health Authority were there - and begged me to work with them. 'Please work with us, Pam, they said. A crisis house is what all the mental health service users say that they want!' Would I work with them? - no! Once you get involved with Health Authorities and Social Services, you get THEIR services, not yours, and not what service users want. Witness the view of former users of the mental health service, 'Reading Your Way' - who now use our services instead. It should be renamed 'Reading THEIR way', they claim. As I said in *This is Madness: A Critical Look at Psychiatry, and the Future of the Mental Health Services*', if you get involved with statutory services, 'You won't get a crisis house. You will get a hospital - masquerading as one!' That is precisely what happened, when the Camden and Islington, mental health service users, planned to set up a crisis house. Once established, the local Health Authority took it over as their flagship project, and it became a statutory service! In this letter, I make yet another plea for crisis houses on the Wokingham model.

'I read Paul Farmer's letter - NHS Mental Health - [21st March]. It brought to my mind a crisis house success story of many years ago. This concerned a man who had made a suicide attempt - because his marriage had broken down, and his Wokingham carpentry business had been failing - the usual situation of more than one, seriously adverse, life event - causing mental breakdown. The man was admitted to the old Fairmile Mental Hospital, under a Section of the Mental Health Act. He had never been in a mental hospital before, and he told me that he was, thus, terrified that he would end up like the broken-down, terribly ill, chronic mental patients - whom he saw around him. So he begged the social worker, to find him somewhere else to go. Under the Mental Health Act, it is legal requirement, that the Sectioned patient be placed, in the least restrictive environment - compatible with effective treatment, and alternatives to a mental hospital, must be considered, so the social worker brought him to us. He stayed in the crisis house for exactly one year - during which time, he re-established his carpentry business, successfully. Fortunately, he was able to park his van outside the crisis

house - this being in the days before the new road was built, and so lost us our parking space. Since his business operated in Wokingham, itself, no location could have been more convenient. Stuck out in hospital, in rural Oxfordshire, or even stuck in Prospect Park, in Reading, such a restoration of successful business, would not have been possible. He found a sympathetic girlfriend - out in the normal world - not among other mentally ill people, and, after a year, they moved into a flat together - recovered, happy, and successful, once again! What did I have to do - to help effect his recovery - apart from making the crisis house available? Sit down to drink a few coffees, and have a few encouraging chats, with him! Did I need numerous degrees in psychology? No! Did I need millions of pounds in funding? No! The excellent Wokingham United Charities have just made us, a most generous donation, of five thousand pounds, and this is, precisely, the kind of grant that we need to keep the Bank Balance up, and keep our services going. Prospect Park Hospital would cease to be in a frantic state - working, under-funded, under- staffed, and under siege, if there were numerous small, volunteer-run crisis houses - accepting, as guests, people like the man I have described. We didn't rehabilitate him; he rehabilitated himself - given the right environment in which to do so. Of course, he COULD have succeeded in a second, suicide attempt. That is the risk you take. But he didn't! They don't - because we show them the light at the end of the tunnel, and the way to crawl through the tunnel - to reach it!'

Getting Back To Normal

In *'The Moving Finger'* - Agatha Christie, Joanna Burton has moved to the country - to look after her brother, Jerry - who is recuperating after being injured in a flying accident. He found Elsie Holland, the Symmingtons' nursery governess, breathtakingly attractive - until she opened her mouth! Agatha Christie writes:

'Joanna suddenly laughed mischievously. 'Bad luck for you about the governess.' 'I don't know what you mean', I, [Jerry Burton], said, with dignity. 'Nonsense. Masculine chagrin was written on your face every time you looked at her. I agree with you. It is a waste.' 'I don't know what you're talking about.' 'But I'm delighted, all the same. It's the first sign of reviving life'.

As always, Agatha Christie has her finger on the pulse. The first sign that one is well on the road to recovery - from any serious illness - mental or physical - is the reviving of interest in the opposite sex.

Everyone acknowledges, and recognises this fact of human nature, and, as the following song avers, 'There isn't any harm in that!'

If a girl and boy should meet,
would you think it, indiscreet,
if they had a friendly chat?
I'm sure, you'd find, there
isn't any harm in that!

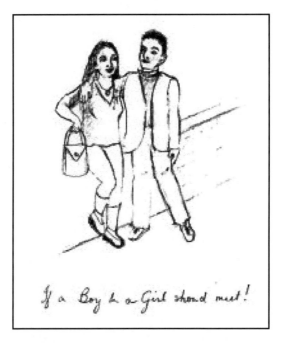

Agatha Christie regarded marriage as the quintessence of normality, and this is apparent in many of her works. For instance, in '*Third Girl*', Hercule Poirot visits the retired headmistress, Miss Battersby, to glean information about her former pupil, who has gone missing. She said;

'Norma, at school, was a perfectly ordinary girl.' 'But Norma showed no signs of mental instability?' Poirot persisted with the question. 'Mental instability! As I said before, rubbish! She's probably run away with some young man to get married, and there's nothing more normal than that!'

Nothing more normal, I would add, if a person with mental health problems is able to form a relationship with a mentally stable partner. Two, mentally unstable, people. getting together, invariably ends in disaster. Our 2020 example is covered in 'Further Funny Stories' - 'Boys Will Be Boys.' Earlier on, our 2019 example of this, is the disastrous situation with Michaela and her estranged partner. [Please see: 'Advocacy - Michaela'.] But it has happened, regularly, throughout the entire history of the crisis house. On Friday 28th February 2020, I was discussing this very subject with some of our befrienders. You may advise until the cows come home. People still do it! Two, mentally ill, people, get together, and it is a problem, compounded! Don't we know it!

Agatha Christie, in her novel, '*Destination Unknown*', also makes some profound statements about suicide attempts. Like the man in my letter - who attempted suicide, because both his marriage, and his business, had failed, Hilary Craven planned to attempt it - because her daughter had died, and her marriage had failed. Restore successful marriage, and successful business, to such people, and they no longer wish to commit suicide.

Hilary was sent to a 'Destination Unknown' - where her life would be in danger - but did that matter - since she had been intending to end it, anyway? Inevitably, after passing through adventures, and new experiences, Hilary found that she didn't want to die, after all. Like the man in my letter, journey ended in lovers meeting.

> *Trip no further, pretty sweeting,*
> *Journeys end in lovers' meeting.*
> *Every wise man's son doth know.*

Attempts on the part of the statutory authorities, to undermine voluntary services, continue - despite their failure to destroy us. I highlight a recent example in the following letter to *The Wokingham Paper*.

'I refer to my letter - 'Toasting Victory' - [25th April]. We have now had a successful Mental Health Awareness Week - with valuable input from Royalty, and other public figures, so I am toasting this, as well. I have always believed mental health education to be of vital importance, so, for many years, I served on the National Schizophrenia Fellowship's National Council, and, as their volunteer, I organised their education

programmes. As well as grass-roots work, I ran international research conferences. The research conclusions were not always as people might expect. I recall bringing Dr. Assen Jablensky over from Bulgaria - to speak at my conference at Imperial College. He headed up the World Health Organisation's Pilot Study into schizophrenia - which, perhaps surprisingly - concluded that the incidence and prevalence of the disorder - do not vary - whatever the culture. Remote Indian village, or New York, its incidence remains at one in a hundred, and its prevalence at four in a thousand! I also brought, Father of Biological Psychiatry, Dr. Seymour Kety, over from America. He conducted an exhaustive, longitudinal, study of all the families in Denmark - where identical twins had been separated from birth - one being raised by the natural parents, and the other by adoptive parents. Where, in later life, one such twin developed schizophrenia, so did the second, in a statistically high, number of cases. He thus demonstrated that schizophrenia runs in the biological family, and is not caused by environmental factors - though these can affect its successful management. Such research findings, can be invaluable for people seeking genetic counselling. The mentally ill and their families certainly need mental health education, but they also need, grass-roots, practical help - so I then went on to set up the Wokingham Crisis House - in order to provide this. I return to the second lady in my letter. After the Wokingham Statutory Mental Health Service declined to complete her Application Form for Universal Credit, she told them that I had done so, instead. 'I hope she knows what she is doing; that form requires medical information!' - they replied. Having, for years, organised education for the mentally ill and their families - delivered by the world's authorities on mental illness - I considered myself to be capable of completing a Benefits Application Form, correctly. I was! More champagne! The lady's application for Universal Credit, proved successful!'

The current campaign for mental health has been widely welcomed, but I have a caveat - which I expressed in the following letter to *The Wokingham Paper* - published 17th October 2019.

'Excellent though the current campaign for mental health and well-being, is - both here, in Wokingham, and headed up by Royalty at National level, I am inclined to agree with the view expressed by the Royal College of Psychiatrists. The current focus is on mental health - rather than on mental illness, while severe mental illness, in particular, should be our priority for more resources. Indeed, many of the current

initiatives apply to people who are not mentally ill at all. These are people who are simply seeking stress-busting activities - to help them cope with the everyday stresses of work, and life, that are experienced by everybody. Putting major resources into such work, is the diametrical opposite, of what used to be the case. Traditionally, virtually all resources went into the old asylums - which provided for the severely, and chronically, mentally ill. Indeed, up until the introduction, of the Mental Treatment Act of 1930, asylums didn't cater for voluntary patients, at all. All mental patients were what was known as 'committed'. Nowadays, this is known as being 'Sectioned' - that is, detained under compulsory medical supervision - and, frequently, this detention was for life. I am not proposing that, in modern times, severely, and chronically, mentally ill people, should be committed to asylums for life; but I am suggesting that greater resources should be put into providing them with services for life - services such as sheltered work, and supported accommodation. I can identify several of our current members, who are living in ordinary flats - where they can't cope. They would be better off in hostels - where staff provide the basics - a bed, a bath, food, and clean clothes. Two of our current members, are now on-the-street homeless. One had, for some time, been provided with a rented flat, and with a Community Care Grant - to buy furniture. Though he had a bed, he slept on the floor, and he sold his white goods - to buy alcohol. Being 'sanctioned' by the Job Centre - for failing to comply with the rules, imposed, as a qualification for receiving Job Seekers' Allowance, he had no money to pay his bills, and so water, and electricity, supplies, were cut off. He relinquished the flat, and went back on the street - relying, for food, upon the sandwiches that supermarkets discard as they exceed their sell-by date. This individual should not have been claiming Job Seekers' Allowance, because he is incapable of regular, open-market, employment. Instead, he should have been claiming the ill re-named, Employment Support Allowance - which was traditionally known as Incapacity Benefit. 'Mentally incapacitated' is exactly what he is. He is capable of doing a small amount of sheltered work, and this should be, required of people, claiming such incapacity benefits. He should not have been provided with a rented flat - where he was incapable of coping. Indeed, a number of our members, are incapable, of organising, and carrying out, regular household routines, and, as a result, live in the most extraordinary chaos, and clutter. Traditional hostel type accommodation - where daily living is organised, and payment, for utilities, included with their rent - is the best thing for them - since they are thus relieved of anxiety. Serious mental illness is here to stay; it won't go away, so we need realistic resources, and services, to provide for it. I recall actually being quoted in the House of Commons - when the Community Care Policy was being debated decades ago - as saying, that community care was only suitable for the less severely ill patients, and this remains my position, now, in the twenty-first century.'

The man described, spent most of the day with us on Friday 18th October 2019. He comes from a Jehovah Witness background - so this - combined with his mental illness, could be described as religious mania. On several occasions I have advised him to try to get into the Salvation Army Hostel, in Reading, before the Winter kicks in. Then one stands no chance at all of getting a place. The hostel then becomes, choc-a-bloc, with tramps who continue with their itinerant lifestyle, throughout the Spring, Summer, and early Autumn, but then seek a roof over their heads for the Winter months. When I try to get his basic needs met, he replies:

'Do not store up for yourself treasure upon earth - where the moth doth corrupt.'

It is always helpful, if you are able to advise people in their own terminology. So I continued the quotation:

'Do not store up for yourself treasure upon earth, where the moth doth corrupt, and the thieves break through, and steal, but store up for yourself treasure in heaven - where the moth doth not corrupt, nor the thieves break through and steal - for where your treasure is, there will your heart be also.'

But I then went on to advise, that meeting one's basic physical needs is not storing up treasure on earth. Did not Jesus Christ, at the last supper, take bread, give it to his disciples, and say, 'Eat ye all of this.'? So God wants us to eat. Did He then not take the cup [of wine], and say, 'Drink ye all of this.' So God wants us to drink. At this juncture, I handed the man a 'fireball'. This is whisky mixed with spices. As its name implies, it burns warmth into a freezing body! Then I continued, by saying, 'Did not St. Paul, the greatest of the Christian saints, and whose church is just up the road from the crisis house, write to Timothy - asking for an extra cloak - to stave off the cold? So God wants us to have warm clothes in the Winter.' Indeed, the Salvation Army, a Christian organisation, is one of the best, and most effective, when it comes to providing for people's basic physical, needs. I believe that this man's mental health is deteriorating fast - because homelessness is getting to him, so I shall go on persevering - difficult though it is when one is up against religious mania!

Homelessness continues, as a worsening problem, with every year that goes by. Wokingham has finally responded with its proposed night shelter, and, as a result, I had the following letter published in *The Wokingham Paper* (14th November 2019).

'Thank goodness that, as I read in The Wokingham Paper *(31st October), Wokingham has finally acknowledged that it is not some kind of wonderland - devoid of social problems - and is to create a night shelter for the homeless - a service which neighbouring Bracknell, and Reading, have already run successfully for some time. When I first read of the proposed night shelter in Wokingham Borough Council's latest Homelessness Strategy Document, my reaction was that I would believe it when I saw it! But, thankfully, it will now, with the support of Christian, and other organisations, actually happen. It is a pity that the shelter doesn't start until January, since the nights are already very cold. If the service could stretch from the beginning of October, until the end of March, this would meet the need more fully. I read that the shelters are to be drugs and alcohol free - an optimistic ambition - since those running the service will certainly meet these problems. Addictions, as well as mental illness, are major root causes of homelessness. I recall, that when we still had beds at the crisis house, I once took a couple of homeless heroin addicts off the street, and, with a lot of work, got them addiction-free, and, eventually, into permanent accommodation. There was - at the time that I was going through this process - a critical suggestion that I was creating the problem! But I wasn't; the problem was already here in Wokingham. I was simply solving it - just as the night shelters will solve problems with their service. I recall telling a former Chief Executive of Wokingham Borough Council, that when a house has drug-addicts living in it, it will have drugs in it. When they leave - addiction-free - to move into permanent accommodation, the house will cease to have drugs in it! The problem was never anything to do with us, and was all water off a duck's back to me. I am interested, only, in providing a service to meet a perceived need. People are always asking me why other areas don't have crisis houses - like ours in Wokingham. Surely all communities have some old 'white elephant' buildings - which can be obtained for a peppercorn rent, and would be*

suitable as crisis houses. But I suspect that those wishing to set them up, get embroiled with systems, hierarchies, and bureaucracies - which I never have, and never will, and so the much-needed crisis houses never happen. The forthcoming Wokingham night shelter, with a number of agencies involved, is certainly a step in the right direction.'

December and Christmas always bring problems for the mentally ill - as I explain in the following letter to *The Wokingham Paper* - which was published on 5th December 2019.

Festive mental health
'Looming, once again, is the annual nightmare for the mentally ill - Christmas! Everywhere is closed; there is no public transport, and all their carefully devised routines, that keep them stable, are disrupted. So they sit in their four walls - lonely and isolated - thinking enviously of all the happy families who are having such a wonderful time. I am not convinced that all families do have such a wonderful time at Christmas, but this is how the mentally ill perceive things to be. I think now, with nostalgia, of the days when we had beds at the crisis house. One Christmas, at the crisis house, a mentally ill man who happened to be a trained Army chef, stayed here. I gave him the money to get a turkey, a Christmas pudding, and some wine. He cooked a splendid Christmas dinner for any service users who would have been alone on Christmas Day. It was a great success, and helped him get his self-confidence back - so that he recovered, and went back to work. I wish that we could have those days back, but, nevertheless, I endeavour to make the ordeal as brief as possible. This year, strictly speaking, the crisis house won't close over Christmas, at all. Our party is to be held on Monday 23rd December. Every year, faithfully, our Patron, Lady Elizabeth Godsal, comes to the party, in order to distribute the Christmas presents - which, sad to say, together with the greetings card from us, are the only ones that some of our service users receive. I am also opening the drop-in centre on Christmas Eve - so that members with no family support at all, can at least get some company then. This year, Christmas Day falls on a Wednesday, and Boxing Day, on a Thursday - which are days when the drop-in centre doesn't, normally, open anyway. We shall re-open on Friday 27th December - thankfully, all back to normal, and it will all be over, once again, for another year!'

Chapter 29

Exchange Of Letters 2020

Well, who would have thought it? There am I - thankful to get, Christmas 2019, over with, and back to normal! Who would have thought, in 2020, that we would all be practising, 'Focussed Protection', going around in masks, socially distancing, and washing our hands, at a rate, to rival Lady MacBeth! It is a week, by week, and, at times, a day by day, existence, so one can only resort, to the sentiments, expressed in this song.

Give Yourself A Pat On The Back

Yesterday was full of
trouble and sorrow.
Nobody knows what's
going to happen, tomorrow.
So, give yourself a pat on the back,
A pat on the back, a pat on the back,
And say to yourself,
'Here's jolly good health,
I've had a good day,
today!'

No words could describe, better, our 2020 situation, than those of the old music hall song, 'Give Yourself A Pat On The Back'. Literally, 'Nobody knows what's going to happen, tomorrow!' Sometimes, circumstances, and advice as to how to cope, changed, daily. The coronavirus pandemic, escalated so rapidly, that our Association had to make some very quick, contingency plans. As I wrote, in the following letter, and in my previous letter to *The Wokingham Paper*, entitled, ''Strictly Carrying On', one can only solve the problems of today! For imminent - even if, only temporary, holding of the fort, one can only work with the people, currently, with us. One can't sigh, nostalgically, for capable people, who were with us, five years ago, nor seek, mistily, for those who might be with us, in five years time! People have to be suitable, but they also have to be, currently available, to do the job. Fortunately, Dan, Patrick, and Elise, are both! On the day that I am writing this, 18th March 2020, I am extremely well, and perfectly capable of continuing to run the crisis house. But, no fewer than four, sets of my neighbours, have offered to help us out, if we have to self-isolate, and I have accepted their kind offers, with gratitude. We could succumb to the virus - anybody could! But those, with whom I have discussed it, agree with my stance. Mental health services are so vital, that they need to continue. Furthermore, I believe the current protective measures, to be, unnecessarily draconian. It is ridiculous to expect, healthy, and active, seventy-year-olds, to self-isolate, for months on end. The age group, selected, should have been those over eighty, where most are likely, in any case, to have some underlying, physical, health problems. Furthermore, as Elise said, healthy seventy-year-olds, won't comply with the measures. For a week of so - maybe - but not for months, on end. I recall my mother, who lived in London during the Blitz, saying the same thing, about people's behaviour, during the War. When the bombing started, people hid, in their air raid shelters, but, as time went on, a return to normality, kicked in. You have to eat, so you have to shop - bombs, or no bombs! You'd go stir crazy - stuck in your four walls - especially since the Second World War, lasted for six years! So you have to go out, and this is what will happen, with this crisis - in due course. Agatha Christie, with her wonderful insight into human nature, was well aware of these facts. In her novel, '*The Pale Horse*', she writes:

'Ginger rang me two hours later. 'He [the doctor]'s been', she said. 'He seemed a bit puzzled, but says it's probably 'flu'. There's quite a lot about. He's sent me to bed, and he's sending along some medicine. My temperature is quite high, but it would be, with 'flu', wouldn't it?' There was a forlorn appeal in her hoarse voice, under its surface bravery. 'You'll be all right,' I said, miserably. 'Do you hear, you'll be all right. Do you feel very awful?' 'Well, fever, and aching, and everything hurts, my feet and my skin. I hate anything touching me, and I'm so hot.' 'That's the fever, darling. Listen, I'm coming up to you! I'm leaving now, at once. No, don't protest!' 'All right. I'm glad you're coming, Mark I dare say, I'm not so brave as I thought.'

The plot of '*The Pale Horse*' revolves around an organisation that specialised in getting rid of unwanted people - supposedly causing them to die - from ordinary diseases, like influenza - induced by remote control! Ginger and Mark set out to solve the mystery - not believing that anything would actually happen, to them, but it did, and their behaviour is exactly as it will be, with the coronavirus. Like Ginger, though she had agreed to do so, they will not be able to tolerate long periods of self-isolation, and will start to mix again, in normal social life.

Our members are, by definition, more anxious, than the average person; some fear that the virus will keep coming back, and that it will be the end of the world. I doubt it! The 1918, Spanish flu pandemic, killed millions, but further millions, survived it. The Second World War killed millions, but further millions, survived it, and it is remarkable, as the following song states, whatever the crisis, 'How life goes on the way it does', eventually - though it is, of course, very sad, that so many people are losing, and will, lose their lives - due to the coronavirus pandemic.

The End of the World

I wake-up in the
morning and I wonder,
Why everything's
the same as it was.
I can't understand,
no, I can't understand,
How life goes on
the way it does.

I was pleased to see my letter, published in *The Wokingham Paper*, on Thursday 28th March 2020.

Yes, Carrying On
'I refer to my letter - 'Strictly Carrying On' - [The Wokingham Paper: 5th March]. With the current, coronavirus, crisis - talk about having quite enough to do, with solving the problems of today! At present, the crisis house drop-in centre, is staying open on its normal, three days per week. Numbers attending, will be reduced, of course - as some of our elderly, and, physically vulnerable, members, need to self-isolate. But our younger members, in particular, are, mentally, rather than, physically, vulnerable, and we don't want to see a spate of suicides - caused by, unnecessarily enforced, social isolation. It now looks as though, my belief, that our services can continue, without me, is to be tested, rather sooner, than I anticipated. If I have to self-isolate, I have arranged for two of our charity's Trustees, to hold the fort. I have

suggested, that they try it out, for one day, per week, at first. Then, if this goes smoothly, progress on, to two, or to our, three, normal days of opening. One Trustee has been with us for twenty-one years, and received a Wokingham Town Council Civic Award, for his work at the crisis house. The second Trustee, has been with us for thirteen years, and has the advantage, of being young. He is aged, only thirty-six. We also have a young volunteer, and car driver, aged only thirty-two, who is on stand-by, to collect, and deliver, shopping, and medication, for any of our members, who are vulnerable. She will also offer any other help that may be needed. We shall be keeping in touch with self-isolating members, by telephone. In extreme circumstances, I have also made arrangements for the crisis house animals to be looked after – during what is, undoubtedly, one of the biggest crises, ever to strike the crisis house!'

Miss Edith Brinton's Curtains

Our eventual resolution, of the continuing of our services, during the coronavirus outbreak, reminded me, of the funny story, that my mother used to tell - of Miss Edith Brinton's curtains. Miss Edith Brinton, was an eccentric old spinster, and my mother, was employed, in her service. One day, Miss Brinton said, to my mother, 'Florence, we need to change, those curtains, in the drawing room'. My mother hastened to obey. Together, the two spent all day - sifting through piles of curtains, hanging them in the drawing room, and then, rejecting, each choice. After twelve hours of labour, Miss Brinton, said to my, by then, exhausted mother, 'Florence, I think that we shall have to put the original curtains up, again' - which they proceeded to do! As I explain, to deal with the coronavirus pandemic, we started, by thinking that we would have to close, completely; then, it was 'reduce the service', and finally, we went right around in a circle, and ended up, with exactly the same service that we had before!

When, on Monday 23rd March 2020, Boris Johnson introduced, stricter measures, for social distancing, even I, began to think that we may have to close the crisis house, after all. But these are times in which to avoid panic, and to use one's head, as well as one's heart. On Tuesday 24th March, I arranged to meet Trustees, and the younger service users who were still coming to the drop-in centre - to discuss things further. None of these people are in the high-risk group. They agreed with my stance, that we should remain open, as usual. Above all, mentally ill people, need stability, security, and an uninterrupted routine. With all the panic, one of these service users - who suffers from a severe anxiety neurosis - reported that she was suffering from nightmares, and panic attacks. She feared that the coronavirus would keep returning, and, eventually, destroy the whole world. I doubt it. The whole world would take some destroying! But one has to accept that this is the kind of agony that neurosis sufferers go through. I telephoned our Patron, Lady Elizabeth Godsal, and she said that, due to her age, she was self-isolating, but that she did, at least, have a large house and garden, as indeed, I do myself. Imagine being stuck, for weeks on end - incarcerated in a tiny bedsitter, with no access to a garden - which are, the living conditions, of some of our service users. We are able, to supply things, that pass the time - such as jigsaw puzzles, but being isolated, with nightmare thoughts and fears, is bound to trigger suicidal feelings - especially where these are already, underlying. This is where using my head, kicked in, and contributed to my decision, to keep the drop-in centre open. Actual suicides are very sad, and affect the heart, but attempted suicides are burdensome, and who has to bear the burden? Answer - the National Health Service. Where patients take overdoses or self-harm, they require physical treatment, in ordinary hospitals, before they are transferred to mental hospitals - so they require the services of ambulances, emergency departments, doctors, and nurses. The last thing that the NHS needs, with the coronavirus pandemic, is an additional spate of overdoses, and self-harm admissions. My stance is, that - where they are able to tolerate, doing so, our service users should self-isolate, but, knowing that we are still open, and physically available to them, will, to some extent, reduce their anxiety, and so prevent suicidal ideation, and attempts. This is my stance in late March, 2020. Things may change again, and our Government may, if necessary, impose total Lockdown, but, for the present, I consider our decision to be logical, and my colleagues, fortunately, agree with me. As I set out for the crisis house, the streets are deserted, and the trains, practically, empty. But, we travellers, who are providing essential services, are greeted with a cheerful message - thanking us for keeping things going, and station staff, such as are still on duty, are very kind - supplying us with, protective, gloves. Through all the panic, I am fortified by the words of my favourite hymn - that old, Quaker, poem, 'Dear Lord, and Father of Mankind'. It could have been written, specifically, for mental health! I like the line - 'Take, from our souls, the strain and stress' - but, particularly relevant, in the current crisis, is the line, 'Speak, through the earthquake, wind, and fire, oh, still, small, voice, of calm.' I have kept my promise to keep in touch, by telephone, with older members, who are, necessarily, isolated. In such circumstances, an ordinary telephone call, makes all the difference to the monotony! Also, as promised, our young volunteer, is doing sterling work, collecting, and delivering, their essential shopping, and medication. She is an, absolute, godsend to them!

The following, poignant, song, expresses exactly, the lonely position that many of our members are in, during Lockdown. Even a simple, telephone call, cam make all the difference to one's mental health, in such circumstances.

All alone
I'm so all alone,
There is no one
else but you.
All alone,
By the telephone.

The Self Isolators. These are some of those, whose response to self-isolation, is not mentioned, elsewhere, in the text.

Chris

Hello! Hello! Who's your lady friend?
Who's the little girlie by your side?

I telephoned, Chris, on Friday 20th March - shortly before the, stricter, self isolating rules, were imposed. He was, of course, discontinuing his visits to the crisis house, for the duration of the pandemic, but he was, just off, for his usual swim. At this juncture, public amenities, such as swimming baths, were still open. I promised to telephone, again, on 27th March. Now, Chris was, almost completely, self-isolating, but he was managing, nevertheless, to keep in touch, with his lady friend. 'And what is your lady friend's name?' I enquired. 'Maria', Chris replied. Chris, has often lamented, that he had never met a person - whom he wanted to marry, though he would have liked to have done so. Now, he says, sadly, that Maria would have been that person - had they met, many years ago. This reminds one of the lawyer - in the novel - '*A Town Like Alice*' Initially, he denied being, in love, with the lady whom he was advising, but then averred, that she was the woman whom he should have met, forty years previously! Well, it's never too late to fall in love!

Although my hair is turning grey.
I still believe it when I say -
It's never too late to fall in love.

I telephoned Chris, once again, on Friday 3rd April, and we had a good chat, and a good laugh. Chris is among those fortunate of our members, who has a number of hobbies, to keep him busy, during the Lockdown. He is painting more pictures, doing some reading, continuing with his writing, and getting out for his daily walk - though he misses his trips to the swimming baths. On Friday 10th April, things were continuing, much the same, but we are all, longing, for a return, to normality, and to, actually, be able, to meet again. Everyone is expressing this sentiment - including Dame Vera Lynn, and Queen Elizabeth The Second! People are pulling out all the stops - to encourage, naturally frustrated, self-isolators, and I was, particularly, impressed, by the Archbishop of Canterbury's discussion with Andrew Marr - broadcast on Sunday 12th April 2020. I have continued to chat over the telephone, with Chris, every Friday morning, since Lockdown, and he said, on Friday 12th June, that he thought we would be able to 'meet again', on Friday 3rd July. It is particularly poignant, that Dame Vera Lynn, passed away, only shortly, after giving this song, as her last, encouraging, message to the nation.

We'll meet again,
Don't know where,
Don't know when.
But I know we'll meet again,
Some sunny day.

Human beings are adapting animals, and will find ways of living with a pandemic - while respecting the rules for public safety.

You meet, not really by chance

You fly down the street,
On a chance that you'll meet,
And you meet, not really by chance.

People are behaving, very well, during the Lockdown, and finding ways of maintaining human contact - without breaking the social distancing rules - that are helping to save lives. You might, 'just happen', to see somebody, when having your daily exercise walk, and speak to them - albeit from a safe distance! But what a relief it was, once the Lockdown started to ease, and people were, at least, allowed out in the fresh air. I have, throughout the crisis, listened carefully to the advice given by doctors. One, very sensible, General Practitioner, said that, even those with underlying health conditions, can't remain walled up, forever, and that exposure to the sun, and the consequent production of Vitamin D, actually boosts the immune system, and thus makes people more able to fight off infection.

While strolling through the park one day,
In the merry merry month of May,
I was taken by surprise,
By a pair of roguish eyes.
In a moment my poor heart was stole away.

Thank God that, during the Lockdown, people were, at least, allowed to take the dog for a walk, and so, thus, get some fresh air, for themselves.

Our continuing service is going well. We are being able to practise the, two metres, social distancing, because far fewer people are attending the drop-in centre, and, not all at once. But those who are, are in desperate need of our services. In the wider picture, I also questioned, the necessity of closing National Parks, such as the Lake District - here, surely, the vast open spaces, are exactly what are needed, to prevent to spread of coronavirus. Are not the highest number of infections to be found in London, and Birmingham, precisely because, these cities are so densely populated? I discussed this view, with our Patron, Lady Elizabeth Godsal, and she said that, the Government, were worried, that, with a rush to places, like The Lake District, there would be, very heavy, traffic on the roads - exacerbating the problems, and this is, indeed, a valid point. The truth is, in these awful times, that there are no perfect answers. Being incarcerated indoors, is extremely deleterious - for both physical, and mental, health, and this becomes, more the case, the longer Lockdown goes on. On Tuesday 23rd June 2020, all those attending the drop-in centre, sat down together, to listen to Boris Johnson's announcement, on the further easing of Lockdown. What a relief! We can go to the pub! We can get our hair cut! We can 'meet again' - at least, for the time being!

Joan Thompson: 'Thou shalt not kill; but needst not strive officiously to keep alive'

I telephoned Joan on Friday 27th March; she is now in her eighty-ninth year! She said that she was going out for her daily exercise walk - accompanied by her son, Nigel. Her other two children were also looking after her. I found her comments on the coronavirus pandemic, interesting. She echoed the views of Lady Elizabeth Godsal. 'Pneumonia' used to be known as 'The old man's disease'. Indeed, I have mentioned, to several people, the fact, that when I was working as a nursing auxiliary - [Please see: 'The Path of Recovery'], one December, on the acute medical ward, where I was working, we had three deaths, from pneumonia, in one night! This was not regarded as being out of the ordinary. All three patients were in their late eighties, or nineties, and it was accepted that pneumonia carried off a large number of elderly people, every winter. In fact, Joan said, that it would have been better for her late husband, Gilbert, if he had died from the bout of pneumonia, which he had suffered at the age of eighty-eight - rather than having to suffer for two more years of dementia, doubly incontinent, having to be fed, lifted, and washed, and not recognising his family! My own position was not dissimilar. My mother contracted pneumonia, and died, in a January - the commonest month, for such deaths. Her doctor said, at the time, that because of her anaemia, she was less able to fight off infection, than were people without, underlying, health conditions. This is, precisely, the situation of those, suffering from coronavirus. At this juncture, my mother was in the early stages of dementia. Give her another two years - and her situation would have resembled that of Gilbert. I agree with Joan; it is better to pass away, naturally, from pneumonia.

Glyn: 'Keep your social distance'

Glyn came to the drop-in centre on Friday 27th March, and a question that I had been asking myself, was answered. 'How can you 'stay at home', if you have no home?' He came towards me, brandishing a letter which he had received from Wokingham Borough Council. I insisted that he kept the required two metres distance. 'It is not only, that you could infect me', I explained. 'I, equally, could infect you - since no testing has yet been made available, to us, I could have the virus, and not know it.' 'The coronavirus wouldn't dare!' quipped Dan Kent. 'No, it dared to infect our Prime Minister, our Secretary of State for Health, and the Heir to the Throne!' The letter, and I was intrigued as to how the Council were delivering them, to the street homeless, explained that temporary accommodation was being organised, in the efforts to control the pandemic, and that Glyn should telephone the Council, in order to find out what was being arranged for him - which turned out to be, a temporary, room, with a microwave oven supplied, but no actual food, provided, so he said. But I discovered, from another homeless man, who had also, been provided, with such a room, that food parcels were being delivered as part of the package of care. Luckily, we remain open, and our facilities remain, available. How does a street homeless person, with no mobile phone, and no money to use a public telephone - assuming that any still exist, locally, and with all public facilities closed, telephone a Council? While Glyn, gave up his room in West Berkshire, and is back, homeless, on the streets of Wokingham, another homeless member, Wes, accepted a place, in a hotel, out in Aldermaston. He visited us, at the drop-in centre, on Friday 29th May, and reported that he went out, and did a lot of, local, walking, but that he was, during the crisis, nevertheless, grateful, for the roof over his head.

Eliza: 'I believe in the 'herd immunity' theory'
I managed to contact Eliza, who now lives in Oxford, by telephone, on Tuesday 7th April. She, and her son, who is also her carer, are managing, to cope, during the coronavirus pandemic. Prior to becoming ill, with paranoid schizophrenia, Eliza was a trained nurse, and she believes in the 'herd immunity' theory - which was our Government's first stance - before 'Lockdown' became their, necessary, option - since this was being followed by all other countries. I telephoned, again, on Friday 24th April - to thank, Elizabeth, for her latest donation - which is mentioned, in the section, entitled, 'Benefactors'.

The numbers attending our drop-in centre, during the crisis, have reduced to six or seven people, at any one time, so we are, easily able, to practise social distancing, of at least, two metres - while at the same time, relieving mental distress, but having some human contact! We will continue to sit, as far apart, as possible, but now that the social distancing has been reduced to, a minimum, of one metre, we will be able to cope, if numbers attending the drop-in centre, start to increase.

Tony and Ethel are self isolating, and are having their shopping delivered, directly, to the house. On Friday 27th March, I telephoned him - not only to see how he was doing, but, also, to tell him about Brendan's newspaper feature on Bi-Polar Affective Disorder. Tony has always been an excellent befriender, for Brendan. [Please see: 'Good

Male Befrienders' – in *'Triumph and Tragedy'*.] I telephoned Tony, again, on Tuesday 14th April. He said that Aileen was in a bad place - please see: 'Poignant Stories - All To Myself, Alone'. She had kept in touch with Tony - who had continued advocacy work, with her. He hoped that I would be able to telephone her, but, whether it would be wise for her to return to our drop-in centre - while Glyn is still attending, is debatable. Glyn is totally dependent upon our services as the following letter which I wrote to *The Wokingham Paper*, on 15th April, indicates.

'I recall, from some time ago, a Wokingham Paper *reader, who was campaigning for extra funding, for Wokingham's schools, and who stated, in the Paper, her belief, in the supreme importance, of education. Our, current, fraught, circumstances, certainly vindicate, her position! One of our, self-isolating, members, can, at least, pass the time - playing the cello. Another, like me, is writing a book. We have one, painting pictures, and another, more prosaically, painting her flat! Yet another, like me, passes the time - doing embroidery. These are all skills - first learned, in school. But for those people, whose only interests are social - going out to pubs, and going to gatherings, of friends, current times, are indeed, very difficult. We have been able to supply, from our large stock, at the crisis house, fiction books, jigsaw puzzles, and table games. Otherwise, social butterflies' only resort - is to watch television. During the pandemic, local councils have been required to find, temporary, accommodation, for the street homeless - in order to help control, the spread of coronavirus. This is, yet another, difficult task, for them. One, destitute, member, was found a room - far out, in West Berkshire. He revealed, that, after his first day out there, he had, like a, latter day, Mary Jones, walked the, full, twenty-four miles, to us, and back, simply in order to continue accessing our coffee, biscuits, and support! He certainly got his bit of daily exercise! Fortunately, on his second day of doing so, another member gave him his fare back, and he was able to obtain a month's supply of food, from the Wokingham Food Bank. I have never done so much telephoning, as in recent weeks. It is, particularly good, to chat with our Patron, Lady Elizabeth Godsal - reminiscing, about the War, and its immediate, aftermath. Nowadays, people are, strictly, vegan. We weren't them. We ate anything, and were grateful, for it. I recall, a particular staple, being rabbit stew, and you saw the little grey, furry, rabbits - hanging up, in the butcher's shop. Chicken every week? Not in those days! Only on Christmas Day; you bought the chicken - straight from a farm, and you had to pluck, draw, and prepare it for the oven, yourself. Such early experiences, have a*

lasting effect. You can eat anything, make do with anything, and cope -
with anything! Due to the stress caused by the current crisis, our
schizophrenia sufferers, are, even more, schizophrenic, those with
anxiety, are, even more, anxious, and those with depression - are, even
more, depressed, but we are carrying on with our, essential work, for
mental health, and every morning, on the train, a cheerful message, from
the Government, is broadcast - thanking us for doing so.'

Our attitude is exactly that, described in the letter. We are making do,
during the Lockdown, and eating any food that we can get. In fact, just
as we used to sing, as young children, immediately after the War,
'Hurrah, Hurrah, We've Sausages For Tea'.

> *Hurrah, hurrah, we've sausages for tea.*
> *Hurrah, hurrah, we've beaten Germany.*

Glyn may have walked his twenty-four miles - just in order to access
our drop-in centre, but the inspiration of the moment, is, undoubtedly,
Captain Tom. We all, certainly, salute him - in gratitude for the, thirty-
three million, pounds that his walking, has raised, for the National
Health Service Charities. Now, with Michael Ball, he has also made a
recording of, 'You'll Never Walk Alone', which has reached, 'Number
One' in the Charts, and this, no doubt, will raise further millions of
pounds, for the Charities. The crowning moment was when, in July
2020, Captain Tom was dubbed 'Knight', by the Queen, in person, at
Windsor Castle.

> *Walk on, walk on,*
> *With hope in your heart,*
> *And you'll never walk alone,*

Compared with the, very sad, circumstances, of those who have lost
their lives, or who, like Rosie, [Please see: 'Further Tragic Stories'], the
lives of their loved ones, or those, who have been heartbroken, to see the
business, that they had worked so hard, to establish, and maintain, go
to the wall, a few minor inconveniences, caused by the pandemic, are
nothing. Nevertheless, one is used to one's creature comforts - such as
having one's hair cut, regularly. At last, in desperation, I have scraped
mine up, into an, unbecoming bun, at the back of my head. Until
normality is resumed, I shall have to grin, and bear it. I have sympathy,
with the sentiments, expressed by Tuppence Beresford, at the beginning

of Agatha Christie's collection of short stories, entitled, *'Partner in Crime'*. Agatha Christie writes:

'Six years ago, continued, Tuppence, I would have sworn, that, with sufficient money to buy things with, and, with you, for a husband, all life would have been, one grand, sweet, song, as one of the poets, you seem to know so much about, puts it'. 'Is it me, or the money, that palls upon you?' inquired Tommy, coldly. 'Palls', isn't exactly the word, said Tuppence, kindly. I'm just used to my blessings, that's all. Just as one never thinks what a boon, it is, to be able to breathe through one's nose, until one has, a cold in the head.'

So we will, walk on, putting up with minor inconveniences, and looking forward to the future, when we can see friends, and family, again, and when life, will be restored, to normal.

It was indeed, good, on 3rd July, to have further restrictions, lifted, so that Chris and Anna could visit the crisis house, once again. It was so good to have them back in our midst, and we had a genuine feeling, as a result, that, we were getting our old life back, with the friendship of dear old pals!

Dear old pals, jolly old pals. Clinging together, in all sorts of weather
Although a degree of normality has thus been restored to our lives, some restrictions, necessarily, continue. We are now wearing masks, on public transport, and, from 24th July, mandatorily, in shops. I think that people are being over-critical of Government advice - claiming that it is confusing. Scientific evidence, as to the value of mask-wearing, has varied, and extra time given, though criticised, for people who had not already done so, to obtain masks, before they became mandatory, was, in my opinion, a sensible measure. Human beings need time to adapt to things, and one of the problems with the coronavirus pandemic, has been, the rapidity, with which people have had to adapt to the new ways of behaving. We are fortunate, at the crisis house, that we have several rooms, in which people can sit, so social distancing hasn't been a problem for us. At one juncture, during the pandemic, I thought that the mandatory wearing of masks, might make people feel complacent, and so, bother, less, with social distancing. Now, I believe that their value, as well as physically reducing infection, is one of keeping people aware. You are wearing a mask; everyone around you, is wearing a mask; so you stay aware, that the virus, still threatens. As we await the visit from

Tommy Warfield's Care Co-ordinator, to look at our Covid Safety Procedures, we think it possible that the wearing of masks, indoors, may be recommended. Up until now, we have made their wearing voluntary. Some do, and some don't. Such a new rule, would not, I believe, present us with too much of a problem.

Occasionally, I write to *The Wokingham Paper*, on a topic which is of more general concern, and not directly connected with our work at the crisis house. Through letters to the Paper, I joined in the current debate about the removal of statues of national heroes. I pointed out, that nothing can be gained by destroying monuments to great figures from history - particularly those, like Admiral Lord Nelson, who achieved such spectacular victories - through his naval prowess. Modern images which inspire us, are those like the picture of the black man - rescuing a white man, from mob violence. In this instance, it wasn't a case of 'White man's burden', but rather, it was a case of 'Black man's burden'. Such should be our memories of 2020 - not the destruction of our history. The following song salutes Admiral Lord Nelson, and other such national, naval, heroes.

> *Sons of the sea–*
> *all British born –*
> *Sailing every ocean –*
> *laughing foes to scorn.*

Rod Stewart, expresses similar sentiments, in a more modern idiom, and, indeed, the Task Force, sang 'Sailing', as they set forth, to liberate the Falkland Islands.

> *We are sailing, we are sailing*
> *Home again,*
> *'Cross the sea.*
> *We are sailing,*
> *Stormy waters,*
> *To be near you,*
> *To be free.*

'I emphasised, that we don't want white supremacy, but we don't want, black supremacy, either, and we most certainly, don't want, mob, supremacy! What is needed, is the equal treatment, of all citizens, under the law, and this is not achieved, by acts of vandalism.'

Certainly, great figures, from history, behaved inappropriately, as the following, comic song, illustrates. Our history is both rich, and colourful, and not to be lightly abandoned!

> *In the tower of London,*
> *large as life,*
> *the ghost of Anne Boleyn*
> *walks they declare.*
> *With her head tucked,*
> *underneath her arm,*
> *she walks the bloody tower.*

On the subject of racism, and the, equal value, of all human lives, we need to learn wisdom 'out of the mouths of babes, and sucklings'. Do not small children, in Sunday School, sing this song?

> *Jesus died for all the children,*
> *all the children of the world.*

Some things, mistaken as racist, are nothing of the kind. Our members say that they were forbidden, by their parents, to watch the television programme, 'Till Death Us Do Part' - because it was racist. Johnny Speight wasn't racist. In his programme, it was the racist bigot who was being ridiculed - not the people of ethnic minorities!

Our campaign for mental health, through letters to *The Wokingham Paper*, continues, as the following letter, published on 30th July 2020, July, illustrates.

Mental Health Awareness
'We persevere, manfully, with our campaign to educate the public about mental health - through 'Wokingham Today'. In particular, we endeavour to show, how common, mental health problems are. Due to the stresses imposed by the coronavirus pandemic, the statistic has actually increased. You only have to read the report in last week's edition, to realise how busy the Wokingham Citizen's Advice has been - dealing with the increased volume of enquiries, and if anyone doubts that a younger person, can take over a service, successfully, as an older person retires, then you need look, no further, than at the Wokingham Citizen's Advice. It WAS one in four people who would, at some time, suffer from a mental health problem - hence our former campaign -

being entitled - 'One In Four'. Now the number is something nearer to 'One In Three'! Psychiatric rehabilitation, is neither speedy, nor magical. On the contrary, it is slow, laborious, painful, and is achieved, not all at once, but in stages. The fourth stage, is returning to full-time paid employment, and thus, getting off benefits, and off dependence upon tax-payers. Not everyone achieves this - though it is always our goal and ambition - particularly for younger people. I tell our members, regularly, 'If you work - then you are normal, in the eyes of society.' It is, indeed, the case, that nothing is worse for mental health, than sitting around, isolated, staring at the wall, and thinking about yourself, and nothing is better for mental health, than being fully, and gainfully, occupied!'

Of course, there have been tragedies, and many sad things, occurring, because of the coronavirus pandemic, but we are determined to look on the bright side, and stay cheerful. The songs - with which this book abounds, help us to keep cheerful, and to keep going!

Look for the silver lining,
Whenever a cloud
appears in the blue.

The British Red Cross, celebrated its one hundred and fiftieth anniversary, on Tuesday 4th August, 2020. We are particularly grateful, to this organisation, so I wrote the following letter, of which I include part, to *The Wokingham Paper* - expressing our gratitude.

'I should like to join the ranks, of all those people, congratulating the British Red Cross, on its recent, one hundred and fiftieth anniversary. We owe a particular, debt of gratitude, to the Wokingham Branch of the British Red Cross - because they helped our Association, to get established. We were founded in 1987, but we didn't have, a regular base, until 1989. when we applied to the British Red Cross - to hire their hall, in Denmark Street, as a drop-in centre. So, we then spent, two, very happy, years, at the British Red Cross - until we moved into Station House, in 1991. Their ladies were very kind, and I have, fond memories, of Joyce, Mavis, and Anne. After leaving them, we kept in touch, and the Wokingham Branch of the British Red Cross, came up trumps, once again, in 2007, when it appeared that we would have to leave Station House, because its electricity supply, was to be disconnected. The Red Cross offered to have us back, if necessary. Fortunately, we were able to solve the electricity problem, but it was good, for our vulnerable

members, to know, that alternative accommodation would be available, if we had to leave, Station House. So we send the British Red Cross, hearty congratulations, on their anniversary. In these times, of the coronavirus, crisis, their services, have never been more necessary - both locally, and, globally.'

The Wokingham Paper, on 27th August 2020, reported that 'Black Lives Matter' was to hold a demonstration, at Elms Field, in Wokingham. This stimulated me to write a letter to the Paper, and this was published on Thursday 3rd September 2020. I point out, that perhaps, it hadn't been such a 'land of hope and glory', for the majority of people, but also, as the song, 'Strolling', avers, people who have had very little, are content with the simple things, and it is those who have lost their former wealth, who suffer most in economic crisis.

> *Land of Hope and Glory,*
> *Mother of the free,*
> *How shall we extol thee,*
> *Who are born of thee?*

> *Strolling, just strolling,*
> *In the cool of the evening air,*
> *I don't envy the rich in their automobiles,*
> *For a motor car is phoney.*
> *I'd rather have Shanks's pony.*

> *Rule, Britannia, Britannia rule the waves.*
> *Britons, never, never, never, shall be slaves.*

There can be no harm in our continuing to sing, traditional, patriotic songs, but our aim, through appropriate laws, is that nobody should be a slave. Even so, the words of John Bunyan's hymn, remain as pertinent, now, as they did when he wrote them, in the seventeenth century.

> *He that is down need fear no fall.*
> *I am content with what I have,*
> *Little be it or much;*
> *And, Lord, contentment still I crave,*
> *Because thou savest such.*

The pandemic has restricted, all but, the most essential, travel, for everyone, but we look forward to the time, when we can travel the world, again, or even, as this letter indicates, make the most of our own, natural, beauty spots. On this subject, my letter, which follows, was published in 'Wokingham Today', on Thursday 8th October 2020.

'I read, in 'Wokingham Today' (1st October), that your reader, Jan Francis, would like letters, on subjects, other than the Wokingham Borough Council, debates. How about the following subject - for something, completely different? We have recruited, a new volunteer, who has come here, recently, from South Africa. She is not familiar with the British Isles, but we have our beauty spots. At present, all travel is restricted, but we are advising her, as to the most beautiful places to visit - once restrictions, lift. I would start with, Wordsworth country, the Lake District, and then, move down, to beautiful Snowdonia. How about, the wild, rugged, beauty, of Cornwall - Daphne Du Maurier, country? In complete contrast, there is the, green, beauty, of the West of Ireland - see, the sun, go down, on Galway Bay! If you want something nearer, you can't beat , the charming, Cotswolds - such gentle, rolling, hills. But, if I have to advise anyone, on the most beautiful place, in the whole of the British Isles, then you'll take the high road, and I'll take the low road - to the bonnie, bonnie, banks, of Loch Lomond! For breathtaking, beauty, you can't beat Scotland! Have you ever visited, the Isle of Iona, and looked out, across the sea, to the Isle of Staffa - wherein is Fingal's Cave? Inspiration for Mendelssohn's composition, 'The Hebrides Overture', both the places, and his music, are, unutterably beautiful.'

The beauty of Scotland, has inspired many songs - of which the following, are, just five, of my favourites.

> *Maxwellton braes are bonnie,*
> *Where early fa's the dew,*
> *And 'twas there that Annie Laurie*
> *Gave me her promise true.*

> *Speed, bonnie boat, like a bird on the wing,*
> *Onward! the sailors cry;*
> *Carry the lad that's born to be king*
> *Over the sea to Skye.*

When the long shadows fall, and the sun goes to rest,
Behind the dark Cuillins, away in the West.
And its beautiful Mary, so lonely for by,
Since you left me, alone, on the Island of Skye.

Mull of Kintyre, oh mist rolling in from the sea,
My desire is always to be here,
Oh Mull of Kintyre.

Oh if I could stay forever,
near to the Sound of Iona.
I would leave you never, never,
lovely Sound of Iona.

PART TEN

Students at the Crisis House

Chapter 30

Students Over The Last Five Years

We greatly enjoy having Reading University's students on Placement at the crisis house. These are second year undergraduate psychology students, and Master's students - specialising in clinical aspects of psychology, or in psychopathology. There is no doubt about it. Education has evolved. When I served on the National Schizophrenia Fellowship's National Council, I had a friend, then, who would be, as I write this in 2019, aged one hundred and eleven - were he alive today. He told me, that in his young days, university degrees were so rare, that, having attended Marlborough Public School - where he had shared a sixth form study with Anthony Blunt, the spy, and then achieved an Oxford University degree, by the age of twenty-six, he was virtually running the Foreign Office! He served in the Diplomatic Service, and was awarded the Honour - CMG - Commander of the Order of St. Michael and St. George - a very high distinction! Even in my young days, though becoming much more commonly held, a good Honours degree guaranteed one, a good, well-paid job. Fifty years on, I am of the opinion that an undergraduate degree, nowadays, is the equivalent of what five 'O' levels would have been, fifty years ago - simply giving one, a slight edge, over those who held no qualifications, at all! In a even earlier, era, the School Certificate gave the same, slight, advantage. A Master's degree, now, in terms of the jobs it will achieve for you, is the equivalent of 'A' Levels, or the former, Matric. A PhD. now gives you the advantage that an undergraduate degree did in my young days, but you practically reach the age of thirty, before you can achieve this qualification, and most of our Master's students don't want to do it!

My views are echoed by those of Patrick Small - [Please see: 'Five Success Stories']. He worked for fifteen years as a technical photographer, at Kew Gardens, and it was his redundancy from this job, that contributed to his mental breakdown - from which he is, now, recovering. When he started there, two 'A' Levels would secure a job, that now requires a Master's degree for entry, and no senior position can now be held by anyone without a PhD.

Chapter 31

Students: 2016 - 2017

Zac

I have told the Student Placement Officers at Reading University that their youngsters do us good - just by walking through the door - and no one could illustrate this, more perfectly, than Zac. Tall, blond, good looking, affable - with such a nice, friendly, approach to people - he would make the perfect therapist. After completing his, Master's Psychology Placement, with us, he took a post with Oxford University's 'Student Counselling Service' - working on social skills training, with undergraduates on the autism spectrum. Since Zac is the personification of social skill - this would be the ideal occupation for him!

Sara

Sara came to Reading University from the Lebanon - where she had taken an Undergraduate Degree, in Psychology, and was now embarking upon her Master's Degree. She fitted in with us, very well, and was popular with our service users. Having achieved her Master's Degree, she went on to take an Assistant Psychologist post - with a Health Authority.

Hadi

Hadi was also from the American University, from the Lebanon, also fitted in very well, and was equally popular with our service users. But there is one thing that intrigues me about these foreigners! What is it that they have - that we don't - so that they are able to master several foreign languages - with such ease? Hadi was fluent in English, French, German, Polish, and Arabic! What a godsend, he must be, to any Health Authority, lucky enough, to recruit him. How do they do it? In school, as well as learning English - throughout my education, I learned French for seven years, Latin for four years, and German, for one year. I am able to struggle around Paris - my French, sufficient, for me to order meals, to ask for things in shops, and hotels, and to negotiate, the geography, of the city! I can find the occasional, apposite, Latin quotation, and my year's German – amounts to '*Guten Tag*', *Auf Wiedersehen*!' '*Bitte*', and '*Danke Schon*!' These are my linguistic limits! Not so, Sara and Hadi, and indeed, the numerous other foreign students, whom we have welcomed, on placement, in the crisis house. Having completed his Placement with us, and achieved his Psychology Master's degree, Hadi also took a post as an Assistant Psychologist with a Health Authority. English people's failure to master other languages, and, the consequent, disadvantages suffered, were noted, by Agatha Christie, in her collection of short stories, entitled, '*The Labours of Hercules*'. Due to ignorance of languages, other than English, Harold Waring, became the victim of a confidence trick. Hercule Poirot, who solved the mystery, and rescued Harold from the tricksters' clutches, said to him:

'You must not go through life, being too credulous, my friend. The Police of a country are not so easily bribed - they are probably not to be bribed at all - certainly not when it's a question of murder! These women trade upon the average Englishman's ignorance of foreign languages.'..... 'Harold Waring drew a deep breath'. He said crisply: 'I'm going to set to work, and learn every European language there is! Nobody's going to make a fool of me, a second time!'

Jeremy

Jeremy was a mature student, and, like so many people, who have recovered from mental health problems, wished then, to qualify in mental health, and so help others to recover. Thus, he had chosen to obtain a Psychology Degree, and then go on to psychotherapy training. He spoke very highly of the Cardinal Clinic in Windsor - where he had received excellent treatment.

Jess

Jess was taking an Undergraduate Degree in Psychology - with a view to going into counselling. Amusingly enough, I remember, the comments that she made, about a Wedding Outfitters, where she worked - in order to cope with her student expenses. She commented, that couples would spend fifty thousand pounds, on a wedding, and then have nowhere of their own to live. We all agreed that, the fifty thousand pounds, would be much more wisely spent, as a deposit on buying a property, and unless rolling in money, it might be wiser to plump for a simpler, and cheaper, wedding. Jess was so pleasant and sensible, that we very much liked having her, as a student, on placement, with us. In 2019, we received an update on Jess. She had been participating in Charlie's research project for his Master's degree, and he was able to tell us that Jess, having successfully completed both her undergraduate, and Master's degrees, is now embarking upon a PhD, in September 2019.

Chapter 32

Students: 2017 - 2018

Anika

Anika was taking her Degree in Psychology, at Reading University - having failed to get into university, in her native Germany. There, higher education is free, but much more difficult to get into. Here, we have adopted, the American system - easy to get into, but very costly. Anika spoke perfect English, as well as perfect German, so she did very well. She obtained a post in, Human Resources, with the German scientific company, Siemens. Able to be interviewed in German, she was a gift to them. Psychology and languages - an excellent combination!

Georgia

Georgia wanted to go into forensic psychology, and, being one of the four hundred applicants applying for such a post at Broadmoor Hospital, and getting down to a shortlist of twelve, we considered that she had done well. She didn't get the post, but it was, nevertheless, a creditable achievement. On graduating, Georgia took a post with the Berkshire Health Authority - working with young people with mood and behavioural disorders. This was not exactly, her first choice, of forensic psychology, but was, nevertheless, excellent experience, to get under her belt.

Lucy

Lucy was a, very pleasant, young undergraduate - with the usual ambition of going into counselling and psychotherapy. I have just given her a glowing reference - to work with children with autism, and I look forward, to hearing, whether she obtains this post.

Niamh

Niamh was, an excellent, undergraduate psychology student, and was actually instrumental, in setting up, an in-house, mental health association, for Reading University students. We all believed that she would, go far, in the field of mental health. Sometimes, we are a trifle sad. Some of these top, dynamic, students would make excellent teachers - Niamh would - but they don't want to do it! Teaching is, no longer, the obvious choice of career, for university graduates, that it once was.

Aimie

Aimie, once she had completed her Undergraduate Psychology Degree, was intent upon a career in mental health nursing. This is always a very sensible choice. The National Health Service is always short of nurses, and they can always get jobs - which is not, sad to relate, the case with psychologists!

Chapter 33

Students: 2018 - 2019

Indiana

Indiana, was a very vivacious, Master's Psychology student. We thought that she would be excellent - working either with adults, or with children. Nevertheless, the competition is so fierce, that she had trouble, getting a job. Prior to taking her degrees, she had some experience of working with children, and, eventually, she was successful in obtaining a post as a Teaching Assistant. Our Lucy Farmer, corresponds with Indiana on Facebook, and reports that she is, having a wonderful time, as a party girl! It is true that Indiana just scraped through her exams, but nevertheless had good social skills - which are valuable in the work with children in which she is now engaged. One's own youth, remains, so vividly, in one's memory, that it is hard to conceive, that the fashions of yesteryear, mean nothing, a generation, or two, on. 'The Beatles - weren't they popular in the nineteen-thirties?' Indiana enquired, in all innocence. I assured her, that for those of us who were there, The Beatles, will remain the quintessence of the nineteen-sixties, to the end of our lives!

Kirsty

I wrote glowing references for Kirsty. She wanted to work with 'excluded' children - helping them to improve their behaviour, and so get back into mainstream education. She didn't obtain the first post, that she applied for, but she did obtain the second. I made them all laugh, because I said that I would not like teaching children with behavioural problems. I would prefer a nice, private school - where they are all well-behaved, and, if they are not, you get rid of them. Apparently, this is not politically correct, but, nevertheless, it is the truth! In September 2019, Kirsty informed us that, having now achieved some experience as a Teaching Assistant, she has embarked upon a Teacher Training Course. This is good news. Then, on Tuesday 16th June 2020, Lucy, who has kept in touch with Kirsty, on Facebook, was able to bring us the good news, that Kirsty, is now, a fully qualified, teacher!

This news is most gratifying, because I have, a poignant memory, of Kirsty - sitting in the crisis house lounge, and saying, bitterly, 'I have done everything that the education system has required of me - GCSE's, A Levels, Undergraduate Degree, and Master's Degree, and now, I can't get a job.' As I have explained, she got one, shortly after this, and now is launching into a worthwhile profession - which justifies all the hard work that she has put in. Kirsty is now teaching psychology, at The Holt School, in Wokingham. The Holt, is a very good school, and one attended, by my own great niece. Kirsty is also, with her partner, buying a house, in Wokingham, so she is, what we want, for all of them - successfully launched, into the adult world!

Cherish

Lucy Farmer, our excellent befriender, groans whenever Cherish's name is mentioned. I think that she is our only student - ever - who had no interest, whatsoever, in the people attending the crisis house, and spent all her time with us, on her mobile phone, bored stiff, and, so obviously, only clocking up the hours, that she was required to do - in order to obtain her Master's Degree. She had taken her Undergraduate Degree in Psychology in Nigeria, and I thought that she might be experiencing, some culture shock - not really understanding what we were about. She had passed her Master's theory exams at Reading, so, in the end, I, reluctantly allowed her to pass - by awarding her fifty percent - the lowest pass mark, for her Placement with us. One mark less, and she would have failed! Lucy believed that I should have failed her! 'But look', I said, 'she has paid a lot of money, for the Course, and has passed her exams. She is never going to be a psychologist, anyway, because she is incapable of communication with people, so why should we deprive her of her bit of paper? She will never be able to use it in any practical way, but, possibly, she might decide to go into research.' The uselessness of 'bits of paper', I described cogently, in the chapter, entitled, 'Give a Dog a Bone' - from 'Twenty-Five Funny Stories' in *Triumph and Tragedy*.

Debbie

Debbie was an undergraduate psychology student, and I can recall her, just like Kirsty, stating, despondently, that everyone has a degree, nowadays, and that it is, not easy, to get into the field of work, that one would like. I was, therefore, delighted, to hear from Debbie, in August 2020. She said that she had achieved, a second class, undergraduate, degree, and had achieved her highest grade for this, with her module for the Placement at the crisis house. As a result of this success, she had been accepted for a Master's course in Sports Psychology, at Staffordshire University. Debbie has, wisely, chosen to combine theory, with practice, so, in addition to pursuing further training, she has applied for a job, as a support worker, for a person, suffering from head injury, and I have supplied a good reference for her - in order for her to obtain this post.

Chapter 34

Students: 2019 - 2020

Charlie

Charlie was a Master's Psychology student, who joined us, on Placement, in 2019. He was very pleasant and affable, and fitted in extremely well. He was very taken with my book, *Triumph and Tragedy*. As well as all the laughs - such as 'five years' out-of-date calendars' on the walls of statutory mental health services, and 'plants dying in their pots - because nobody had been funded to water them' - he was amazed that Wokingham Borough Council could sacrifice four mental health crisis beds - for the sake of two thousand pounds per year! How wonderful, to be twenty-two, to be young, to think that the world is a good place, and human beings full of good will! In fact, there are no limits to the destructive powers, of jealous, and vindictive, human beings. As Miss Marple says in the short story - 'The Blood-Stained Pavement' from Agatha Christie's, *The Thirteen Problems*':

'There is a great deal of wickedness in village life. I hope you dear young people will never realise how very wicked the world is.'

Similarly, in the short story, 'Sing a Song of Sixpence' - by Agatha Christie - in the collection of short stories, entitled, *'The Listerdale Mystery'*, Sir Edward Palliser, K.C., had been very captivated by the young, and innocent, Magdalen Vaughan, when they had met, on a trip home from America. He had said, then, that if ever she needed help, and if there was anything, in the world, that he could do for her, he would do it. When she approached him for such help - some nine or ten years later - Agatha Christie writes:

'He flashed a quick glance at her - she was still a very good-looking girl, but she had lost what had been to him her charm - that look of dewy, untouched, youth. It was a more interesting face now . . . but Sir Edward was far from feeling the tide of warmth and emotion that had been his at the end of that Atlantic voyage.'

I actually told, the Placements Officer, from Reading University, when she attended one of our Open Days, that her students do us good - by just walking through the door! We share the feelings, of Sir Edward Palliser, for the young and beautiful. Mature students may be equally conscientious, and equally, helpful, but, like Magdalen Vaughan, they have lost that look of dewy, untouched, youth - and thus the ability to brighten up our lives!

Charlie completed his Placement, with us, on Friday 31st August. I had recommended to him, that he apply to the Maudsley Hospital - London University's, top, mental health, teaching hospital - for a position as Assistant Psychologist. He did this, and also applied to St. George's Hospital, Tooting. His girlfriend is working in London, so Charlie wants to be near her, and has also arranged to share a flat with a friend - in order to share the high rent. We believe that Charlie will get a job in London, and are confident that he will have, a successful career, in clinical psychology. In January 2020, Charlie had applied for a post - supporting patients with head injuries, and we were able to provide a good reference for this.

Valenka

Valenka completed her Placement, with us, in August 2019. She fitted in very well, was very pleasant, and also had achieved some very useful experience - working at St. Andrew's Forensic mental health hospital, working with children, and also working in elderly health care. She applied for posts - both in Bristol, and, nearer her, Swindon home - at Devizes. We are confident of her success - wherever she is employed.

Vasiliki

Vasiliki had taken her, Undergraduate Degree in Psychology, at the University of Athens, and had then come, to Reading, to complete her Master's Degree. She proved to be not quite so fluent, in English, as some of our other foreign students, on Placement, have been. In May 2019, she expressed anxiety - because she was having to sit her first exam – writing answers in English. We encouraged her. 'You'll be able to write it, in English, a whole lot better, than we could do, in Greek!' we said. This encouragement was quite sincere. How do they do it - these foreigners? Psychology requires good mathematical, and statistical skills, scientific knowledge, and linguistic skills. Imagine us, having to bone up, on all that stuff - and then have to write about it - in Arabic or in Greek! These foreign languages don't even use the same alphabet as ours! Vasiliki applied to King's College, London, to undertake, a second Master's Degree, in family therapy. They placed her on their waiting list, for a place, and, if successful, she arranged to share accommodation, with two fellow students, who were also planning to work in London. Vasiliki is aged twenty-seven, so it is a fact that, when she completes this second Master's degree, she will be approaching the age of thirty, before her career commences!

This is why, so few of our students, wish to proceed to PhD studies. It takes up too much life. Charlie, in particular, was champing at the bit, to be done with it all, and to get on with, normal, working life!

I have high-lighted this current situation where all jobs require a degree, and some require three, in the following letter to *The Wokingham Paper*.

'Local Police have told me that the Thames Valley Force is having difficulty in getting people to join - now that their Recruitment Budget has been slashed, and that new entrants must hold a degree. The Lincolnshire Police Force have taken a step further. They are questioning, the new qualification requirement, in Court - arguing that

Policing skills are better learned on the job. It is true that - in these days - where every second person has a degree - youngsters often end up, with having lots of qualifications that they can't use, and not having the qual - ifications, that they actually need! This debate takes me back sixty years - to when I was a youngster in school, and we were given Careers Talks. On one such occasion, the career being suggested, was mental health nursing. 'You don't have to have 'O' Levels, [then, the equivalent of a modern degree], for entry', said the Speaker. The Headmistress of the school - who was, herself, an M.A. [Oxon], interposed immediately. 'That doesn't apply to any of us', she said, patronisingly. Then, the Speaker took her to task - not something that one did with impunity! 'The qualities that are needed for passing examinations, are not, necessarily, the qualities that are needed for mental health nursing', she retorted! That Careers Adviser, of sixty years ago, had put her finger on the nub of the matter. I, personally, happen to be academic. I can write for England, and it flows from me, like a stream - without effort, but this doesn't mean that I fail to appreciate people who are not academic – but have other skills. We won't go back to the system, where very few people held formal qualifications. It is like cars. Everybody agrees, that it would be better, to have fewer cars on the road, but nobody wants to give up their own! So what is the solution? I happen to believe that a good education is a good thing in itself - whatever occupation it leads to, so I have nothing against a person being an M.A. [Oxon]. But what we need to do, is to value the vocational qualifications as highly as the academic ones. This is already the case in Germany, and explains why their technical skills are unrivalled - throughout the world. But this parity of esteem must be genuine. Institutions that provide vocational courses and practical training, should be renamed - 'Technical Universities', and the certificates that they award, should be renamed - 'Vocational Degrees'. Only then, will people accept their equality of status, with those of academic institutions. Even with such a reform, I have long held the view, that with some occupations - typically, teaching and nursing - you either are one, or you're not one, and all the training, and degrees, in the world, will not make you into one, if you're not one! Our best qualified member has three degrees - one in philosophy, from Trinity College, Cambridge, one in Physics, from King's College, London, and then, a Master's Degree in Engineering. His favourite aphorism is - 'It takes a really clever person to be a perfect fool!'

Boris Johnson's commitment, in August 2019, to pumping considerable extra funding into vocational training, does, at least, indicate that the Government is aware of the skills shortage, and that 'Mickey Mouse', university degrees, are precisely that - bits of paper! Nevertheless, we greatly enjoy having students on Placement with us - academic or not.

Chapter 35

Students: 2020 - 2021

Exactly as predicted, we had, about a dozen, Reading University students express an interest in a Placement, at the crisis house, during 2020, and, as usual, five - two undergraduates, and three Master's Psychology students, eventually, availed themselves, of the offer. Also, as in all previous years, all proved to be charming, and to fit in with us, perfectly!

Lucy is an undergraduate student - taking, a basic, degree in psychology Her studies continue, but on-line - due to the coronavirus pandemic.

Toni is an undergraduate student - also taking a basic degree in psychology Her studies also continue, on-line.

Unfortunately, due to the coronavirus pandemic, Lucy and Toni's Placements, with us, had to be truncated, as Reading University, like everyone, entered Lockdown, and both students returned home.

Danae, whose home is in Cyprus - has come to England to study. She is a Master's psychology student. Again, Danae's Placement, had to be suspended. Nevertheless, I was determined that her time, with us, would be properly appreciated, and I submitted, a glowing, 'exit report', to the university, on her behalf, in August 2020, and sent to her, now back in Cyprus, all our good wishes for her future. In her 'exit' report, I explained how useful, it was, for Danae to get practical experience of conditions, such as acute schizophrenia - as a basis for her future career in clinical psychology.

Nerisha, whose home is in Kuala Lumpa - in Malaysia - but who has come to England to study - is also a Master's Psychology student. Nerisha stayed in England throughout Lockdown, but, as I have explained, has been supporting one of our self-isolating members, by telephone. However, she is intending to return to Malaysia, to complete her degree. Nerisha duly returned to Malaysia on 30th June 2020 and, on 9th July, I completed, for the University, her Exit Report - which was glowing, and recommended her, strongly, for a career in mental health. In this Report, I explained, that a career in mental health, resembles, those in teaching, and in nursing. Some teachers only like teaching very able, pupils, while some will, happily, teach slow learners. Some nurses prefer acute medicine, and surgery, while some will nurse in hospices. Similarly, some mental health workers prefer working with those who, with support, will recover completely, while some are happy to work with the chronically mentally ill. Placements with us, help students to make their choice.

Sarina is also a Master's Psychology Student, and also had to discontinue her Placement with us, due to the coronavirus pandemic. I also heard from her on 9th July, and agreed, happily, to be a referee - since she has applied for a post of Assistant Psychologist, with the NHS. In August 2020, I also submitted a glowing 'exit report', for Sarina - explaining how useful, her experience, on Placement with us, had been. Then, in November 2020, I submitted a further glowing reference for Sarina. She is one of the few who has decided to embark on a PhD Course - for which, I wish her every success.

One invaluable contribution that students, on Placement at the crisis house, make - is their ready mastery of technology. They are easily able to get 'on line' with service users, and so access information, for them. My technological abilities, just about match those of my driving abilities - [Please see, the chapter in *'Triumph and Tragedy'*, entitled - 'Paddle Your Own Canoe']. Not having become familiar with mobile phones, I was, particularly challenged, during January and February 2020. Open Reach were upgrading the telephone technology, and the old service was made redundant, by them, before the new technology was fully in place. So for seven weeks, we were without internet, and without, land-line, telephone contact. This didn't cause problems for our service users - all of whom have smart phones, but new people, in crisis, who needed to contact us, were, unfortunately, unable to do so. It was a great relief to have the service restored on 19th February 2020. For an amusing description of our plight, - [|Please see: 'More Funny Stories - The Political Telephone!'].

The dangers of over-reliance on technology, were identified, as early as half a century ago, by Agatha Christie, in her novel, 'The Pale Horse'. Agatha Christie writes:

'Even the minor domestic noises of today, beneficial in action, though they may be, yet carry a kind of alert. The dishwashers, the refrigerators, the pressure cookers, the whining vacuum cleaners - 'Be careful,' they all seem to say. 'I am a genie, harnessed to your service, but if your control of me, fails. . .' A dangerous world, that was it - a dangerous world.'

The way that I perceive our reliance on technology, is not so much that of danger, as that of our total helplessness - when a technology, which we have taken for granted, and become, totally reliant, upon, suddenly, is no longer there! I confess to being a dinosaur. Indeed, I have much, in common, with Inspector Neele, who appears in Agatha Christie's novel, 'A Pocket Full of Rye'. Inspector Neele is visiting Yewtree Lodge - in the pursuit of his murder investigation. Agatha Christie writes:

'Inspector Neele, surveying the house, was saying to himself, 'Call it a lodge, indeed! Yewtree Lodge! The affectation of these rich people.' The house was what he, Inspector Neele, would call a mansion. He knew what a lodge was. He'd been brought up in one. . . Mrs. Neele had never discovered the pleasures of electric irons, slow combustion stoves, airing cupboards, hot and cold water, from taps, and the switching on of light, by a mere flick of a finger. In winter, the Neeles had an oil lamp, and, in summer, they went to bed when it got dark. They were a healthy family, and a happy one, all thoroughly, behind the times.'

Roll time forward, and, in the twenty-first century, I am the same. I live without, mobiles, smart phones, videolinks, wi-fi, WhatsApp, and streaming. I rely on an old, landline telephone, in order to communicate, with people, and I am, perfectly happy, the way I am.

Due to the coronavirus pandemic, Reading University closed, in March 2020, and all tuition was to be provided, on line. This also meant that our 2020 students could not continue with their Placements - for the time being. I have been able to organise some telephone contact, between students, and our service users, and this will count towards Placement hours. Fortunately, on 13th April, the Placements Officer, from Reading University, contacted me - to thank me for arranging telephone contact, and saying that, in the exceptional circumstances, they were reducing the number of Placement hours that students would be required to complete - in order to obtain their degrees. Great relief, for all concerned!

PART ELEVEN

Chapter 36

Annual Reports: 2015 - 2020

I am happy to report on excellent years throughout 2015 to 2019, and on an excellent, if somewhat, unusual year, for 2020 - during which, all the Wokingham and West Berkshire Mental Health Association services, have been very well-used. All the history, written in the 2015 - 2019, Reports, is covered, elsewhere, in this narrative. The history for 2020, follows.

Annual Report: 1st November 2019 - 31st October 2020

Drop-In Centre

The decision, which we charity trustees, took, in March 2020, to keep the drop-in centre open, as usual, was based on what is now known, in the new jargon, as 'focussed protection'. The very old, and physically vulnerable, must shield, and be supported, by telephone and videolink. For younger, physically healthy, but mentally vulnerable people, the mental health risks of social isolation, outweigh, the physical risks of coronavirus, so the drop-in centre has been kept open for them, and we have formed, what is known in the new jargon, as a 'bubble'. We have support, for our decision, from very august, quarters. Prince William, has announced, that to deprive human beings of social interaction, is to cause a mental health catastrophe. We have been able to keep all the rules – hand-washing, social distancing, and face coverings, where appropriate, and these have been facilitated, by reduced numbers, attending the drop-in centre. Despite all, from November 2019 to October 2020, attendance at the drop-in centre, and people receiving help, from our services, reached a total of one thousand, seven hundred, and twenty-two.

Crisis Intervention, Information, and Advocacy
This service expanded greatly, throughout the year, and is covered, in detail, in our chapter, on Advocacy.

Befriending
This service also continued, successfully, and is described, in our chapter on Befriending.

Station House
Throughout 2019 to 2020, we have stuck to our policy, of carrying out, only essential repairs to Station House, which, nevertheless, continues to serve our purposes, well.

Pets as Therapy
Old Ferris, the cat, continues to delight our service users. Early in 2020, our budgie passed away, at the ripe old age, of sixteen. I had intended to obtain a new pair of budgies, but put this, on hold, due to the coronavirus crisis. Our goldfish continue to be a popular feature of the drop-in lounge - with their soothing, and calming, effect.

Finances
It has been a good year for finances, and this has been described, in detail, in our chapters on 'Benefactors'. As a result, we have been able to continue, the private treatment, for one service user, whose Health Insurance had expired, to pay for another to attend Counselling Training, and also, to buy carpets, and pay the removal expenses, for a service user who was moving into a new flat, and had no other means of support.

Obituaries
We were sorry, this year, to hear that Gary Gardiner, [Gee-Gee], had passed away, and that Ethel Heyes had died - after a battle with cancer. Gary is remembered, in our chapter, entitled, 'Further Tragic Stories', and Ethel, is remembered, in our chapters, entitled, 'Obituaries at the end of long lives'.

Students on Placement
Unfortunately, student placements had to be curtailed - due to the pandemic, but, for the time that they were with us, 2020 students are

described, in our chapters on 'Students at the Crisis House'.

Publication of Book
This was submitted to the Publisher in November 2020 - for publication, in March 2021 - the thirty-year anniversary, of the crisis house.

Thirty Year Anniversary of the Crisis House
We hope to have a proper celebration, and a Book Launch, as we did for the twenty-five year anniversary, but, in these uncertain times, one is unable to plan ahead, as one would like. If a vaccine becomes available in early 2021, then normality can return.

Christmas
Our Christmas 2019, party, included our usual happy throng, with Lady Elizabeth, and her daughter, attending, and distributing the presents, as has always been our tradition.

Unfortunately, due to social distancing restrictions, we cannot hold our regular, big, Christmas Party, in 2020, but we will still have a Christmas Tree, cards, and presents. So a 'mini' party will be held, on Tuesday 22nd December. I shall come over on Thursday 24th December, to see to the animals, and we shall re-open on Monday 28th December. This is a Bank Holiday, in lieu of Boxing Day, but we always open on Bank Holidays, and are closed, only, on Christmas Day and Boxing Day, itself.

Vote of Thanks
Gratitude and thanks, to all our supporters, our expressed, warmly, throughout this, entire book - to which I just add, a Vote of Thanks, for the year, 2019 to 2020.

PART TWELVE

Benefactors

'You've got to have something in the Bank, Frank'!

*'You've got to have something
in the bank, Frank,
You've got to have something,
to start,*

*When you have something
in the bank Frank,
I'll give you my heart.*

Chapter 37

Money In The Bank

*There's a place for Us, a time and a place for Us.
Hold my hand and we're halfway there.
Hold my hand, and I'll take you there.*

Never were truer words spoken, than those of that song - 'You've got to have something in the bank.' Without the generosity of our benefactors, the crisis house would never have been able to continue for thirty years. Every year, we experience their financial support for us, and we are most appreciative of it. In her novel, '*The Man in the Brown Suit*', Agatha Christie writes - of Ann Beddingfeld:

'I've always longed for adventures. My father, Professor Beddingfeld, was one of England's greatest living authorities on Primitive Man. Papa did not care for modern man. Unfortunately, one cannot entirely dispense with modern men. One is forced to have some kind of truck with butchers, and bakers, and milkmen, and greengrocers.'

I am in full sympathy with Professor Beddingfeld! I am very happy to 'have truck' with those who support us, financially, and with people whom we need, for practical assistance, in running the crisis house. But I have no desire, whatsoever, to form any other networks, nor liaisons. Separatist, I shall always be! We can only continue our vital service, if we can continue to pay the bills, so 'Money, Money, Money', is something that is always in our thoughts, and on our agenda!

*Money, money, money,
Must be funny,
In the rich man's world.*

259

Chapter 38

Benefactors: 2016 - 2017

Our first major fund-raiser in 2016 was, of course, the money raised from the sale of '*Triumph and Tragedy* - The Twenty-Five Year History of the Wokingham Crisis House'. We did very well initially, but continue to sell the books - years after first publication. I am hoping that the forthcoming sale of '*There's a Place for Us* - The Thirty Year History' - will be equally profitable. In 2016, we also raised money from a successful Street Collection, and Chris, and student, Zac, raised funds from a second, successful, Swimathon. We also received a generous donation from 'Curves', a Wokingham Ladies Gym, and another, from the local Sainsbury's Token Scheme. Our annual Agatha Christie Quiz was, also successful, in raising funds. At Christmas 2016, the Wokingham Lions' Club made its usual donation of Christmas goodies. We benefit from their generosity every Christmas.

Chapter 39

Benefactors: 2017 - 2018

In January 2017, we received a generous donation of five thousand pounds from the Berkshire Community Foundation - funding from their campaign to relieve isolation and loneliness. In 2017, we also received a generous donation of five hundred pounds from The Wokingham Singers. Our member, Philip Worthing donated five hundred pounds from a legacy that he had received during the year, and then, a further, one hundred pounds at Christmas 2017. The parents of one of our service users also donated eighty pounds - to swell our funds at Christmas. In 2017, we received a small donation in memory of our former volunteer, Catriona, who. Sadly passed away in September 2017. [Please see: 'Obituaries'].

Chapter 40

Benefactors: 2018 - 2019

In 2018, I made applications for funding from three major funding bodies - 'United Way UK - Give Local', a national funding organisation, Wokingham United Charities, and the Postcode Lottery. We were successful with the first two of these applications. 'United Way UK - Give Local', select annually, one small charity in each of thirty towns in the UK to receive a donation of one thousand pounds. We received this money for our work for the mentally ill of Reading. In 2018, we were also successful in our application to the local Funder - Wokingham United Charities; we received from them a generous donation of two thousand pounds. Also, in 2018, our member, Howard, made us a generous donation of five hundred pounds, and our member, Elizabeth, who used to live in Wokingham, and who, though she now lives in Oxford, always keeps in touch, made a generous donation of one hundred and fifty pounds, and a further, single donation, of fifty pounds.

Chapter 41

Benefactors: 2019 - 2020

2019 proved to be a particularly successful year for donations. In March 2019, we received a further generous donation of five thousand pounds from the Wokingham United Charities - from their funding to relieve isolation and loneliness. We also received a generous donation of seven hundred and fifty pounds from the rich relatives of one of our long-standing service users. A local organisation, the Wokingham Burial Grounds, also made us a generous donation of five hundred pounds in 2019. In April 2019, our volunteer Tony, and I, attended a meeting of the West Forest Townswomen's Guild - to receive a donation of one thousand pounds - the proceeds of all their fund-raising events for the past year. Most surprising, but, nevertheless, extremely welcome, was the occasion in 2019, when a lady walked through the door, and made a generous donation of one thousand pounds to our charity. Would that such could happen every day! During 2019, we have received some small donations from the PayPal Giving Fund - Internet Giving. All donations, large or small, help keep our services going, and we are most grateful to all our benefactors. Ever since we received our major legacy, from Gillian Homer, which is now twelve years ago, we have refused to rely on our laurels! We are a self-help organisation, and can never afford to stop making an effort - and, particularly, not to stop making a fund-raising effort! Each year, we continue with our Agatha Christie Quizzes - which are, invariably, profitable. In 2019, Dave H ran another half-marathon for us, and this raised extra money for our services. Dave K is also now producing some more sweat-shirts for sale. These are both, a fund-raiser, and, with their logo, 'One in Four - Fighting Back' also contribute to eliminating the stigma of mental illness. In 2019, we continued to receive our monthly direct payments - that go straight into the charity's bank account - from Dennis, Tony H, Tony W, Mark, and Chris. These donations are most valuable, because they provide us with predictable income. Not to be forgotten is the humble collection box, that sits on the table in the Drop-In Centre. In October 2019, alone, I banked two hundred poundsworth of donations from this box - so one can easily estimate an annual income of around two thousand pounds from this source alone.

Christmas is always a good time for us to receive generous donations, and Christmas 2019 was no exception. The Wokingham Lions' Club, gave us Christmas goodies, and food parcels, and cash contributions to our Collection Box, also proved particularly generous this year. The relative of one of our service users made a donation of two hundred and fifty pounds, and one of our long-term supporters, Joan, made a donation of one hundred pounds - particularly for the relief of the mentally ill homeless. As a result of our benefactors' generosity, I was able to bank six hundred pounds - the total of their Christmas 2019 donations. I include a copy of the letter that the relative sent me.

'Please find the enclosed donation to support your invaluable work with people struggling with mental ill-health and its knock-on impacts to so many of aspects of life.

I am sister to one of your clients - Pamela. I can vouch for the fact that the work you do is literally life saving at times. I know she has been able to turn to you in many very bleak moments and able to rely on your total support and expertise. Living so far away from her makes it very hard to offer on the spot support, so your support has been vital as she has been beset with so many financial issues to tackle on top of the ongoing emotional challenges.

For this reason I wanted to make a small but I hope helpful donation of £250.00 to support your work, a token - both of my appreciation for your commitment to Pamela, gratitude for the many extra miles you go to try and smooth problems and difficulties. I can confirm that this donation is eligible for Gift Aid as I am a UK taxpayer.

My hope is that 2020, will be a start of new positive things, for Pamela, than another year of looking backwards. I am sure with your continued support (and that of family, friends and other professionals) this is possible.

May I take this opportunity to wish you, and your team, a restful break, over Christmas, to recharge the batteries for the new year and its new set of challenges.'

Chapter 42

Benefactors: 2020 - 2021

On the afternoon of Friday 24th January 2020, our service user, Philip Worthing, walked into the crisis house drop-in centre, and said that he wanted to make a donation to the crisis house. He then handed me two rolls of bank notes - which totalled - two thousand pounds! Philip has been involved with our association, for almost a quarter of a century, and actually stayed in the crisis house in the summer of 1995. He is a very lonely, and isolated, schizophrenic, and so the likelihood is, that the crisis house drop-in centre, is the most precious thing in his life. Other service users wondered that he could afford this, most generous, donation, but, some time ago, he received a large legacy, and spends very little money on himself. He always wears the same outfit, and apparently, sleeps in a tent in his bedsitter, and sits on a fishing chair - rather than going in for conventional, and comfortable, furniture. I explained to our service users, that I must, of course, accept this donation - because we are totally reliant upon such donations, and our own, modest, fund-raising efforts, to keep our services going, and our services are vital for people like Philip. My favourite hymn, 'Dear Lord, and Father of Mankind', expresses, perfectly, the human need for asylum. Interestingly, this hymn was chosen, both by Chris, for his sister's funeral, and by Rosie, for her son, Carl's funeral. 'Take from our souls, the strain, and stress' - what words could be more appropriate, for current times?

On Tuesday 14th April, Phil was, fortunately, able to get into the drop-in centre, by taxi. He was urgently in need of our support. Generous, as always, he donated a further one hundred and forty pounds to our charity – a most welcome donation, as all are. Also, in April 2020, Elizabeth, from Oxford, made, yet another, generous donation, of one hundred pounds, to the crisis house.

On Monday 24th February 2020, I attended the event, 'Strictly Charity'. This was a new initiative - organised by the Wokingham United Charities. These charities are among the most ancient in the United Kingdom, and specialise in providing almshouses. At one juncture, Wokingham Borough Council, wanted to buy some of their land - for their own building purposes - and so demolished some almshouses, bought the land on a Compulsory Purchase Order, and had to pay the charities, ten million pounds, in compensation. The United Charities' Trustees. took the view that there was no point in sitting on so much money, when a number of local organisations needed grants – hence the 'Strictly Charity' Event. Twelve local charities, including ours, were selected to pitch for the prize, of fifteen thousand pounds, but each of us was to receive five thousand pounds - just for attending the Event, and putting our case. I explained our services, and pointed out that we were very lucky to have a house, as our base, since some of those present, had only, very restricted, hired space. Station House may be old, and dilapidated, but it is our 'everything'!

> *It's only a shanty, in old Shanty Town,*
> *the roof is so slanty,*
> *it touches the ground.*
> *But my tumbled down shack,*
> *by an old railroad track,*
> *like a millionaire's mansion,*
> *is calling me back.*

Obviously we are grateful to organisations like the Wokingham United Charities, and are willing to attend their events - since they are making us generous donations. But, as a general rule, I don't attend meetings. On the rare occasions that I do - which is, generally, about once in every five years - the situation is always the same, and is most amusing. Having finally appeared, it is their one chance, in five years, to nail me. 'Could the crisis house be used differently? Could some of the other organisations use our rooms on the days that we don't open the drop-in centre? Could we pool resources, and all work together?' In addition, invariably, that hoary old chestnut comes up - 'Who will take over running the crisis house, when I am no longer able to do so?' As I explained, at the 'Strictly Charity' event, the crisis house is - a leaky old roof, crumbling old walls, and creaky old floors. It needed a fairy godmother - who would take a pumpkin, wave a magic wand, and turn it into a golden coach. Certainly, without continued effort, the golden coach could well turn back into a pumpkin, and, with everything that we have paid for, removed, a squashed pumpkin, at that! But I'm optimistic for the future. We have, recently, been fortunate, in recruiting, some, very able, and, much younger, volunteers - people still in their twenties, and early thirties. And even among our middle-aged helpers, we have, for instance, a recently retired, headmistress - who has a good twenty years of voluntary service - yet to contribute. Furthermore, we have also, recently, appointed a new, additional Charity Trustee, who has volunteered with us, for thirteen years. He is highly intelligent, and is aged - just thirty-seven! In addition, we have our, regular, crop of psychology students - the younger generation - who, most certainly will, take over the mental health services, as the older generation retires. 'Triumph and Tragedy' devoted an entire section to them - as does this book! Our service users are very happy with our services, and we achieve excellent results - in terms of getting people back to work, and in restoring quality to their lives. Nevertheless, I always get this impression, that people, outside, would like to change us! Furthermore, often, their suggestions for doing so, are not, properly thought through, and would result in chaos. Take this suggestion - of allowing other organisations to use the crisis house, on the days that our drop-in centre, doesn't open. For starters, they would need seven separate keys - cost, about one hundred pounds a bunch, creating additional expense, for us, before they can even get through our doors! Then, they would use electricity, create a need for more cleaning, cause wear and tear, and, generally, make a lot more work for us! So we are definitely NOT allowing other groups to use the crisis house. I have always maintained, that we do not need bigger crisis houses; we need more of them, and there is no reason why other groups cannot set up such facilities for themselves. So we, very firmly, intend staying 'As sweet as we are'.

Stay as sweet as you are,
Don't let a thing
Ever change you.
Stay as sweet as you are,
Don't let a soul
rearrange you.

Richard and Jane

In June 2020, Richard, and Jane, who manage the McColl's supermarket, in Priestwood Square, Bracknell, donated a most generous gift of biscuits, cakes, sugar, coffee, and tea, to the crisis house. They said that they wanted to do something to support the NHS, and that since we had supported local mentally ill people, by keeping open, throughout the crisis, they would like to donate something to our service. We were most grateful, and I have thanked them, for this gift, in a letter to *The Wokingham Paper*.

Des

On Monday 22nd June, 2020, Des handed me a cheque for one hundred sounds, as a donation to our Association. He said, 'I am all right when I am here, but when I am at home, alone, I am, terribly, depressed. Here, I can talk with people, who have been through, what I have been through.' 'This, I replied, is what is known as 'fellowship', and nothing can be more therapeutic.'

Sadie

On Monday 29th June, Sadie handed me a donation of three hundred pounds. She had received a legacy, from an old aunt, who had died, and so wished to contribute some money to the crisis house. This type of donation, is precisely what we need, to keep our coffers, replenished, and so enable us to keep going, independently. We are most grateful, but there is a bitter/sweet, sequel, to this narrative. Sadie had inherited twenty-one thousand pounds, and, a fortnight later, had not one penny left! Another version of Hippie-Jack. [Please see: 'Further Poignant Stories' - 'The Parable of the Talents']. Sadie gave a considerable amount of her legacy to her boyfriend, and then, had to ask for some back! She paid off her numerous debts, and completely refurnished her house. Well, at least she has the, new furniture, to show for the money - though I doubt that there was, anything wrong, with the furniture that she threw out. As I said, poignantly, to Chris Hoskin. 'The redistribution of wealth - stuff and nonsense! God's truth, lies, invariably, in The Parable of the Talents!' I also admonish our members, regularly; 'You can stop people being silly with your money, and you can stop them, being silly, with the charity's money. But you can't stop them, being silly, with their own money!'

The crisis house is always full of surprises. On Monday 27th July 2020, three traffic wardens visited, and handed us, a generous, cash donation. They said that they had organised a collection, for Wokingham charities, and we were one, chosen to benefit. Such generous gestures, hearten us, greatly.

Reg
Reg always makes generous donations, whenever he visits, and Tuesday 28th July 2020, was no exception. He never fails to produce banknotes - to help swell our coffers.

Don
Don, as well as being a regular service user, is also, a regular, giver. Every week, he hands me a ten pound note, and I explain, gratefully, that it is precisely such regular donations, that enable me to keep the crisis house, going.

Maurice
Maurice, had been obliged, to discontinue, his regular donations, made directly into the bank, because his benefits had been axed, but, fortunately, in September 2020, he was able to re-instate this. We are most grateful, for such, regular, direct payments. As well as being made by Maurice, these are now, being made regularly, by Chris, Dennis, Tommy, and Tony.

On Tuesday 6th October 2020, I received a telephone call, from a local branch of Waitrose. The redoubtable, Dan Kent, had put our name forward, and we had been selected, as one of three charities, which are chosen, by them, each month, to share, equally, a donation, of one thousand pounds. A most welcome, injection of cash!

On Friday, 9th October, Anna, who has provided the illustrations, for this book, visited the crisis house, with Chris. She brought a donation, of twenty Christmas presents. We won't be able to have our usual, big party, this year - having to restrict attendance - due to social distancing rules. Nevertheless, we are determined to be as normal, as possible. We will have a party, for our small bubble - with a Christmas tree, and lovely presents, thanks to Anna!

On Friday 16th October, Dan Kent brought in a gift of biscuits and tea - a, very welcome, donation. He had asked the Wokingham Branch of Tesco's for a donation, in kind, and they, responded, most generously.

On 21st October, Tony e-mailed to say that he was increasing his monthly subscription, from twenty pounds, to fifty pounds, per month, because he was impressed, that we had been able to keep our services open, during the pandemic. This is a most generous, and welcome, gesture.

PART THIRTEEN

Visitors To The Crisis House

Chapter 43

Comments Of Visitors: 2016 - 2017

David Crepaz-Keay, (User Involvement Director, The Mental Health Foundation). - 'So lovely to be back. Thanks for all your support.'

Kerry-Ann Leslie and Valerie Leslie. - 'Wishing you the very best of luck with your book. Great to see you.'

Christopher Charles Hazell, and David Millward, (Rethink Mental Illness). - 'What a lovely house and home! Rethink will be telling all our clients about this wonderful service.'

Sandra Nolan, (Smart Drugs and Alcohol Rehabilitation Service). - 'Lovely, homely, feel. Excellent, safe place - to have company and warmth.'

June Rubens, (Wokingham). - 'Lovely to be shown around the lovely house. I will be offering my help.'

Clive Bate, (Bracknell and Wokingham College). - 'Great house and facilities to support those in need.'

Katherine Beatty, (Bracknell and Wokingham College). - 'Very insightful - seeing how the house works. Beautiful décor and ethos. I hope it continues to run for many more years!'

Kerry Johnson, (Student Deacon, Wokingham Methodist Church). - 'God bless you all! I will think of you, and hold your work, as precious, in my prayers.'

Thirty year anniversary of Association - 7th March 2017

Gaye Pottinger, (The Berkshire Community Foundation). - 'Congratulations on a great thirty years!'

Lady Elizabeth Godsal, (Association Patron). - 'Lovely to be here again. Congratulations.'

David Dunham, (Wokingham Town Mayor's Attendant). - 'Here's to a long future!'

Gwynneth Hewetson, (Wokingham Town Mayor). - 'Congratulations - an amazing place.'

Joan Thomason, (Wokingham). - 'Nice welcome. Thank you.'

Phil Creighton, (*The Wokingham Paper*). - 'Happy Anniversary!'

Chapter 44

Comments Of Visitors: 2017 - 2018

Anne-Marie Gawen, (Brighter Berkshire). - 'Unlock your wellbeing.'
Graeme Morrish, (Victoria, Australia). - 'Bonza Blue!'

Chapter 45

Comments Of Visitors: 2018 - 2019

Rod Sears, (Wokingham United Charities). - 'Very worthwhile support.'

Julian McGhee-Sumner, (Wokingham Town Mayor). - 'Great visit!'

Jude Humphries, (Birmingham, West Midlands). - 'Thank you for making me so welcome. A lovely, homely, house.'

Steve Wright, (Caversham, Reading). - 'It's nice to feel at home.'

Chapter 46

Comments Of Visitors: 2019 - 2020

Angela, (CMG, Local Carers' Agency). - 'Lovely place.'

Graeme Morrish and Blake, his son, (Fleet, Hampshire). - 'Excellent. See you soon!'

PCSO Bryant and PCSO Saunders, (Thames Valley Police). - 'Brilliant facility. Excellent centre for mental health.'

Heloise Sykes, - 'Lovely to meet you. See you soon.'

Nerisha Nur Malek, - 'Really nice people to talk and listen to.'

Charne Buissinne, - 'Can't wait to get more involved. What a lovely homey, and welcoming centre!'

Councillor Lynne Forbes, (Town Mayor - Wokingham Town Council). - 'Lovely visit. Thank you.'

Lady Elizabeth Godsal, - 'Thank you, and have a lovely Xmas.'

Lucy Zeal, (High Sheriff of Berkshire, and High Steward of Wokingham). - 'Happy Christmas to Everyone.'

Chapter 47

Comments Of Visitors: 2020 - 2021

Tracey Simons, (Wokingham). - 'Lovely home for everyone who comes. Pam is lovely.'

Rod Sears and Tracey H., (Wokingham United Charities). - 'Visiting Pam.'

Courtney Harris, (CMG). - 'Best place in Wokingham. Love it!'

David Wickens, (Reading). - 'Very nice company, and helpful, adults.'

PCSO Natalie Beeches, and PCSO N.A. Simmonds. - 'Visiting Pam and Dave, regarding latest vandalism. We were welcomed, with a virtual tour of the crisis house, with an account of its history.' [Our Trustee, Dave, arranged this visit, in order to achieve greater Police surveillance

- following a spate of vandalism - targeting Wokingham churches, and charities].

CPN, Louis Webb, (Wokingham Community Mental Health Team). - 'Welcoming atmosphere, visiting Pam and House.' [As I explained in the chapter, 'Success Stories Maintained', this visit was arranged, in order to enable Tommy Warfield, to resume attendance at the drop-in centre].

Susan Eaglestone, (Wokingham). - 'I was very welcome, and warm, and cosy.'

Marianne Petty, (Wokingham). - 'Very nice welcome; like home from home; will come again.'

PART FOURTEEN

Reminiscences

Chapter 48

Thanks For The Memory
The following songs express, just how important, memories are, to people - especially when they have more life behind them, than in front of them.

Memories, memories,
Dreams of love so true.
O'er the sea of memory,
I'm drifting back to you.
Childhood days, wild wood days,
Among the birds and bees.
You left me alone, but still you're my own,
In my beautiful memories.

The, sweet, sweet memories, you gave me,
You can't beat the memories, you gave me.
One girl, one boy, some grief, some joy.
Memories are made of this.

Mental illness, brings a lot of tragedy to people's lives - not just for the sufferers, themselves, but for their families, as well. I remember,

Pamela, a friend of my Schizophrenia Fellowship days, who told me that, in later life, she could not bear going on trips to the seaside. Her daughter, Catherine, suffered from, very severe, schizophrenia, and, even in the nineteen seventies, and nineteen eighties, was still, permanently resident, in a mental asylum. Pamela said that, the seaside, reminded her of happy times, when Catherine and her brother, were young children - enjoying idyllic holidays by the seaside, with their parents. To be reminded of such happy times, and then have to face the present, and future, nightmare, was, Pamela explained, unbearable.

However, memories - of happy times, and funny times, can also, bring enjoyment, to people's lives, and the following songs, express this perfectly.

> *Thanks for the memory,*
> *Of sentimental verse,*
> *Nothing in my purse,*
> *And chuckles*
> *When the preacher said,*
> *'For better or for worse.'*
> *How lovely it was.*

The drop-in centre is used, regularly, by a number of older people - who - because they have retired from working life, have the time, to get to us, on all the days that we are open. A favourite occupation for them, is reminiscing. They like recalling successes in their careers, girlfriends of the past, idyllic holidays, and the doings of their children, and grandchildren. These reminiscences, are augmented by the exchange of photographs. In Agatha Christie's novel, *'Mrs. McGinty's Dead'*, the whole murder plot, revolves around photographs, and recognition of faces, from the past. How true, is what Agatha Christie writes:

"Poirot said, in an almost casual tone of voice, 'Why do people keep photographs?' Because they just don't throw things away. Or else, because it reminds them - Poirot pounced on the words. Exactly, 'it reminds them.' Now, again, we ask, why? Why does a woman keep a photograph of herself, when young? And I say that the first reason is, essentially, vanity. She has been a pretty girl, and she keeps a photograph of herself to remind her of what a pretty girl she was. It encourages her when her mirror tells her unpalatable things. She says, perhaps, to a friend, 'That was me, when I was eighteen.' And then she sighs. 'Then that is reason No. 1. Vanity. Next reason, No. 2. Sentiment.' 'That's the same thing.' 'No, no, not quite. Because this leads you to preserve, not only your own photograph, but that of someone else'."

Hercule Poirot, and Superintendent Spence, could have been sitting in the crisis house drop-in centre. Regularly, we reminisce about the past, and pass around photographs - not only of ourselves, when we were young, and beautiful, or handsome, but also of other people who have featured, importantly, in our lives. If these lives, have been blighted, by mental illness, or other misfortunes, evidence of success, and happier times - revealed in photographs, are all the more important, to us. Successful careers, may have ended now, but they WERE successful. Marriages may have broken down, but there WAS a honeymoon period. Babies may have grown up, and left you, but there WAS a time, when the baby was on your knee. Agatha Christie writes, in her novel, '*A Murder Is Announced*', describing an investigative visit, by Inspector Craddock, to Belle Goedler, invalid widow of the multi-millionaire, Randall Goedler - to whom Letitia Blacklock, had been secretary. Belle spoke, with affectionate contempt, of the professionally efficient, but spinster, Letitia, whom, she believed, had missed all the fun of life.

"Craddock thought it was odd, the real pity, and indulgent contempt, felt by this woman, a woman whose life had been hampered by illness, whose only child, had died, whose husband had died, leaving her to a lonely widowhood, and who had been a hopeless invalid, for years. She nodded her head, at him. 'I know what you're thinking. But I've HAD all the things that make life worthwhile - they may have been taken from me, but I have had them. I was pretty and gay, as a girl, I married the man I loved, and he never stopped loving me . . My child died, but I had him for two, precious years. . . I've had a lot of physical pain – but, if you have pain, you know how to enjoy the exquisite pleasure of the times when pain stops. And everyone's been kind to me always . . . .I'm a lucky woman really'."

Belle Goedler was already, terminally ill, when this visit took place, and passed away, shortly afterwards - leaving the Goedler millions to Pip and Emma. Due to mental illness, most of our members, have never been, in a position, to accumulate, any wealth, to leave to anyone. Sadly, those who suffer from bi-polar affective disorder, may indeed, have made millions, but, due to this devastating illness, they have lost them! So, for most of our members, it is a case, of leaving, 'the sunshine to the flowers': At least, everyone, is in a position to do this! I recall that this song, was a particular favourite, of my mother's, and she would sing it, as she went around the house, cleaning.

> *I leave the sunshine, to the flowers,*
> *I leave the spring time, to the trees,*
> *And to the old folk, I leave a memory,*
> *Of a baby upon their knees.*
> *I leave the nighttime, to the dreamers,*
> *I leave the songbird, to the blind,*
> *I leave the moon above, to those in love,*
> *When I leave the world behind.*

> *I remember you..*
> *You're the one who made*
> *My dreams come true.*

Dan Kent, in particular, likes talking about all the girlfriends of the past, and how, like most people, he had one, who was special, the one 'who made his dreams come true'. He is also, currently, in March 2020, engaged in the, arduous, task of sorting out his late parents' house, and possessions. In the process, many family photographs, stored, for years, under a bed, are now coming to light. Old wedding photographs, old family gatherings, memories of happy times. He finds it, therapeutic, to show these to people in the drop-in centre, and, to reminisce, about old times. I have advised him, that it would be, a good idea, to sort them all out, and then, to place them in an album. Finally, in August 2020, he said that he was, intent upon obtaining, such an album, from W.H. Smith's, and getting the old photographs, organised. As Tommy Steele, would have it, 'Stick it in your family album!'

> *Clap hands, stamp your feet,*
> *Banging on the big bass drum.*
> *What a picture, what a picture,*
> *Um-tiddly-um-pum-um-pum-pum.*
> *Stick it in your fam'ly album.*

I recall enjoying, Tommy Steele's songs, and films, way back, when I was a young teenager, so it was good to see him, now as a, somewhat ancient, rocker, receive a Knighthood, in the 2020, Queen's Birthday Honours. The following song was played, regularly, on the radio of the day, and we all used to sing along, with it.

Well, I never felt more like singin' the blues,
'Cause I never thought that I'd ever lose,
Your love dear.
Why'd you do me this way?

Phil, also has good memories of the happy days that he spent - with a Metal Detecting Group, and is eager to share his photographs of their activities - including many of the, breathtakingly, beautiful, West Berkshire countryside.

Tragically, for Dan, Don, Pamela, Lucy, and numerous others, who have used the crisis house, it is always their former partner's inability to cope with mental health, that has led to the breakdown of the relationship. It is a statistical fact, that bi-polar affective disorder, causes the highest rate of relationship breakdown, and divorce, than any of the other mental illnesses. True, with some of the other illnesses, such as schizophrenia, from, which, Phil, suffers, their sufferers may not enter into relationships, in the first place, but, the facts are, nevertheless, significant. Interestingly, as well as reminiscing about former girlfriends, and career successes, our members like to go back, even further, and talk about the sweets, that they used to enjoy, as children – everything – from sherbert dips, liquorice allsorts, liquorice bootlaces, fruit gums, and sticky toffees. They love to recall, the, literally sweet, innocent, days, of childhood! The following song, 'Sweets For My Sweet', is actually, bittersweet - since mental health problems, frequently prevent, love, from lasting forever.

Sweets for my sweet, sugar for my honey,
Your first sweet kiss thrilled me so.

Dan feels, acutely, the loss of his self esteem - having lost, both his career, and his long-term partner. I reassure, him, constantly. 'You have HAD the success. You have BEEN, a top Quality Engineer - travelling, abroad, for the Company. You have HAD a, successful, long-term relationship.' And, I have reassured, Dan, further, that once he has, recovered more, from, the bereavement, of losing his parents, there is no reason for him, not to seek, a new partner - someone, a bit younger, and, in good health. Like Belle Goedler, he has HAD the things, that make life, worthwhile, but, unlike, Belle Goedler, there is still, a future life, ahead of him. Dan still keeps, amicably, in touch with his former partner, but she now has a new boyfriend, and this can lead to difficulties - including wistfulness, and jealousy - this being experienced, by both men! Recently, Dan's former partner, offered him some candelabra, as a gift, but he politely declined to accept them - saying, whimsically, 'They remind me of you!' Dan says, how nice it would be, if he had someone - just to speak to him - on the telephone - hence, 'A telephone, to ring, but who's to answer?' - that features, so poignantly, in the following song.

> *A cigarette that bears a lipstick's traces*
> *An airline ticket to romantic places*
> *And still my heart has wings*
> *These foolish things, remind me of you.*
> *The winds of March, that made my heart a dancer,*
> *A telephone that rings, but who's to answer?*
> *Oh, how the ghost of you clings,*
> *These foolish things,*
> *Remind me of you.*

As well as poignancy, 'These Foolish Things', brings me, a humorous memory. Many years ago, I used to run, a social group, for a large number of, institutionalised, mental patients. We used to get them, out of hospital, for the evening, and arrange entertainments, for them. On one occasion, the hired singer, failed to turn up, so I had to improvise. Among other songs, I sang, for them, 'These Foolish Things', and my colleagues reported, that they had never seen these patients, so bright, and laughing, so much!

In addition to bringing in, personal, family photographs, on Tuesday 16th June, Dan brought in some photographs of, earlier, and happy days, at the crisis house. There was one photograph, of us, all enjoying Christmas dinner, at the pub, next door. Since these photographs included, former minibus driver, Ralph, his girlfriend, June, volunteers, Janet, Frances, Carol, and Gilbert - all of whom have, since, passed away, to have pictures, in their memory, is, particularly, precious, to us.

> *When I grow too old to dream,*
> *I'll have you to remember.*
> *When I grow too old to dream,*
> *Your love will live in my heart.*

On Friday 3rd July, it was good to see Des and Don join in the exchange of nostalgic photographs. Don displayed those of himself, in his days of sporting prowess, and Des showed photographs of happy days - with June and Jenny - before he became the sad, and isolated, man that he has become - since June died, and he has been, unwillingly, excluded from supporting Jenny. It was particularly, poignant, since he had just received a letter from the social services - apologising for the fact that he felt, unappreciated, but, nevertheless, dismissing him, from any further involvement with them. He asserts, continually, that something should be done about them, and I respond, continually, that they should be, abolished, not reformed. I explained that, in 1984, I attended a House of Lords Debate, on the case of Jasmine Beckford. This was chaired by the late, Baroness Lucy Faithfull, former Head of Oxfordshire's Children's Services. She said that social work training, needed to be improved. Getting on for forty years, and the cases of Tyra Henry, and Baby P. - to name but two - later, social work has not improved. Enough said!

Berkshire Born, and Berkshire Bred

Both Don and Des, are Berkshire born, and Berkshire bred, with the most extreme version of the Berkshire accent. This is, actually, quite unusual, because so many people come from other parts of the UK, and beyond, to work in the Thames Valley's high tech. industry, that one doesn't encounter, that many, who are, original, Berkshire countrymen. These two swap reminiscences. They remember the primitive conditions of rural life - some of their families' cottages - not even having running water, and sanitation. In her novel, '*Death on the Nile*', Agatha Christie describes the intention of, the wealthy, Linnet Ridgeway, to get rid of some cottages on the estate that she was now redeveloping. This was described, whimsically, for the inhabitants of these cottages, as 'Compulsory benefit.' Agatha Christie writes:

'Linnet shook her head impatiently' . . . 'I must go and see Mr. Pierce about those plans . . . Some dreadful, insanitary old cottages. I'm having them pulled down, and the people moved.'

Evidently, in rural Berkshire, insanitary old cottages, still existed, in the latter part of the twentieth century. It is so good for Don and Des, to be able to talk, and to share life experiences, together - especially if their memories are alien to most people. City life is always so much ahead of rural life - when it comes to modernisation. It is always good, in mental health, if you can find a companion, of similar background - someone, with whom you can converse, naturally, without having to enter into detailed explanations.

Conclusion

I am perfectly happy with, the work, to which I have devoted, my life. I loved teaching, but not in the way, that I love mental health - because one can't, love anything, in the way that one loves, mental health. So, as Edith Piaf sings, '*Je ne regrette rien.*'

> *No, nothing at all,*
> *Non, rien de rien,*
> *No, I do not regret anything.*
> *Non, je ne regrette rien.*

Of course the day will come when I have to give up running the crisis house. It may be sooner; it may be later. Whichever way, I have taken, the advice, of the greatest of all the saints, St. Paul - whose church is just a short way, up the road, from the crisis house. I have had a good go, or, as he would express it, I have fought a good fight.

> *Fight the good fight*
> *with all thy might.*

As a bewildered adolescent, I enquired, of a Christian Church, 'What should one do?' Their reply was in the words of the following hymn.

> *Long as my life shall last, teach me Thy way!*
> *Where'er my lot be cast, teach me Thy way!*
> *Until the race is run, until the journey's done,*
> *Until the crown is won, teach me Thy way!*

In concluding this sequel to '*Triumph and Tragedy*', I can only reiterate, the points that I have made, throughout both books. You don't need, bigger, crisis houses; you need more of them. Small, effective, meeting the needs of the mentally ill - thus, I regard the Wokingham Crisis House, as one of my 'trophies'!

So I'll cherish the
old rugged cross,
Till my trophies, at last,
I lay down.

    The burden needs to be light - in order for the service to be sustained. Services that are overwhelmed by bureaucracy, cannot deliver, the care and support, that human beings need.
As you can read, in St. Matthew's Gospel;

'Come unto Him, all ye that labour,
come unto Him that are heavy laden,
and He will give you rest.
Take his yoke upon you, and learn of Him,
for He is meek and lowly of heart,
and ye shall find rest unto your souls.

'Come unto Me, and
I will give you rest;
Take My yoke upon you,
hear Me and be blest;
I am meek and lowly,
come and trust My might;
Come, My yoke is easy,
and My burden's light.'

Afterword

By Dan Kent

'This is the story of a moderately successful, and well qualified, engineer. I worked in Wokingham, UK, Europe, the USA, China, and Singapore. I worked hard, and was in charge of a small team. After a while of work, I stressed out. Enter the crisis house – Frances, Pam, the cats, and other fellow sufferers, were now helping me. I converted the old lean-to at the crisis house into the wonderful Lady Balfour Suite. A few of us chipped in our time to paint, and decorate, the new room. Recognition! I got a Civic Award for my efforts. Then I needed a new job. I went from one company to another; then came a low point. I went back to Prospect Park Hospital. By now, my girlfriend, had had enough, so I went back to mum. My mates had stuck by me, and I now spent long hours at the crisis house. My aging parents were getting ill. First, dad died - aged ninety, and then mum got dementia. I looked after her for about twelve months - bad time, and not too much of a life. Eventually, she gave up, and joined dad in St. Paul's graveyard. Then, I went downhill for a year. Eventually, I sorted myself out, and came back to the crisis house. I am now a Trustee, and doing my best for the house. We go on, day to day, week in, week out - taking our pills, and helping each other, as best we can. Life isn't wonderful, but a cosy room, and plenty of tea and biscuits, somehow, help. Even though life is hard, we exist - remembering all the past people, and wonderful helpers. Hopefully, more people understand mental health, now, but you can't understand fully, if you haven't been there!

Dan Kent is a long-standing service user, Trustee, and Civic Award winner, for his work at the Wokingham Crisis House.

From Agatha Christie's Works

Agatha Christie: 'A Fairy In The Flat' -
from 'Partners in Crime': 1929.

Agatha Christie: 'A Murder Is Announced': Collins: 1950.

Agatha Christie: 'An Autobiography': Collins: 1977.

Agatha Christie: 'A Pocket Full of Rye: Collins': 1953.

Agatha Christie: 'Appointment with Death': 1938.

Agatha Christie: 'At Bertram's Hotel': Collins: 1965.

Agatha Christie: 'By the Pricking of my Thumbs': Collins: 1968.

Agatha Christie: 'Cards on the Table': Collins: 1936.

Agatha Christie: 'Crooked House': Collins: 1949.

Agatha Christie: 'Curtain': Collins: 1975.

Agatha Christie: 'Death in the Clouds': Collins: 1935.

Agatha Christie: 'Death on the Nile': Collins:1937.

Agatha Christie: 'Destination Unknown': Collins: 1954.

Agatha Christie: 'Dumb Witness': Collins: 1937.

Agatha Christie: 'Five Little Pigs': 1942.

Agatha Christie: 'Four-Fifty From Paddington': Collins: 1957.

Agatha Christie: 'Hickory Dickory Dock': 1955.

Agatha Christie: 'Jane in Search of a Job' –
from 'The Listerdale Mystery': 1934.

Agatha Christie: 'Miss Marple's Final Cases: Collins: Collins: 1929.

Agatha Christie: 'Mrs. McGinty's Dead': Collins: 1952.

Agatha Christie: 'Murder at the Vicarage': Collins: 1930.

Agatha Christie: 'Murder in Mesopotamia': Collins: 1936.

Agatha Christie: 'N or M': Collins: 1941.

Agatha Christie: 'One, Two, Buckle My Shoe': 1940.

Agatha Christie: 'Peril at End House': 1932.

Agatha Christie: 'Sanctuary' –
> from 'Miss Marple's Final Cases': 1979.

Agatha Christie: 'Sing a Song of Sixpence' –
> from 'The Listerdale Mystery': 1934.

Agatha Christie: 'Sparkling Cyanide': Collins: 1945.

Agatha Christie: 'Taken at the Flood': Collins: 1948.

Agatha Christie: 'The ABC Murders': Collins: 1936.

Agatha Christie: 'The Blood-Stained Pavement' -
> from 'The Thirteen Problems': Collins: 1932.

Agatha Christie: 'The Case of the Perfect Maid' -
> from 'Miss Marple's Final Cases': Collins: 1979.

Agatha Christie: 'The Clocks': Collins 1963.

Agatha Christie: 'The Flock of Geryon' -
> from 'The Labours of Hercules': Collins: 1947.

Agatha Christie: 'The Girl in the Train'
> from 'The Listerdale Mystery: Collins: 1934.

Agatha Christie: 'The Hollow': Collins: 1946.

Agatha Christie: 'The Listerdale Mystery': Collins: 1934.

Agatha Christie: 'The Manhood of Edward Robinson' -
> from 'The Listerdale Mystery': 1934.

Agatha Christie: 'The Man in the Brown Suit': The Bodley Head: 1924.

Agatha Christie: 'The Mousetrap' from 'Three Blind Mice plus other stories': US Only: 1950.

Agatha Christie: 'The Moving Finger': Collins 1943.

Agatha Christie: 'The Pale Horse': Collins: 1961.

Agatha Christie: 'The Secret Adversary': The Bodley Head: 1922.

Agatha Christie: 'The Stymphalian Birds' - from
                   'The Labours of Hercules': 1947.

Agatha Christie: 'The Sunningdale Mystery' –
            from 'Partners in Crime: Colins: 1929.

Agatha Christie: 'The Unbreakable Alibi' –
            from 'Partners in Crime': 1929.

Agatha Christie: 'They Do It With Mirrors': Collins: 1952.

Agatha Christie: 'Third Girl': Collins: 1966.

Agatha Christie: 'Three Act Tragedy': Collins: 1936.

Agatha Christie: 'Towards Zero': Collins: 1944.

Agatha Christie: 'Wasps' Nest' - from 'Poirot's Early Cases': 1974.

Agatha Christie: 'Who's Who': 1980.

Songs

1. From West Side Story: There's a Place for us.

2. Herb Magidson/Allie Wrubel: Music, Maestro, Please.

3. Cole Porter: Don't Fence Me In.

4. Frank Loesser: Have I Stayed Away Too Long?

5. Frank Sinatra/D. Fields/J. McHugh: The Sunny Side Of The Street.

6. From My Fair Lady: With a Little Bit of Luck.

7. From My Fair Lady: I Could Have Danced All Night.

8. George Formby: Bless 'Em All'.

9. From South Pacific: Happy Talk.

10. Bing Crosby/Peggy Lee/Lesser: On a Slow Boat to China.

11. Judy Garland/Harold Arlen/E.Harburg: Somewhere, over
the Rainbow.

12. Traditional Nursery Rhyme: Little Bo Peep.

13. T.W. Connor: She was a sweet little dicky-bird.

14. The Beatles: I Want To Be Under The Sea, In An Octopus's Garden.

15. Dooley Wilson/Herman Hupfield: As Time Goes By.

16. Nat King Cole: Rambling Rose.

17. Traditional Hymn: Here, In The Country's Heart.

18. From the Twenty-Third Psalm: The Lord's My Shepherd.

19. Henry Francis Lyte: Abide With Me.

20. Isaac Watts: O, God, Our Help In Ages Past.

21. John Scott: Immortal, Invisible, God, Only Wise.

22. Monty Python: Always Look On The Bright Side Of Life.

23. Arabella Catherine Hankey: Tell me the old, old, story.

24. Walter Donaldson: Howya gonna keep 'em down on the Farm?

25. Gilbert and Sullivan: Forty-seven years.

26. Lionel Bart: Oom - pah pah.

27. From The Jungle Book: The Bare Necessities.

28. Tommy Steele: I'm the only man on the island.

29. Ginger Rogers: We're in the money!

30. Aled Jones: We're Walking In The Air.

31. Johnson: What Do You Want To Make Those Eyes At Me, For?

32. Eddie Cantor: Ma, He's Making Eyes At Me.

33. Florrie/Forde: Hold Your Hand Out, Naughty Boy.

34. Patti Austin/Harbach/Kern: Smoke Gets In Your Eyes.

35. James Brockman: I'm Forever, Blowing Bubbles.

36. Goldsboro/Russell: Honey.

37. Cecil Sharp: On Yonder Hill There Stands A Creature.

38. Popular Song: There's A Good Time Coming.

39. Viola Wills: Gonna Get Along Without You, Now.

40. Ted York: Abe, Abe Abe, My Boy.

41. Fred Gilbert/Tom Gilbert: At Trinity Church I Met My Doom.

42. W. Baker: The King Of Love, My Shepherd Is.

43. Charles Wesley: Love, Divine, All Loves, Excelling.

44. Wilfred Pickles: Have A Go, Joe!

45. Popular Great War Song: Whiter Than The Whitewash On
    The Wall.

46. Judy Garland: Keep Your Sunny Side, Up, Up!

47. Cecil Frances Alexander: All things bright, and beautiful.

48. Harry Secombe: If I ruled the world.

49. Children's Hymn: There's a friend for little children.

50. Children's Hymn: Jesus, Friend of Little Children.

51. Slim Whitman: Rose Marie.

52. Eleanor Farjeon: Morning has broken.

53. Mary Hopkin: Those were the days.

54. Bob Lind: The Elusive Butterfly.

55. William Blake: Jerusalem.

56. E.W. Rogers/Vesta Tilley: I'm following my father's footsteps.

57. Children's Comic Song: Don't Like School, Don't Like Work.

58. Arthur Colahan: Galway Bay.

59. Glen Daly: The Sky Is Bluer In Scotland.

60. Oliver George Wallace: Loch Lomond.

61. Robert Wilson: Scotland, the brave.

62. Leslie Stuart: The Soldiers of the Queen.

63. Bill Dees/Roy Orbison: Pretty Woman.

64. Teresa Brewer: Music, Music, Music.

65. Nat King Cole/Livingston/Evans: Mona Lisa.

66. Traditional Music Hall Song: We've All Been Doing A Bit.

67. Judy Garland: I'm Always Chasing Rainbows.

68. Children's Church Chorus: Draw Your Swords.

69. The Beach Boys/Wilson/Lowe: I Get Around.

70. Willie Nelson: Let The Rest Of The World, Go By.

71. John Denver: Home On The Range.

72. The Rolling Stones: I Can't Get No Satisfaction..

73. From Pursuit to Algiers: There isn't any harm in that.

74. William Shakespeare: O, Mistress Mine.

75. The Shalom Fellowship: There's A Fight To Be Fought.

76. Florrie Forde: Give Yourself A Pat On The Back.

77. Irving Berlin: All Alone By The Telephone.

78. Worton David: Hello, Hello, Who's Your Lady Friend?

79. From The Boyfriend: It's Never Too Late To Fall In Love.

80. Vera Lynn: Well Meet Again.

81. Perry Como: Hello, Young Lovers!

82. Ed Haley: While Strolling in The Park, One Day.

83. G.W. Hunt: Dear Old Pals.

84. Skeeter Davis: It's The End Of The World.

85. Comic Children's Song: Hurrah, Hurrah, We've Sausages For Tea.

86. Felix McGlennon: Sons Of The Seas.

87. Rod Stewart: Sailing.

88. Children's Hymn: Jesus Died For All The Children.

89. Lee/Harris/Weston/Weston: With Her Head Tucked Underneath Her Arm.

90. Edward Elgar: Land of Hope and Glory.

91. Thomas Arne: Rule Britannia.

92. Flanagan and Allen: Strolling.

93. John Bunyan: He Who Is Down, Need Fear No Fall.

94. The Corries: Annie Laurie.

95. Traditional Scottish: The Skye Boat Song.

96. Callum Kennedy: Mary of Skye.

97. Paul McCartney And Wings: Mull Of Kintyre.

98. From 'Over The Main': The Sound Of Iona.

99. Judy Garland: Look For The Silver Lining.

100. Frankie Vaughan: You've got to have Something in the Bank.

101. Abba: Money, Money, Money.

102. John Greenleaf Whittier: Dear Lord, and Father of Mankind.

103. Doris Day: A Shanty in Old Shanty Town.

104. From Carousel: You'll Never Walk Alone.

105. Nat King Cole: Stay as Sweet as you are.

106. Dean Martin: Memories Are Made Of This.

107. Gus Kahn: Memories, Memories.

108. Bob Hope: Thanks for the Memory.

109. Irving Berlin: I Leave The Sunshine To The Flowers.

110. Frank Ifield: I Remember You.

111. Tommy Steele: Flash, Bang, Wallop.

112. Tommy Steele: Singing The Blues.

113. The Searchers: Sweets For The Sweet.

114. Ella Fitzgerald/Louis Armstrong: These Foolish Things.

115. Oscar Hammerstein: When I Grow Too Old To Dream.

116. Edith Piaf: Rien, *Je Ne Regrette Rien*.

117. John Samuel Bewley Monsell: Fight The Good Fight.

118. Benjamin M Ramsey: Teach Me Thy Way.

119. George Bennard: The Old Rugged Cross.

120. The King's Singers: Come Unto Me.

Quotations, Rhymes, and Poetry

George William Russell: When My Time Is Come.

G.K. Chesterton: I Tell You Naught For Your Comfort.

Harold Munro: Nymph, Nymph, What Are Your Beads?

Horace: *Dulce et Decorum est Pro Patria Mori.*

Jean Ayer: Everyday Things.

John Betjeman: Come, Friendly Bombs, and Fall On Slough.

Joyce Grenfell: If I Should Go Before The Rest Of You.

Pam Jenkinson: 'Triumph and Tragedy': June Press: 2016.

Pam Jenkinson: 'This is Madness; A Critical Look at Psychiatry, and the Future of the Mental Health Services': PCCS Books: 1999.

Percy Bysshe Shelley: Adonais.

Racine: *Ce n'est plus, une ardeur.*

Racine: *Elle flotte; elle hesite; en un mot, elle est femme.*

Randle Toye: The Agatha Christie Who's Who, [Published: Frederick Muller, Ltd: 1980]

Sir Arthur Conan Doyle: *The Red Headed League.*

Sir Winston Churchill: The churchyards are full of people,

                who thought that they were indispensable.

The Bible: Do not store up, for yourself, treasure, on Earth.

The Bible: Words From The Last Supper.

W.B. Yeats: The Lake Isle Of Innisfree.

W.B. Yeats: Turning, and turning, in the widening gyre.

William Brighty Rands: Clean Clara.